Behavioral Disorders in CHILDREN

Behavioral Disorders in CHILDREN

Editors

BD Gupta MD (Pediatrics) FIAP
Editor-in-Chief
Former Professor and Head
Department of Pediatrics
Dr SN Medical College
Former Superintendent and Head
Regional Institute of Maternal and Child Health Institute
Umaid Hospital for Women and Children
Jodhpur, Rajasthan, India
brahmadgupta@hotmail.com

RK Maheshwari MD (Pediatrics) FIAP
Senior Pediatrician and (Retd) Additional Director
Medical and Health Department
Govt of Rajasthan, Barmer, Rajasthan, India
Former PMO and Consultant Pediatrician
Barmer, Rajasthan, India
drrkmbam@gmail.com

Anil Kumar Arora MD (Pediatrics)
Senior Consultant (Pediatrics) and Neonatal Intensivist
Jeevan Jyoti Nursing Home
Jodhpur, Rajasthan, India
anilarora_53@yahoo.co.in

Pankaj Agrawal MD (Pediatrics)
Assistant Professor
Department of Pediatrics
Government Medical College
Barmer, Rajasthan, India
drpankajbarmer@gmail.com

Adarsh Purohit MD (Pediatrics)
Senior Consultant and Head
Department of Pediatrics
Dr Adarsh's Kids Clinic and Medipulse Hospital
Jodhpur, Rajasthan, India
dr.adarshpurohit@yahoo.co.in

Shivji Ram Choudhary MD (Pediatrics)
Junior Specialist
Department of Pediatrics
Government Medical College
Barmer, Rajasthan, India
choudhary.shiv26@gmail.com

Foreword

Piyush Gupta

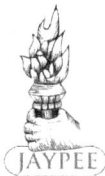

JAYPEE BROTHERS MEDICAL PUBLISHERS
The Health Sciences Publisher
New Delhi | London

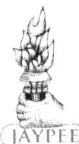
Jaypee Brothers Medical Publishers (P) Ltd

Headquarters
Jaypee Brothers Medical Publishers (P) Ltd
EMCA House, 23/23-B
Ansari Road, Daryaganj
New Delhi 110 002, India
Landline: +91-11-23272143, +91-11-23272703
+91-11-23282021, +91-11-23245672
Email: jaypee@jaypeebrothers.com

Corporate Office
Jaypee Brothers Medical Publishers (P) Ltd
4838/24, Ansari Road, Daryaganj
New Delhi 110 002, India
Phone: +91-11-43574357
Fax: +91-11-43574314
Email: jaypee@jaypeebrothers.com

Overseas Office
JP Medical Ltd.
83, Victoria Street, London
SW1H 0HW (UK)
Phone: +44 20 3170 8910
Fax: +44 (0)20 3008 6180
Email: info@jpmedpub.com

Website: www.jaypeebrothers.com
Website: www.jaypeedigital.com

© 2024, Jaypee Brothers Medical Publishers

The views and opinions expressed in this book are solely those of the original contributor(s)/author(s) and do not necessarily represent those of editor(s) or publisher of the book.

All rights reserved. No part of this publication may be reproduced, stored or transmitted in any form or by any means, electronic, mechanical, photocopying, recording or otherwise, without the prior permission in writing of the publishers.

All brand names and product names used in this book are trade names, service marks, trademarks or registered trademarks of their respective owners. The publisher is not associated with any product or vendor mentioned in this book.

Medical knowledge and practice change constantly. This book is designed to provide accurate, authoritative information about the subject matter in question. However, readers are advised to check the most current information available on procedures included and check information from the manufacturer of each product to be administered, to verify the recommended dose, formula, method and duration of administration, adverse effects and contraindications. It is the responsibility of the practitioner to take all appropriate safety precautions. Neither the publisher nor the author(s)/editor(s) assume any liability for any injury and/or damage to persons or property arising from or related to use of material in this book.

This book is sold on the understanding that the publisher is not engaged in providing professional medical services. If such advice or services are required, the services of a competent medical professional should be sought.

Every effort has been made where necessary to contact holders of copyright to obtain permission to reproduce copyright material. If any have been inadvertently overlooked, the publisher will be pleased to make the necessary arrangements at the first opportunity.

Inquiries for bulk sales may be solicited at: jaypee@jaypeebrothers.com

Behavioral Disorders in Children

First Edition: **2024**

ISBN: 978-93-5696-858-5

Dedicated to

*Our parents and esteemed teachers,
our wives and other family members,
and above all our patients and their parents,
who have encouraged us to complete this task.*

—**Editors**

Contributors

Aakash Mahesan MD (Pediatrics)
Senior Resident
Centre of Excellence and
Advanced Research for Childhood
Neurodevelopmental Disorders
Child Neurology Division
Department of Pediatrics
All India Institute of Medical Sciences
New Delhi, India
aakash191293@gmail.com

Adarsh Purohit MD (Pediatrics)
Senior Consultant and Head
Department of Pediatrics
Dr Adarsh's Kids Clinic and
Medipulse Hospital
Jodhpur, Rajasthan, India
dr.adarshpurohit@yahoo.co.in

Adhiraj Singh MPH
PG Student
Maulana Azad University
Jodhpur, Rajasthan, India
adhirajresearch@gmail.com

Anil Kumar Arora MD (Pediatrics)
Senior Consultant (Pediatrics) and
Neonatal Intensivist
Jeevan Jyoti Nursing Home
Jodhpur, Rajasthan, India
anilarora_53@yahoo.co.in

Ankit Kumar Meena
MD DM (Pediatric Neurology)
Assistant Professor, Department of
Pediatrics, ESIC Medical College and
Hospital, Faridabad, Haryana
ankit.aiims.meena@gmail.com

Anurag Singh MD (Pediatrics)
Senior Professor
Department of Pediatrics
Dr SN Medical College
Jodhpur, Rajasthan, India
singhjodhpur@gmail.com

Archana Vyas MD (Pharmacology)
Assistant Professor
Department of Pharmacology
Dr SN Medical College
Jodhpur, Rajasthan, India
shauryarchana@gmail.com

BD Gupta MD (Pediatrics) FIAP
Editor-in-Chief
Former Professor and Head
Department of Pediatrics
Dr SN Medical College
Former Superintendent and Head
Regional Institute of Maternal and
Child Health Institute
Umaid Hospital for Women and Children
Jodhpur, Rajasthan, India
brahmadgupta@hotmail.com

BS Karnawat MD (Pediatrics) FIAP
(Retd) Senior Professor and Head
Department of Pediatrics
Former Principal and Controller
JLN Medical College
Ajmer, Rajasthan, India
bskarnawat@live.com

Bhanu Pratap Rathore MD (Pediatrics)
Assistant Professor
Department of Pediatrics
Dr SN Medical College
Jodhpur, Rajasthan, India
dr.bhanurathore@gmail.com

DR Dabi MD (Pediatrics)
Former Professor and Head
Department of Pediatrics
Dr SN Medical College
Jodhpur, Rajasthan, India
dhanrajdabi@gmail.com

GD Koolwal MD (Psychiatry)
Consultant Psychiatrist
Senior Professor and Former Head
Department of Psychiatry
Dr SN Medical College
Jodhpur, Rajasthan, India
gdkoolwal@gmail.com

Gautam Kamila MD DNB DM
Senior Research Associate
Centre of Excellence and
Advanced Research for Childhood
Neurodevelopmental Disorders
Department of Pediatrics
All India Institute of Medical Sciences
New Delhi, India
gautam_kamila@yahoo.com

Harshna Aseri MBBS
CRH
Lokmanya Tilak Municipal Medical
College and General Hospital
Mumbai, Maharashtra, India
harshnaaseri@gmail.com

Indraja Sharma MBBS
Resident
Department of Psychiatry
Dr SN Medical College
Jodhpur, Rajasthan, India
indraja.sharma95@gmail.com

JS Tuteja MD DCH PGDAP FIAP
Consultant Teenager's Counsellor
Senior Consultant Pediatrician
Indore, Madhya Pradesh, India
Chairperson AHA 2012–2015
drtuteja@gmail.com

Kapil Jetha
MD Fellowship in Pediatric Neurology
Associate Professor
Department of Pediatrics
Rajkot, Gujarat, India
Jetha.kapil88@gmail.com

Kaushik Ragunathan MD (Pediatrics)
Senior Resident
Centre of Excellence and
Advanced Research for Childhood
Neurodevelopmental Disorders
Department of Pediatrics
All India Institute of Medical Sciences
New Delhi, India
kaushikmedic@gmail.com

KS Multani MD (Pediatrics)
Senior Consultant Pediatrics
11 AF Hospital, Hindon
Ghaziabad, Uttar Pradesh, India
kawaljit000@gmail.com

Lokesh Saini
MD DM (Pediatrics Neurology)
Assistant Professor
Department of Pediatrics
All India Institute of Medical Sciences
Jodhpur, Rajasthan, India
drlokeshsaini@gmail.com

Contributors

Mahesh Hemnani
MD (Pediatrics)
Senior Resident Pediatrics
JLN Medical College
Ajmer, Rajasthan, India
drmicky.ajm88@gmail.com

Manish Parakh
MD (Pediatrics) Clinical Fellowship in Pediatric Neurology (Toronto)
Senior Professor and Head
Department of Pediatrics and
In-charge, Pediatric Neurology Services
Dr SN Medical College
Jodhpur, Rajasthan, India
manparkh@hotmail.com

Monica Juneja MD (Pediatrics)
Director Professor and Head
Department of Pediatrics
Maulana Azad Medical College and
Lok Nayak Hospital
New Delhi, India
drmonicajuneja@gmail.com

Neeraj Gupta
MD DM (Neonatology)
Additional Professor
Department of Neonatology
All India Institute of Medical Sciences
Jodhpur, Rajasthan, India
neerajpgi@yahoo.co.in

Nimish Khatri MD (Pediatrics)
Consultant Pediatrician
Sunshine Hospital
Bikaner, Rajasthan, India
nimish@gmail.com

Pankaj Agrawal
MD (Pediatrics)
Assistant Professor
Department of Pediatrics
Government Medical College
Barmer, Rajasthan, India
drpankajbarmer@gmail.com

PC Khatri MD (Pediatrics)
Former Professor and Head
Department of Pediatrics
SP Medical College
Barmer, Rajasthan, India
pckhatri2@gmail.com

Piyali Bhattacharya MD (Pediatrics)
Pediatrician
General Hospital
Sanjay Gandhi Postgraduate Institute of Medical Sciences
Lucknow, Uttar Pradesh, India
drpiyali@gmail.com

Prahbhjot Malhi PhD
Former Professor and
Unit In-charge (Child Psychology)
Department of Pediatrics
Postgraduate Institute of Medical Education and Research
Consultant (Child Psychology)
Department of Mental Health and Behavioral Sciences
Fortis Medcentre
Chandigarh, India
pmalhi18@hotmail.com

Pradeep Jain MD (Pediatrics)
Senior Consultant Pediatrics
Balaji Hospital
Jodhpur, Rajasthan, India
drpradeepjain70@gamil.com

Pradeep Kumar Gunasekaran MD
Senior Resident
Department of Pediatrics
All India Institute of Medical Sciences
Jodhpur, Rajasthan, India

Pragya Chitlangia Somani
MD (Pediatrics)
Consultant Pediatrician
Mahesh Hospital
Bhilwara, Rajasthan, India
drpragyasomani1@hotmail.com

Pramod Sharma MD (Pediatrics)
Senior Professor and Unit Head
Department of Pediatrics
Dr SN Medical College
Jodhpur, Rajasthan, India
drpramodsha@hotmail.com

Priyanshu Mathur MD (Pediatrics)
Associate Professor
Pediatric Medicine
SMS Medical College
Jaipur, Rajasthan, India
priyanshu82@gmail.com

Puneet Choudhary MD (Pediatrics)
Senior Resident
Centre of Excellence and
Advanced Research for Childhood
Neurodevelopmental Disorders
Child Neurology Division
Department of Pediatrics
All India Institute of Medical Sciences
New Delhi, India
shinepuneet@gmail.com

Richa Tiwari
MD Pediatrics
Senior Resident
Centre of Excellence and
Advanced Research for Childhood
Neurodevelopmental Disorders
Child Neurology Division
Department of Pediatrics
All India Institute of Medical Sciences
New Delhi, India
richatiwari.dr@gmail.com

RK Maheshwari
MD (Pediatrics) FIAP
Senior Pediatrician and
(Retd) Additional Director
Medical and Health Department
Govt of Rajasthan
Barmer, Rajasthan, India
Former PMO and Consultant
Pediatrician
Barmer, Rajasthan, India
drrkmbam@gmail.com

S Sitaraman
MD (Pediatrics) FNNF FIAP Fellow Pediatric Neurology (UK)
Director
Newton Institute of Child and
Adolescent Development
Jaipur, Rajasthan, India
drsraman.jp@gmail.com

Sanjay Gehlot
MD (Psychiatry)
Professor and Head
Department of Psychiatry
Dr SN Medical College
Jodhpur, Rajasthan, India
gehlotsanjaydr@gmail.com

Shaina Raheja MD (Pathology)
Senior Demonstrator
SP Medical College
Bikaner, Rajasthan, India
shainaraheja@gmail.com

Sharanpreet Kaur MBBS
Resident
Department of Pediatrics
SMS Medical College
Jaipur, Rajasthan, India
sharanpreet3110@gmail.com

Sheffali Gulati
FRCPCH (UK) FAMS FIAP FIMSA
Chief
Centre of Excellence and
Advanced Research for Childhood
Neurodevelopmental Disorders
Child Neurology Division
Department of Pediatrics
All India Institute of Medical Sciences
New Delhi, India
sheffaligulati@gmail.com

Shivji Ram Choudhary
MD (Pediatrics)
Junior Specialist
Department of Pediatrics
Government Medical College
Barmer, Rajasthan, India
choudhary.shiv26@gmail.com

Shreyance Jain MD (Psychiatry)
Medical Officer
Umaid Hospital for Women and
Children
Jodhpur, Rajasthan, India
jainshreyance@gmail.com

Smitha Sairam MD (Pediatrics)
Specialist Pediatrician
Centre of Excellence—Early
Intervention Centre
Department of Pediatrics
Maulana Azad Medical College and
Lok Nayak Hospital
New Delhi, India
smithasairam@gmail.com

Srikant Sharma
MD (Psychiatry)
Consultant Psychiatrist
Anandam Psychiatry Centre
Centre of Excellence in Mental Health
Atal Bihari Vajpayee Institute of
Medical Sciences and
Dr Ram Manohar Lohia Hospital
New Delhi, India
anandampsychiatrycentre@gmail.com

Swati Ghate
MD (Pediatrics) MA (Psychology)
Consultant Adolescent and
Developmental Pediatrician
Newton Institute of Child and
Adolescent Development
Jaipur, Rajasthan, India
ghateswati19@gmail.com

Foreword

I am delighted to learn that the organizing team of "Desert PEDICON 2023" is coming out with a book on *Behavioral Disorders in Children*. Behavioral disorders in children have been on the rise over the last few years with the easy accessibility of and overuse of smartphones by children, overuse of social media and online videogames, and decreasing social connections and outdoor activities. Changing social scenarios and lifestyles have also led to rise in genetic disorders many of which are associated with behavioral problems.

There has been a great vacuum of books and literature about these disorders in children and at times it is difficult to identify these problems at an early age and even when identified clinicians find themselves dumbstruck on how to practically deal with these challenged children. This book is a great addition and compilation of the latest literature available on various behavioral disorders in children and provides a practical approach on how to approach these cases.

The aim of this book is to provide a comprehensive resource for parents, caregivers, educators, and healthcare professionals, offering insights, strategies, and guidance on understanding, managing, and ultimately helping children with behavioral disorders to thrive. Separate chapters on *Mobile Phone Addiction in Children*, *Pharmacology of Behavioral Disorders*, *Teenage and Adolescent Behavioral Issues*, and *Counseling of Parents and Children with Behavioral Disorder* are valuable additions. The fact that it is written by leading experts of the country makes it an indispensable tool. I am sure it will find a place on the office desk of every clinician dealing with such patients.

I am fully aware of the expertise, experience of the editorial team and their insights in the highest regard, and it is my sincere belief that their unique perspective would greatly enhance the value and credibility of this book. Your profound contributions to the field of pediatrics, particularly in dealing with behavioral issues in children, make you an ideal candidate to come out with this book. I am sure the book will fill the gap which has been there regarding managing various behavioral issues in children.

I wish you all the success for this venture.

Piyush Gupta MD FIAP FNNF FAMS FRCPCH
Principal and Professor
Department of Pediatrics
University College of Medical Sciences
New Delhi, India
prof.piyush.gupta@gmail.com

Preface

Many scientific researches and technological advancements have led to all the developments we see in the modern world. On one hand, man has landed on the south pole of Moon while on the other hand, he has developed many vaccines and drugs so as to control morbidity and mortality from infectious diseases. These developments have led to a steady decline in infectious diseases, increased survival of "high-risk neonates" and better control of so many incurable diseases. Together with these, changes in social structure like smaller and nuclear families, increased number of workers and rising family income have led to overall increase in aspirations towards quality of life. Also, the availability of modern amenities in homes like TVs, mobile phones, tablets, and other gadgets have created possibilities of learning, entertainment, and social interaction.

But, with these changes we have also invited some unseen problems related to behavior, anxiety and depression among all ages including children. We have all evidenced increasing number of suicides among students, and experienced behavioral disorders in children. All this scenario has given insight to visualize these problems in detail. The chapters incorporated in the book provide in-depth knowledge about individual conditions.

The chapters in the book have been organized to create interest among all students and teachers of pediatrics, psychiatry, and internal medicine. Practicing pediatricians and physicians, who are seriously concerned for the welfare of these innocent patients, will also find it useful to help these kids. We also believe that the book will be able to quench the thirst of serious students of this subject who are practicing developmental and behavioral pediatrics solely. We will be delighted if patients as well as parents are benefitted by readings of this book. We welcome all the suggestions and positive criticism regarding all the chapters of the book.

Albert Einstein has rightly pointed that *Education is not learning of facts but the training of mind to think.*

BD Gupta
RK Maheshwari
Anil Kumar Arora
Pankaj Agarwal
Adarsh Purohit
Shivji Ram Choudhary

Acknowledgments

We are heartily thankful to all the authors for contributing the chapters for the book. We sincerely appreciate the help rendered to us by Drs Rakesh Jora, Jagdish Goyal, Daisy Khera, Vikas Katewa, Mohan Makwana, Nagaram, Suresh Verma, Sandeep Choudhary, Vishnu Goyal, Siyaram Didel, Mukesh Choudhary, Avinash Bansal and Susheel Choudhary, for editorial assistance.

We are thankful to our publishers, M/s Jaypee Brothers Medical Publishers (P) Ltd, New Delhi, India, for their painstaking and cooperative attitude, speedy and excellent publication of the book.

Contents

1. **Introduction to Behavioral Disorders in Children** 1
   BD Gupta, Adarsh Purohit

2. **Autism Spectrum Disorders: Etiopathogenesis and Diagnostic Evaluation** 8
   Aakash Mahesan, Puneet Choudhary, Gautam Kamila, Sheffali Gulati

3. **Management of Autism Spectrum Disorder** 21
   Kaushik Ragunathan, Richa Tiwari, Gautam Kamila, Sheffali Gulati

4. **Attention-deficit Hyperactivity Disorder in Children** 33
   Monica Juneja, Smitha Sairam

5. **Anxiety Disorders in Children and Adolescents** 41
   Prahbhjot Malhi

6. **Exogenous Depression in Children** 54
   GD Koolwal, Shreyance Jain

7. **Nonsuicidal Self-injury and Suicide in Adolescence** 61
   RK Maheshwari, Shivji Ram Choudhary

8. **Obsessive-Compulsive Disorder** 69
   Sanjay Gehlot, Indraja Sharma

9. **Phobias and Hallucinations** 78
   BS Karnawat, Mahesh Hemnani

10. **Oppositional Defiant Disorder** 87
    Adhiraj Singh, Anurag Singh

11. **Conduct Disorders in Children** 92
    Pragya Chitlangia Somani

12. **Substance Abuse in Children: A Growing Concern** 98
    PC Khatri, Nimish Khatri, Shaina Raheja

13. **Feeding and Eating Disorders** 106
    Kapil Jetha, Neeraj Gupta

14. **Hysterical Conversion Disorder in Children** 114
    Pradeep Kumar Gunasekaran, Lokesh Saini

15. **Somatic Symptom and Related Disorders in Children** 119
    Adarsh Purohit

16. **Sleep Disorders in Children** 127
    Manish Parakh, Ankit Kumar Meena, Bhanu Pratap Rathore

17. **Learning Disorders in Children: Intellectual Disability and Specific Learning Disability** 137
    KS Multani

18. **Fluency Disorders** 142
    S Sitaraman

19. **Habit Disorders in Children**..147
    Anil Kumar Arora, BD Gupta

20. **Aggressive Behavior** 160
    Pramod Sharma

21. **Rumination Disorder** 170
    Shivji Ram Choudhary, RK Maheshwari

22. **Enuresis and Encopresis**...173
    DR Dabi, Harshna Aseri

23. **Gratification Disorder in Children** 179
    Pankaj Agrawal

24. **Mobile Phone Addiction in Children** 183
    Srikant Sharma

25. **Teenage and Adolescent Behavioral Issues**..193
    Piyali Bhattacharya

26. **Counseling of Parents and Children with Behavioral Disorder**..................................200
    JS Tuteja

27. **Mobile and Behavioral Disorders in Children**...210
    Pradeep Jain, BD Gupta

28. **Pharmacology of Behavioral Disorders** 217
    Archana Vyas

29. **Genetics and Behavioral Disorders** 231
    Priyanshu Mathur, Sharanpreet Kaur

30. **Cognitive Behavior Therapy** 239
    S Sitaraman, Swati Ghate

Index *245*

Chapter 1

Introduction to Behavioral Disorders in Children

BD Gupta, Adarsh Purohit

INTRODUCTION

Behavior of a child keeps changing from the time of birth to adulthood and thereafter. Behavior of a child depends upon many factors, such as age, sex, educational status, any genetic or neurological disorder or deformity, long-term illness, familial harmony and bonding, influence of the peer group, and so on. To label a behavior as abnormal, we pediatricians have to take into consideration multiple factors and must have thorough knowledge of all the age-appropriate behaviors. *Any persistent behavior which is beyond the expected norm for age and level of development is labeled as abnormal behavior or behavioral disorder.*

THEORY OF MIND[1-5]

Our mind is responsible for most of our thought patterns which in turn affects our behavior. According to theory of mind (ToM), "it is the ability to understand that everyone has feelings, desires, and intentions which are different from one's own feelings, desires, and intentions". ToM was first coined in 1970s by Premack; since then, ToM has been considered to be one of the crucial factors responsible for thought pattern, cognitive development, and social adaptivity in a child. It prepares a child for future social interactions, makes him ready for school and college, and improves mental faculties and reasoning. Beliefs affect the thoughts of a person which in turn can direct the behavioral pattern of that person. ToM is shaped by many factors, such as bonding with parents, harmony in the home, upbringing and education, influence of the peer, and social group. Many neurodevelopmental disorders, such as autism spectrum disorders (ASDs), attention-deficit/hyperactivity disorder (ADHD), expressive speech disorders, and psychiatric disorders such as schizophrenia, impair the ToM which in turn leads to behavioral disorders. Children with poor ToM have been reported to have a higher incidence of conduct disorders, childhood maltreatment, Tourette's syndrome, and other behavioral disorders such as anorexia nervosa. Development of ToM is a complex phenomenon involving structural part of brain pathways as well as socioenvironmental factors. ToM is fully functional only in humans and to some extent in some primates. In humans, it starts developing around 18 months of age and achieved by 3-4 years of age. It is vital for social adaptive ability in any child or adult. Memory and language are two important mental faculties, which are closely connected with formation and development of ToM. ToM space is further divided into seven main mental states: (1) emotions, (2) intentions, (3) desires, (4) knowledge, (5) beliefs, (6) mentalistic understanding of nonliteral communication, and (7) perceptions which are further subdivided into 39 subabilities. Multiple tools and measures have been developed over the years to understand ToM which have a contribution in fundamental science behind different behaviors as well as are useful for clinical practice.

PREVALENCE OF BEHAVIORAL DISORDERS[6-8]

Behavioral disorders in children are fairly common and have been on rise over the last few years due to rise in use of gadgets such as mobile, laptops and videogames, multiple lockdowns during COVID-19, and increasing influence of social media sites. Many of the cases go unnoticed or are not reported and although there are not many studies demonstrating the exact prevalence of these problems in children, yet as per the available studies their prevalence ranges from 29 to 40% among children of various ages. Disruptive behavioral problems, such as conduct disorders, oppositional defiant disorders (ODDs), and ADHD are the most common followed by mood disorders such as anxiety and depression.

RISK FACTORS AND ETIOLOGY BEHIND BEHAVIORAL DISORDERS[9-11]

A child's behavior is one of the most important areas of concern for its parents. A slight deviation from the perceived normal worries them. A slightest of change in pattern makes them bring the child to the pediatrician. As a pediatrician, we must be well aware of the range of normal behavior and be able to catch the slightest clue indicating toward any behavioral disorder. A number of factors are responsible for guiding a child's behavior. The process starts in utero and continues lifelong. The risk factors can be divided into antenatal, perinatal and fetal, and postnatal/environmental.

Antenatal Factors

When child is in utero, factors which can affect a child's behavior are mental state of mother such as maternal depression or anxiety or any other psychiatric illness during pregnancy, use of alcohol or smoking during pregnancy (higher chances of externalizing problems such as hyperactivity and conduct disorders in offsprings), exposure to any teratogenic agent during antenatal period (prenatal phthalate exposure), exposure to heavy metals such as mercury, lead or manganese, gestational diabetes, maternal overweight, or obesity [babies from mothers who have pre-pregnancy body mass index (BMI) of >25 kg/m^2 have been reported to have a higher risk of ADHD], and infection during perinatal period (leads to higher incidence of internalizing problems). Intimate partner violence (IPV) during pregnancy has also been considered as an important risk factor by World Health Organization (WHO). Externalizing as well as internalizing problems have been reported during early childhood in offspring of mothers who have faced IPV during pregnancy.

Perinatal and Fetal Factors

Prematurity and low birth weight are newborn risk factors for development of behavioral and emotional problems later in life, which are more prominent in male children. Excessive blood loss during pregnancy, cesarean section, and prolonged admission in the neonatal intensive care unit (NICU) are some of the perinatal risk factors for the development of behavioral problems. Interestingly, multiple birth has been reported to have some protective effect against development of behavioral problems, especially in moderately preterm babies. Congenital, neurological, metabolic, and genetic disorders are the causes behind many behavioral disorders and such behavioral disorders may be associated with other neurological or systemic diseases in such cases.

Postnatal/Environmental

During developmental phases of life, boys have been found to have more of externalizing problems while internalizing problems are more common in girls making gender difference also an attributable risk factor. Family harmony, school environment, and relationship with the peer groups are the leading factors which affect the mental and emotional condition of a child during the later stages of childhood. Children exposed to bullying in school have higher incidence of behavioral problems. Substance or Drug Abuse and alcoholism are also common during adolescence, which have a cause and effect relationship with the behavioral disorders in these children. Loss of a loved one or separation can trigger change in behavior of the child.

NEUROBIOLOGY OF BEHAVIORAL DISORDERS[6,10-12]

It has been a matter of research over the years that—is there any specific neuro-organic problem behind behavioral and emotional problems in children. Researchers have been trying to pinpoint the area of brain which makes some of the children more prone to various behavioral disorders than the others. Multiple studies have reported that many of these children have reduced gray matter volume (GMV) of various areas of brain, particularly in amygdala, cingulate gyrus, anterior insula, and frontal and prefrontal cortices. There have been reports of dysregulation of hormones during prenatal period (hormonal hypothesis), especially mediated by glucocorticoids associated with reduced hypothalamic-pituitary-adrenal axis (HPA axis) in children with disruptive behavioral disorders. Higher levels of prenatal testosterone have also been hypothesized in many children with disruptive behavioral disorders. Prenatal exposure to alcohol and tobacco has been reported to disrupt HPA axis by cortisol attenuation, which further lead to increased incidence of externalizing behavior in these children later in life. Furthermore, the epigenetic modulation of the human glucocorticoid receptor gene, *NR3C1,* in offspring can be related to maternal depression, anxiety, and IPV which can lead to several behavioral problems. Such modulation leads to increased methylation disrupting the stress response in these children making them vulnerable for emotional and behavioral problems. Besides, there have been reports that immune dysregulation in mother due to any factor may lead to increased level of proinflammatory cytokines affecting the fetal brain development and chances of abnormal behavioral and emotional response in such children.

CLASSIFICATION OF BEHAVIORAL DISORDERS[12-15]

Broadly, childhood behavioral disorders can be divided into externalizing and internalizing problems. Externalizing disorders account for those behavioral problems where the child becomes overtly eccentric, aggressive, violent, or conduct disorders, which are harmful to others or himself. On the other side, internalizing disorders are those where a child develops inwardly negative behaviors, such as depression, anxiety, autism or attention deficit, or psychosomatic disorders. However, there is considerable overlap of both the conditions in an affected child and there may be exhibition of both internalizing and externalizing behaviors, but at different points of time. The Diagnostic and Statistical Manual of Mental Disorders, Fifth Edition (DSM-5) **(Box 1)** and eleventh revision of the International Classification of Diseases (ICD-11) **(Box 2)** are the two internationally accepted classifications of various mental health and behavioral disorders. DSM-5 has been prepared by the American Psychiatric Association (APA) while ICD-11 is the international coding of diseases developed by WHO. DSM-5 was published in May, 2013 while ICD-11 has been in use since 2022. Below are mentioned both the classification system meant to categorize various behavioral and mental health problems into a valid group meant for research purpose as well as for treatment and medicolegal purpose. These classification systems encompass various mental, behavioral, and neurodevelopmental disorders seen in pediatric as well as adult population.

Thus, pediatric behavioral disorders can be broadly divided into following categories although there may be a bit of overlapping of behavioral disorders with some neurodevelopmental or psychiatric disorders:[16-20]

- *Mood/emotional disorders:* Depression, generalized anxiety disorder (GAD), panic disorder, social phobia and other phobias, post-traumatic stress disorder (PTSD), and obsessive-compulsive disorder (OCD).

BOX 1: DSM-5: Diagnostic and Statistical Manual of Mental Disorders, Fifth Edition.

- Neurodevelopmental disorders
- Schizophrenia spectrum and other psychotic disorders
- Bipolar and related disorders
- Depressive disorders
- Anxiety disorders
- Obsessive-compulsive and related disorders
- Trauma- and stressor-related disorders
- Dissociative disorders
- Somatic symptom and related disorders
- Feeding and eating disorders
- Elimination disorders
- Sleep-wake disorders
- Sexual dysfunctions
- Gender dysphoria
- Disruptive, impulse—control, and conduct disorders
- Substance-related and addictive disorders
- Neurocognitive disorders
- Personality disorders
- Paraphilic disorders
- Other mental disorders

BOX 2: ICD-11 for Mortality and Morbidity Statistics (Version: 01/2023).

- Neurocognitive disorders
- Disorders due to substance use or addictive behaviors
- Schizophrenia or other primary psychotic disorders
- Catatonia
- Mood disorders
- Anxiety or fear-related disorders
- Obsessive-compulsive or related disorders
- Disorders specifically associated with stress
- Dissociative disorders
- Disorders of bodily distress or bodily experience
- Feeding or eating disorders
- Mental or behavioral disorders associated with pregnancy, childbirth, or the puerperium
- Psychological or behavioral factors affecting disorders or diseases classified elsewhere
- Impulse control disorders
- Personality disorders and related traits
- Paraphilic disorders
- Factitious disorders
- Insomnia disorders
- Hypersomnolence disorders
- Circadian rhythm sleep-wake disorders
- Gender incongruence
- Disorders of intellectual development
- Neurodevelopmental disorders
- Elimination disorders
- Disruptive behavioral or dissocial disorders
- Secondary mental or behavioral syndromes associated with disorders or diseases classified elsewhere

- *Disruptive behavioral problems:* Oppositional defiant disorder, conduct disorder, and ADHD
- *Pervasive development and autism spectrum disorder:* Autism, Asperger syndrome, childhood disintegrative disorder (CDD), Rett syndrome, pervasive developmental disorder not otherwise specified (PDD-NOS), and pathological demand avoidance (Newson's syndrome).
- *Social (pragmatic) communication disorder*
- *Feeding and eating disorders:* Anorexia nervosa, bulimia nervosa, avoidant/restrictive food intake disorder, binge-eating disorder, and pervasive refusal syndrome.
- *Somatic symptom and related disorders:* Conversion disorder, factitious disorder imposed on another (previously known as Munchausen syndrome by proxy), factitious disorder imposed on self, illness anxiety disorder, and somatic symptom disorder.
- *Sleep disorders:* Insomnia, hypersomnolence, sleep-related movement disorders, circadian rhythm sleep-wake disorders, sleep-related breathing disorders, and parasomnias
- *Disorders of intellectual development:* Learning disabilities
- *Disorders of speech development:* Stuttering and stammering
- *Habit disorders:* Head banging, temper tantrums, thumb sucking, nail biting, body rocking, tics, breath holding, gratification, or infantile masturbation.

ROLE OF EARLY IDENTIFICATION OF BEHAVIORAL PROBLEMS[6,21,22]

Behavioral problems in children are fairly common and it is important to identify them at the earliest possible chance. Many of the children with these behavioral disorders go unnoticed and never seek any treatment. With passing time, these disorders decrease their scholastic performance, hamper their intellectual growth, divert these children toward delinquency and substance abuse, and disturb the familial harmony. Depending upon the type of problem, the child may either become too internalized landing into severe depression, develop suicidal tendencies, or if having externalizing problems may develop severe criminal behaviors. Such children may frequently face rejection from their peer group causing social isolation. One problem may lead to other psychobehavioral issues making the original problem complex. Identification, diagnosis, and early intervention can prevent these problems to a large extent, improve their sociofamilial harmony, can help them get better academic results and achievements in life.

There are many ways to increase the detection of these children depending upon the resources available. One of the earliest chances to identify the problem is to have a developmental and behavioral screening at each vaccination visit by a pediatrician. Whenever a child comes for vaccination, a good amount of time should be dedicated for the assessment of the development and behavior of the child by the medical practitioner. The children who are at high risk with history of any of the risk factors discussed above should be given extra emphasis and must be frequently followed at regular intervals, at least every 3 months during the pretoddler period and then twice every year during the early school years. However, in a vast country like India many children do not get a chance to be assessed by a medical practitioner, here primary teachers can be of great help. Primary teachers can be trained regarding the normal developmental milestones and behavior of a toddler and whenever they note any deviation from the normal, they can refer the child to the nearest medical practitioner for further assessment and intervention.

ASSESSMENT OF CHILDHOOD BEHAVIORAL PROBLEMS[6,16,23,24]

It is of utmost importance to diagnose children with a behavioral disorder at the earliest possible chance. There is no specific investigation with the help of which we can establish a diagnosis, and at times there is amalgamation of multiple disorders which mask the basic problem, so we pediatricians have to rely on our clinical skills to find out the index problem as well as its cause before moving toward the treatment part. As in any other disease in childhood once again history taking has a great importance to know about the disease in a given child, however in behavioral disorders, we sometimes need to take history from different sources as at times parents may exaggerate the problem or may hide the gravity of problem considering it to be a taboo. Therefore, we need to elicit history from parents, other family members living under the same roof and if it is a school going child teachers' description of child's behavior can be of great help. Sudden change in behavior reported by family member, teacher or friends should alert a clinician and should enquire deeply into the events going around the child. History of familial disharmony, sudden loss of a dear one, unexpected results in a recent examination, exposure to bullying at school, or in neighborhood are important points to look for. History taking must be followed by thorough physical examination looking specifically for any clue indicating toward any neurological disorder, facial dysmorphism, vision and hearing assessment, development of the child, signs of any injury indicating if child has ever been exposed to violence, subtle signs of needle stick injuries suggesting intravenous drug use and so on.

Many psychometric tools have been developed to assess these children of which commonly used are:
- Behavioral and Emotional Screening System (BESS) for children from age 3 to 18 years
- Behavior Assessment System for Children, 2nd Edition
- Pediatric Symptom Checklist (PSC)
- Ages and Stages Questionnaire-Social Emotional (ASQ-SE) for children between 0 and 5 years
- Achenbach System of Empirically Based Assessment (ASEBA) for children starting from 1.5 years through adulthood
- Rutter Children Behavior Questionnaire (RCBQ).

PREVENTION OF BEHAVIORAL PROBLEMS IN CHILDREN[6,18]

Prevention of behavioral problems is a multifaceted approach which starts from prenatal period and continues through adulthood. Emphasis on physical and psychological health of a pregnant lady is one of the most important steps toward preventing long-term behavioral and emotional issues in the offspring. Proper nutrition during pregnancy, preventing or early control of any infection during pregnancy, avoiding alcohol use and smoking, and proper rest, and sleep are some of the key components during pregnancy which help mother in turn helping offspring. Any psychological stress in mother must not be taken lightly and must be addressed with love and compassion and if required by proper professional psychological counseling.

Child delivered prematurely or those who have a stormy early newborn period are at high risk of developing behavioral problems later in life. Similarly, those children who have an elder sibling with some behavioral issues are also a high-risk candidate for such problems. Such children must be followed up frequently preferably by a pediatrician acquainted with developmental and behavioral problems. Anything that can aggravate or trigger these problems in these children must be strictly avoided such as use of mobile phones, long screen times, poor social exposure to peer group and isolation, and sleep deprivation. Providing proper nutrition and sleep, good sociofamilial harmony, and exposure to peer group go long way in establishing proper emotional development of the child. At the earliest clue of any problem, immediate intervention in form of structured behavioral management must be started in such kids. Positive reinforcement must be preferred over negative reinforcement in such children.

Adolescence is again a very critical phase where the child goes through multiple emotional and behavioral changes, is emotionally labile and prone to such problems. Adolescence clinics in school with presence of a counselor can be of utmost help to recognize if child is going through any significant problem which can affect the emotional or mental health; here early identification of the problem and providing emotional support in a friendly manner is the key. Sometimes, the child may develop wrong or challenging behaviors under peer-pressure, so it is necessary for the parents to keep talking with the child at a regular basis and too in a friendly manner earning his/her trust. Overstrictness can sometimes prove detrimental and should be avoided. Therefore, the role of parents and teachers is of great importance during this phase of a child.

MANAGEMENT OF BEHAVIORAL DISORDERS[6,18,25]

Although, management of every kind of behavioral disorder and even every case has to be individualized and cannot be the same yet broadly it consists of behavioral management strategies and pharmacotherapy. Pharmacotherapy is not the treatment of choice and behavioral management programs form the core of managing such problems. Yet, pharmacotherapy is an adjunct where there is slow or poor response, or in severe behavioral problems. Among behavioral management strategies, there are parent skills training to help parents learn how to tackle these challenging behaviors, cognitive behavioral therapy (CBT) especially for children with ASD and mood disorders, self-esteem building strategies, differentiated educational strategies in school such as TEACCH program (Treatment and Education of Autistic and Related Communication Handicapped Children), positive behavioral interventions and support (PBIS), response to intervention (RTI), applied behavior analysis (ABA) for classroom behavioral management, individualized approach to children with learning disabilities, psychotherapy, and so on. The main purpose of these behavioral management therapies is to improve social communication skills of these children, help them learn their moods and teach them coping skills, and help them achieve academic qualifications so as to make them independent.

CONCLUSION

Behavioral and emotional problems are quiet a common problem roughly affecting more than one-third of kids at different phases of childhood. Apart from the child, the whole family is affected by it and it definitely affects the quality of life of the child as well as everyone around him. We need to have a structured national program to address this problem starting right from the antenatal period till the child achieves adulthood. Early identification and intervention through proper behavioral management strategies is the key and for this we need to have specialized teams consisting of counselors, child psychiatrists, speech therapists, occupational therapists, audiologists, and social workers. Involvement and education of parents as well as school teachers are also of vital importance as they are the ones who are in consistent contact with the child. A national universal screening program to identify these children is also the need of the hour.

REFERENCES

1. Suway JG, Degnan KA, Sussman AL, Fox NA. The relations among theory of mind, behavioral inhibition, and peer interactions in early childhood. Soc Dev. 2012;21(2):331-42.
2. Korkmaz B. Theory of Mind and Neurodevelopmental Disorders of Childhood. Pediatr Res. 2011;69(5):101R-8R.
3. Beaudoin C, Leblanc É, Gagner C, Beauchamp MH. Systematic Review and Inventory of Theory of Mind Measures for Young Children. Front Psychol. 2020;10:2905.
4. Nonnenmacher N, Müller M, Taczkowski J, Zietlow AL, Sodian B, Reck C. Theory of Mind in Pre-school Aged Children: Influence of Maternal Depression and Infants' Self-Comforting Behavior. Front Psychol. 2021;12:741786.
5. Rix K, Monks CP, O'Toole S. Theory of Mind and Young Children's Behaviour: Aggressive, Victimised, Prosocial, and Solitary. Int J Environ Res Public Health. 2023;20(10):5892.
6. Ogundele MO. Behavioural and emotional disorders in childhood: A brief overview for paediatricians. World J Clin Pediatr. 2018;7(1):9-26.
7. Barman N, Khanikor MS. Prevalence of Behavioural Problems among School Children: A Pilot Study. Int J Health Sci Res. 2018;8(12):95-101.
8. Preeti, Dua K. A review of behavioral disorder in school going children. Pharma Innov J. 2021;10(8):207-9.
9. Den Haan PJ, de Kroon MLA, van Dokkum NH, Kerstjens JM, Reijneveld SA, Bos AF. Risk factors for emotional and behavioral problems in moderately-late preterms. PLoS One. 2019;14(5):e0216468.
10. Chiu YN, Gau SS, Tsai WC, Soong WT, Shang CY. Demographic and perinatal factors for behavioral problems among children aged 4-9 in Taiwan. Psychiatry Clin Neurosci. 2009;63(4):569-76.
11. Tien J, Lewis GD, Liu J. Prenatal risk factors for internalizing and externalizing problems in childhood. World J Pediatr. 2020;16(4):341-55.
12. James R, Blair R. The neurobiology of disruptive behavior disorder. Am J Psychiatry. 2016;173(11):1073-4.
13. Gozi A. Highlights of ICD-11 Classification of Mental, Behavioral, and Neurodevelopmental Disorders. Ind J Priv Psychiatry. 2019;13(1):11-7.
14. Gaebel W, Stricker J, Kerst A. Changes from ICD-10 to ICD-11 and future directions in psychiatric classification. Dialogues Clin Neurosci. 2020;22(1):7-15.
15. Center for Behavioral Health Statistics and Quality. (2016). 2014 National Survey on Drug Use and Health: DSM-5 Changes: Implications for Child Serious Emotional Disturbance. [online] Available from: https://www.samhsa.gov/data/sites/default/files/NSDUH-DSM5ImpactChildSED-2016.pdf [Last accessed September, 2023].
16. Yousif MK, Almuhyi AA, Abood SA, Abid AA. Prevalence of common habit disorders in children aged 3-13 years. Int J Med Sci Adv Clin Res. 2018;1(3):1-6.
17. Nicholls D. Eating disorders in children and adolescents. Adv Psychiatr Treat. 1999;5:241-9.
18. Perrotta G, Fabiano G. Behavioural disorders in children and adolescents: Definition, clinical contexts, neurobiological profiles and clinical treatments. Open J Pediatr Child Health. 2021;6(1):5-15.
19. Ophoff D, Slaats MA, Boudewyns A, Glazemakers I, Van Hoorenbeeck K, Verhulst SL. Sleep disorders during childhood: a practical review. Eur J Pediatr. 2018;177(5):641-8.
20. Nechay A, Ross LM, Stephenson JB, O'Regan M. Gratification disorder ("infantile masturbation"): a review. Arch Dis Child. 2004;89:225-6.
21. Eklund K, Renshaw TL, Dowdy E, Jimerson SR, Hart SR, Jones CN, et al. Early Identification of Behavioral

and Emotional Problems in Youth: Universal Screening versus Teacher-Referral Identification. Calif Sch Psychol. 2009;14:89-95.
22. Koegel LK, Koegel RL, Ashbaugh K, Bradshaw J. The importance of early identification and intervention for children with or at risk for autism spectrum disorders. Int J Speech Lang Pathol. 2014;16(1):50-6.
23. Joseph N, Sinha U, D'Souza M. Assessment of determinants of behavioral problems among primary school children in Mangalore city of South India. Curr Psychol. 2021;40:6187-98.
24. Child Behavior Checklist (CBCL). Available from: URL: https://aseba.org/school-age/ [Last accessed September, 2023].
25. Undiyaundeye, Florence A. Management of Behaviour and Emotional Disorder for Child Integration in Societal Functioning: Implication for Teaching and Learning. J Afr Interdiscip Studies. 2019;3(1):21-8.

Autism Spectrum Disorders: Etiopathogenesis and Diagnostic Evaluation

Aakash Mahesan, Puneet Choudhary, Gautam Kamila, Sheffali Gulati

INTRODUCTION

The neurodevelopmental disorders (NDDs) are characterized by a failure to reach cognitive, emotional, and motor milestones. More than 3% of children worldwide are affected by NDDs and they constitute a serious health problem. There is a disruption of the tightly coordinated events in brain development. The etiologies are heterogeneous affecting cognition, communication, adaptive behavior, and psychomotor skills. Autism spectrum disorder (ASD), intellectual disability (ID), attention-deficit/hyperactivity disorder (ADHD), and epilepsy constitute these NDDs.[1] Usually ID, ASD, and epilepsy are reported together as a combination in individual patients. Among these NDDs, abnormalities in social relationships and repetitive or restricted behavioral patterns characterize ASD.[2]

EPIDEMIOLOGY

The global prevalence is estimated to be around 28.3 million, with an incidence of 603,790 individuals and 4.3 million disability-adjusted life years (DALYs) in 2019. The prevalence and incidence of autism have been increasing sharply. Since 1990 to 2019, the increase in prevalent cases, incident cases, and DALYs were 39.3, 0.1, and 38.7%, respectively. Another study indicated the worldwide ASD prevalence to be 0.6% with prevalence in Asia, Africa, America, Europe, and Australia to be 0.4, 1, 1, 0.5, and 1.7%, respectively.[3,4] In 2023, the Centers for Disease Control and Prevention (CDC) estimates based on data from 11 Autism and Developmental Disabilities Monitoring Network sites gave a prevalence of 27.6 per 1,000 which would mean 1 in 36 children had autism and 3.8 times more prevalent in boys than girls.[5] The INCLEN study in 3,964 Indian children from five different regions of India estimated the overall prevalence of NDDs to be around 12% in children between 2 and 9 years of age with ASD prevalence estimated around 1 in 89 overall. 20% of the children with NDD had more than one associated comorbid conditions and autism was the most common among them receiver operating characteristic (ROC). All racial, ethnic, and socioeconomic groups have more or less similar incidences of ASD, but is consistently identified more in Caucasian children which could be explained by better access to healthcare services, lesser stigma, etc. Down syndrome, tuberous sclerosis, fragile X syndrome, and Rett syndrome are few of the most commonly and consistently associated syndromes with ASD.[6,7]

ETIOLOGICAL RISK FACTORS

Parental Age

One of the well-established risk factors for chromosomal aberrations and psychiatric/neurodevelopmental conditions is advanced parental age. There is a cumulating risk for mutations during spermatogenesis possibly leading to increased risk of ASD.[8,9] Some NDDs, such as ADHD, due to psychosocial factors, might be associated with a young parental age. A meta-analysis found a reduced risk of autism in offspring with lowest parental age, while increased risk was with highest parental age.[10]

Fetal Microenvironment

Diabetes, maternal obesity, sex hormone alterations, hypertension, and infections are various environmental prenatal exposures that have been linked to ASD etiology. A recent meta-analysis found a 1.35 pooled odds ratio for ASD risk in offspring of mothers with hypertensive disorders of pregnancy. Maternal immune activation hypothesis is supported by antibodies and elevated inflammatory markers in pregnant women with autistic offspring. There is higher risk of ASD in children born to obese as well as underweight mothers. Excess weight gain during pregnancy may increase the risk of autism. Evidence for smoking as a risk factor in ASD is inconsistent although it is associated with increased risk for autism and ID. In addition to maternal smoking, paternal second hand smoking exposure should also be investigated for the risk of ASD. These risks may be due to genetic disposition and environmental interactions that compromise the maternal-fetal-placental system.[8] These risks can lead to adverse neurodevelopmental outcomes in offspring including altered deoxyribonucleic acid (DNA) methylation patterns, impaired cognitive function, and psychiatric outcomes.

Perinatal Risk Factors

Perinatal risk factors, such as hypoxia, prematurity, low birth weight, and hypoxia may contribute to autism risk. Complications resulting from hypoxia are consistently associated with ASD risk, while no other complication of pregnancy is consistently connected to ASD. Abnormal presentation, low birth weight, feeding difficulties, cesarean section, and birth spacing <12 months or >60 months have increased risk. Medication use during pregnancy and lactation lacks sufficient evidence for safety. Valproic acid (VPA) poses risks for offspring including cognitive dysfunction and neural tube defects. Selective serotonin reuptake inhibitors (SSRIs) have a positive association with ASD but the absolute risk is small. Neurological and psychiatric disorders due to smoking and alcohol use during pregnancy are known, but evidence for ASD is inconsistent. Maternal nutrition during pregnancy determines nutrients available for fetal development (e.g., short intervals between pregnancies) and deficiency can adversely impact outcomes, and increases autism risk for offspring. Vitamin D deficiency during early development may predispose to ASD with little evidence supporting that it may have therapeutic benefits in reducing autism symptomatology. The association between iron and ASD is conflicting although iron is crucial for neural function and fetal development. Maternal zinc and copper deficiency during pregnancy may contribute to ASD risk.[8]

Vaccination

Despite evidence to the contrary, the MMR (measles, mumps, and rubella) vaccine has been falsely linked to autism, leading to reduction in vaccination with outbreaks of measles. Large-scale epidemiological studies have refuted this notion.[11]

Toxic Exposures

The modern world has produced around 80,000 environmental chemicals with approximately 1,000 being neurotoxic and the rest unstudied.[9] Heavy metals, air pollutants, organic pollutants, and pesticides all constitute the neurotoxins that can alter neurodevelopment through diverse pathophysiological pathways. A recent meta-analysis of 23 studies found evidence of toxicity of air pollution during early development, supporting government health policies to limit their exposure.[11] Exposure to toxic metals, such as mercury and lead, can negatively impact bodily functions and may contribute to the development of autism. A systematic review and meta-analysis found that ASD cases had significantly higher levels of lead and mercury in their blood and erythrocytes as well as higher concentrations of lead and antimony in their hair.[12] Pesticides, including herbicides and insecticides, are designed to harm and kill organisms and have been associated with an increased risk of ASD, particularly during pregnancy. Nonpersistent organic pollutants, such as phthalates and bisphenol, are used in plastics and can negatively affect reproductive, respiratory, and endocrine systems as well as neurodevelopment.[8] Persistent organic pollutants, such as dichlorodiphenyltrichloroethane (DDT), polybrominated diphenyl ethers (PBDEs), and polychlorinated biphenyls (PCBs), accumulate in the environment and food chains and have been linked to adverse neurodevelopmental, endocrinological, and immunological effects including cognitive skills and gene expression.

Psychosocial Causes

The psychosocial environment plays a critical role in modifying outcomes and could have long-term behavioral and biological effects on the child.[9] Maternal immigration, as a cause of stress, has been studied but results on its association with autism are mixed. The Project Ice Storm, QF2011 Queensland Flood Study, and a study on tropical storms in Louisiana found that exposure to prenatal maternal stress during gestation can affect autistic symptoms and theory of mind skills in children.[13] Adopted children from deficient orphanages could exhibit atypical behaviors due to severe early deprivation. Nonetheless, only a minority develop quasi-autism with the rest making a recovery.

Genetic Factors

A study revealed that when a male was associated with risk in the family, ASD was diagnosed in 4.2% of female siblings and 12.9% of male siblings. When a female was associated with risk in the family, ASD was diagnosed in 7.6% of female siblings and 16.7% of male siblings. Even cousins showed a two-fold increase in the risk, suggesting a genetic component.[14,15] The autistic traits are highly variable in the general population and are highly heritable similar to the genetic influence to autism itself. Subjects from simplex families had higher prevalence of de novo chromosomal rearrangements when compared with subjects from multiplex families. This suggests a differential mechanism of genetic transmission of autism. Environmental factors can interact with genetic components to increase the risk of ASD. Epigenetic mechanisms, such as DNA or histone modifications, play a critical role in neurodevelopment and can be affected by environmental risk factors. Genetic mechanisms, such as mutations and polymorphisms, can make individuals susceptible to the effects of certain environmental risk factors. Methylenetetrahydrofolate reductase (*MTHFR*) gene polymorphism leading to folate deficiency, might impair methyl donation and subsequently lead to impaired epigenetic regulation.[8]

Hypoxic Damage and Oxidative Stress

Autism spectrum disorder is linked to altered immune status, increased oxidative stress, and neuroinflammation, which may be caused by environmental factors such as mercury and lead. Mitochondrial dysfunction and impaired methylation are also associated with ASD. Hypoxic/ischemic insult can lead to oxidative damage, inflammation, and excitotoxicity, which can exacerbate neuronal damage and death, and may be related to ASD through disruption of the fragile X mental retardation protein (FMRP) signaling pathway. Cerebral palsy, ID, and seizure are associated with perinatal hypoxia and hypercarbia which could also increase the risk of ASD.

Endocrine Factors

Autism spectrum disorder affects genders differently with higher prevalence in boys and differences in psychopathological, biochemical, and genetic aspects. The extreme male brain theory suggests that ASD reflects an extreme male pattern, which may be influenced by hormonal imbalances caused by endocrine-disrupting chemical.[15] Endocrine-disrupting chemicals can alter steroid balance and thyroid function, which have been linked to an increased risk of ASD. Prenatal maternal thyroid dysfunction in prenatal period and ASD in the child has also been hypothesized.[8]

PROTECTIVE FACTORS

Emerging research suggests that prenatal vitamin supplementation, particularly with folate, may reduce the risk of autism in offspring by supporting neural and neurobehavioral development. Folate may buffer additional risks in mothers or infants with gene variants impacting folate-dependent one-carbon metabolism by acting as a methyl donor during early embryogenesis. Omega-3 fatty acids are important for neurodevelopment and cognitive functioning, but studies on the effect of maternal supplementation on autism outcomes have been inconsistent.[9] The role of the gastrointestinal tract and probiotics in autism protection is a promising area.

MODERN THEORIES OF ASD DEVELOPMENT

Neural Connectivity

Neural connectivity refers to the ability of neurons to communicate with each other through synapses. Impaired neural connectivity is one of the proposed theories for the pathogenesis of the disorder. Neural connectivity is essential for the proper functioning of the nervous system. It allows different parts of the brain to communicate with each other and coordinate their activities. The formation of neural connections begins during embryonic development and continues throughout life. In ASD, there is evidence of altered neural connectivity, which may contribute to the characteristic features of the disorder, such as impaired social interaction and communication. Some studies have suggested that individuals with ASD have fewer connections between various brain regions, while others have suggested that there may be an overgrowth of connections in certain areas of the brain. During the building of connectivity in a normally developing brain, the number of neurons is decreased, which seems to be impaired in ASD.[16] Interhemispheric connectivity, mini-column abnormalities with increased density creates noise in the circuit. This disables efficient processing of information and is proposed as one of the mechanisms of impaired connectivity and imperfect synaptic plasticity leading to ASD. Abnormalities in the amygdala include rapid and early increases in size, greater spine density, and an initial overabundance of neurons in young ASD subjects.[17] However, the exact mechanisms underlying impaired neural connectivity in ASD are not yet fully understood. It is important to understand the complex interactions between different parts of the brain and the role they play in the development of the disorder.

Impaired Neural Migration

Neural migration is a process that occurs during embryonic development, where neurons move from their place of origin to their final destination in the brain. This process is essential for the proper formation and functioning of the nervous system. During neural migration, neurons undergo a series of complex movements guided by a variety of molecular signals. These signals help to direct the neurons to their correct location in the brain, where they will form connections with other neurons. In ASD, there is evidence of disrupted neural migration, which may contribute to the characteristic symptoms of the disorder.[16] Some studies have suggested that individuals with ASD may have abnormalities in the structure and organization of the brain, which may be related to disruptions in neural migration. One example is *Reelin* gene mutation which is involved in proper positions of neurons in the neocortex and their migration.[18] Increased thickness of the cortex especially in the temporal and frontal lobes might be explained by this. The peak overgrowth corresponds to 1–2 years of age which is the age of first clinical symptom onset usually. Additionally, exposure to certain environmental toxins during pregnancy may also disrupt neural migration and increase the risk of ASD. 5-hydroxytryptamine (5-HT) receptors, such as 5-HT3A and 5-HT6, play a role in neuronal migration and dendritic differentiation during embryonic development and disruptions in 5-HT-dependent neurogenic processes can occur due to maternal inflammation during pregnancy.[17]

Impaired Synaptogenesis and Dendritic Morphogenesis

The overabundance of initial synapse formation with selective synaptic elimination is noted early in the CNS development.[16] Impaired synaptogenesis is important in ASD with evidence of abnormal dendritic morphology and reduced developmental spine pruning. This is best explained in Rett syndrome with mutated *MeCP2* protein playing a crucial role in synaptic maturation and pruning which gets disrupted.[19] Autophagy plays a crucial role in regulating synaptic strength and connectivity of neurons with reduced neuronal autophagy [regulated by mammalian target of rapamycin (mTOR)] consistent with increased mitochondrial mass in ASD brains. Impairments in both pre- and postsynaptic membranes including scaffolding proteins NLGN3, NLGN4, and SHANK support ASD pathogenesis.

Excitation/Inhibition Imbalance

The excitatory/inhibitory (E/I) balance is crucial for proper brain function and is maintained through regulated mechanisms and is closely related to other theories of ASD. Glutamatergic and gamma-aminobutyric acid-ergic (GABAergic) receptor disturbances contribute to E/I imbalance. Excessive glutamatergic excitation can propagate neuroinflammation by causing excitotoxic cell death.[20]

Broken Mirror Theory

Learning by imitation and understanding others' actions and emotions without cognitive mediation are carried out by mirror systems in the brain. These functions are enabled by neural networks located in the parietal lobe, premotor cortex, insula, and anterior cingulate cortex. It is closely related to the theory of mind, which is the capability of understanding subjective mental states, including thoughts and desires, no matter how real or unreal the circumstances may be.[21] Limited development of the mirror mechanism may contribute to core aspects of ASDs and affect communication skills. While some studies support the role of the mirror neuron system in ASD, others challenge this hypothesis.[16]

Impaired Immunity and Neuroinflammation

Immune system alterations, both acquired and innate immunity, are commonly studied in ASD, but their role in the disorder's etiology is still unclear. Immune dysregulation is present in ASD with an imbalance in T cell subpopulations and natural killer cells. Neuroinflammation involving neuroglia is a consistent finding in ASD, and immune dysfunction may contribute to central nervous system (CNS) dysfunction. Astrocytes, microglia, perivascular macrophages, and endothelial cells play important roles in neuronal function and homeostasis, cortical organization, neuroaxonal guidance, and synaptic plasticity.[22] Astrocytes maintain the blood–brain barrier integrity, detoxify excitatory amino acids, and facilitate neuronal survival by producing growth factors. Postmortem brain tissue analysis of autistic patients shows active and ongoing neuroinflammatory processes characterized by astroglial and neuroglial activation in the cerebral cortex and white matter.[16] Further, exploration is needed to understand the specific neuropathology and behavioral disturbances in ASD related to the neuroinflammatory response.

Unifying Theory

Three contributory features of autism are identified: (1) an autistic personality dimension, (2) cognitive compensation, and (3) neuropathological risk factors as per the unified theory. It describes a common pathophysiological process through which a variety of endogenous and exogenous risk factors contribute to autism through the restriction of neurodevelopment and cognitive impairment.[23] The theory's key conclusions are that the overall autism phenotype is presented as a nonpathological core personality component that is shared by the population and uncoupled from concomitant characteristics such as poor cognitive function and immunological dysfunction. It suggests that contributing risk factors and findings of immune and autonomic dysfunction are clinically ascertained rather than part of the core autism construct. The theory can serve to inform reasoning regarding future research, interpretation of findings, and development of classification methods.

GENETIC MODELS

Epigenetics

Deoxyribonucleic acid methylation and histone modification are the two main molecular epigenetic processes involved in regulating gene expression. Another significant role in the control of chromatin shape and gene expression is noncoding ribonucleic acid (RNA). DNA hydroxymethylation has been implicated in ASD and studied in animal models with mutations in ASD-related genes, resulting in ASD-like behavioral phenotypes. 5-hydroxymethylcytosine (5hmC) is found abundantly in many genes, *GAD1* (glutamate decarboxylase 1) and *RELN* genes, which are associated with neural development in ASD and supported by animal models. Rett syndrome is always associated with ASD symptoms and is caused by a mutation in the *MeCP2* gene, which is important for brain development. Dysregulation of proteins controlling histone modifications, such as H3K4me3 and KDM5C, is associated with ASD and ID. Mutations in chromodomain helicase DNA-binding (CHD) protein are frequent in autistic individuals, particularly those with CHD8 mutations. MicroRNAs (miRNAs) are short RNA molecules that regulate gene expression and control functional pathways in the brain, and their deregulation can lead to NDDs. As miRNAs can be delivered into cells and either downregulated or replaced to compensate for low-expressing miRNAs, miRNA-based therapy is promising. Epigenetic regulation, including alterations in gene expression, may contribute to ASD. The microbiota–gut–brain axis may also play a role in ASD pathogenesis through the production of short-chain fatty acids and potential epigenetic effects mediated via noncoding RNAs and RNA splicing factors.[24] Further research is needed to fully establish the role of epigenetics and the microbiota–gut–brain axis in ASD.

Single Gene Disorders

Genetic etiology with contribution of environmental factors constitutes ASD. Investigatory approach in ASD studies looks for similarities in gene function rather than a single "autism gene" as in arterial hypertension being caused by multiple genes. Finding a common function for all of the offending genes is challenging. A few genes that affect synapse function are *NLGN3/4*, *SHANK3*, and *NRXN1*. Genes fit into clusters related to synaptic transmission, abnormal cellular/synaptic growth rate, and gene transcription/translation. Tumor suppressor genes are having negative regulatory role in neuronal hypertrophy which is proposed to be crucial in synaptic pruning. TSC1/2, PTEN, and NF1 are potential pathways. Inhibitors of mTOR pathway may show promising effects in ASD also. Specific pathomechanisms for ASD are not yet clear, but unique spatiotemporal characteristics may produce ASD. Several genes including *IMMP2L*, *DOCK4*, *FOXP2*, and *RAY1/ST7* have been associated with ASD, but further research is needed to determine their exact role in the disorder.[25]

Copy-number Variations

De novo copy-number variations (CNVs) contribute to 7% of ASD families with specific duplications and deletions associated with ASD. *KCTD13* gene deletion affects brain development leading to cognitive impairment and brain abnormality in ASD. Neurocognitive impairments, cognitive deficits, behavioral autistic symptoms, language, and social communication problems are associated with genetic deletions in SHANK3 and 22q13 regions as well as alterations in neurexin superfamily and cadherin genes. Deletion at the 17q12 region is a strong candidate for ASD and schizophrenia, affecting brain development and function. Autism may arise as a result of defects in neuronal maturation and long-term potentiation that were seen in KALRN and PLA2G4A deletion animal models.[26] The FMRP controls polyribosome-mediated translation at synapses by interacting with ASD-related genes. Splicing factor nSR100/SRRM4 regulates neural microexons and reduced levels of nSR100 are associated with misregulated microexons in ASD patients. Epigenetic dysregulation can cause ASD by altering the fine-tuning of development-related genes and the development of the brain.

Mitochondrial Dysfunction

Numerous animal models of ASD have been discovered to have mitochondrial abnormalities according to studies. Studies of mitochondrial oxidative stress and function in ASD have also been carried out in vitro. Mitochondrial DNA (mtDNA) deletions were found in up to 16.6% of ASD patients. Uncertainty exists regarding the association between chromosomal defects and ASD or mitochondrial dysfunction.[27] When compared to healthy controls, ASD patients' serum includes a considerable amount of mtDNA and mtDNA from extracellular vesicles, which may be an alarmin-inducing proinflammatory mediator secreted by immune cells. There is also an increased prevalence of comorbidities linked to ASD and the reduced mtDNA presence in ASD when compared to healthy controls. Patients with ASD may have oral mucosa that has significantly more mtDNA for the genes *MFN1*, *MFN2*, and *OPA1*. All of the researches up to this point emphasize how crucial it is to investigate and draw clear conclusions about the relationship between these genes and ASD and their appropriateness as ASD biomarkers.

ANIMAL MODELS

Animal models are important for understanding ASD, but no commonly accepted model exists yet. The current models are models for autism rather than models of autism. Most of these models fall into one of the four categories: (1) neuro-biological models, (2) genetic models, (3) lesion models, and (4) environmental models. Environmental models involve exposing pregnant animals or neonates to certain chemicals or infected/inflamed individuals during pregnancy. Models must meet criteria for construct, face, and predictive validity to be useful in developing treatments.[16]

MODELS INDUCED BY ENVIRONMENTAL FACTORS

Biological Agents

Maternal infection during pregnancy can lead to early immune dysregulation and activation of microglia and astrocytes in the brains of autistic patients, as well as upregulation of proinflammatory cytokines, such as tumor necrosis factor α (TNFα), interleukin 6 (IL-6), and IL-1β. Pregnant rat models are usually employed as animal model for this theory.[28]

Chemical Agents

Over 200 chemicals have neurotoxic effects on the adult brain, and some are potential teratogens. VPA is widely used for ASD modeling but has a teratogenic effect that increases the risk of ASD by threefold when used during early pregnancy. Oxidative stress, histone deacetylase (HDAC) inhibition, and decreased antioxidant system activity leading to the manifestation of teratogenic effects and ASD-like symptoms can be caused by VPA exposure. HDAC modulation in different cell types at different time points may lead to different outcomes.[16]

Brain Lesion/Damage

Because most brain lesions are irreparable, animal models are employed to create brain dysfunctions that are analogous to neurological illnesses. Brain tissue can be damaged using a variety of techniques, such as mechanical lesion, electrolytic and radio frequency lesions, excitotoxic or neurotoxic lesions, and intraventricular injection of short-chain fatty acids.[29] A significant disadvantage is that it would be challenging to attribute causality because damage to one single brain region would affect the entire CNS.

Genetic Modifications

Several human syndromes caused by gene mutations increase the risk of ASD leading to genetic animal models of ASD development. Single gene knock out mouse models do not represent the whole complexity of behavioral alterations.[17] However, these models have limitations in representing the complexity of the disorder, and combining genetic and environmental factors may provide us with a better holistic model.

EARLY CLINICAL FEATURES

The initial signs of autism in children are understated and typically come to attention and assessment when parents observe delays in language development and unusual behaviors. Numerous research studies have indicated that the clinical signs of autism may become apparent and recognizable as soon as a child reaches 6 months of age.[30] Based on early clinical features, two major groups have been identified: one with early delay and another with regression after a period of relatively normal development. Both groups exhibit similar severity of symptoms by the age of 24 months.[31] Various early clinical features are:[30]

- Lack of social smile
- Absence of stranger anxiety
- Absence of direct eye contact with parents
- Absence of response to name
- Impaired communication gestures
- Delayed onset of babbling
- Feeding problems.

DIAGNOSTIC CRITERIA AND CLINICAL FEATURES

The clinical diagnosis of ASD relies on both the child's behavioral observations and their medical history. The Diagnostic and Statistical Manual of Mental Disorders, Fifth Edition (DSM-5), published in 2013, provides the diagnostic criteria for this disorder.[2]

A revised edition, known as DSM-5-TR (Text Revision), was published in 2022.[32]

The DSM-5 guidelines for ASD consist of two main categories: (1) Challenges in social communication and (2) interaction, as well as limitations in behavior, activities, and interests that are repetitive and restricted. Moreover, these symptoms should negatively impact a child's functioning, emerge during the early stages of development, and not be more appropriately attributed to ID or global developmental delay.[2]

DSM-5 diagnostic criteria and the associated clinical features are depicted in **Box 1**.

BOX 1: DSM-5 diagnostic criteria for autism spectrum disorder and clinical features.[2]

1. Persistent challenges in social communication and interaction across multiple settings and manifested currently or by history. All three of the following must be present:
    i. *Deficits in social-emotional reciprocity:* The spectrum of difficulties can include abnormal social approaches and a failure to engage in typical reciprocal conversations, as well as a decrease in sharing interests, emotions, or expressions. Additionally, it may involve challenges in initiating or responding to social interactions
    ii. *Impairment in nonverbal communicative behavior:* The range of challenges can include difficulties in integrating verbal and nonverbal communication effectively, abnormalities in eye contact and body language, as well as deficits in understanding and utilizing gestures. At the extreme end, it may involve a total lack of facial expressions and nonverbal communication
    iii. *Challenges in forming, sustaining, and comprehending relationships:* The challenges can range from finding it difficult to adapt behavior to different social contexts, facing difficulties in participating in imaginative play or building friendships, to displaying a lack of enthusiasm in interacting with peers

2. Restricted, repetitive patterns of behavior, interests, or activities as manifested by at least two of the following, currently or by history:
    i. Engaging in repetitive motor stereotypies, object manipulation, or speech, such as simple motor stereotypies, arranging toys in a line, flipping objects, echoing speech, or using unique phrases
    ii. Demonstrating a pronounced insistence on sameness, inflexibility toward routines, or participating in ritualized patterns of verbal or nonverbal conduct. This might include experiencing significant distress over minor changes, encountering challenges with transitions, inflexible thinking patterns, adhering to specific greeting rituals, or maintaining the same daily routes and dietary preferences
    iii. Displaying highly limited and fixated interests that are unusually intense or focused. This could involve a strong attachment to or preoccupation with uncommon objects, exceedingly narrow or persistent interests
    iv. Showing heightened or diminished responsiveness to sensory stimuli or revealing an unusual fascination with sensory aspects of the environment. This could encompass apparent indifference to pain or temperature, adverse reactions to particular sounds or textures, excessive smelling or touching of objects, or a visual captivation with lights or motion

3. The symptoms described should be evident or observed during the early developmental period
4. The outlined symptoms result in notable hindrance in current social, occupational, or other crucial domains of functioning
5. These disturbances cannot be attributed to intellectual disability or global developmental delay as the primary cause

(DSM-5: Diagnostic and Statistical Manual of Mental Disorders, Fifth Edition)

SEVERITY ASSESSMENT AND SPECIFIERS

The severity levels of social communication difficulties and restricted and repetitive behaviors are outlined in the DSM-5 criteria and should be evaluated separately for each domain as shown in **Table 1**. It is important to note that the severity may change over time. Additionally, it is possible for individuals with ASD to have coexisting neurodevelopmental or behavioral conditions, such as ID, anxiety disorders, ADHD, depressive disorders, bipolar disorders, tics, Tourette's syndrome, sleep disorders self-injury, or feeding disorders. Furthermore, genetic or medical conditions such as Down syndrome, Rett syndrome, neurofibromatosis, tuberous sclerosis, or epilepsy may be present alongside ASD. Severity and coexisting conditions must be evaluated and noted in the diagnosis as specifiers.[2]

SCREENING TOOLS

The various ASD screening tools are brief; standardized tools appropriate in different socioeconomic contexts. It is advised to conduct screenings for ASD in children who display delayed language or communication milestones. It is also recommended for children who experience a regression in social or language skills, as well as for those whose caregivers express concerns about ASD at any point in their development. The American Academy of Pediatrics suggests conducting ASD screening at both 18 and 24 months of age.[33]

The M-CHAT-RF (Modified Checklist for Autism in Toddlers, Revised with Follow-up) is one of the most widely used screening tools for ASD. It is a two-stage parent-report screening tool validated for toddlers aged 16–30 months. The first stage comprises a set of

TABLE 1: Severity assessment in autism spectrum disorder (ASD).

Severity level	Deficits in social communication and social interaction	Restricted and repetitive patterns of behavior
Level 1 (requires support)	Without assistance, deficiencies in social communication give rise to noteworthy hindrances. Individuals might encounter challenges in initiating social interactions and display unconventional or ineffective reactions to the social signals of others. They could also seem to exhibit diminished enthusiasm for social engagements. As an illustration, an individual capable of speaking in full sentences and participating in conversations might struggle to engage in two-way exchanges, and their efforts to establish friendships could be odd and frequently unproductive	The rigidity of behavior leads to significant disruption in functioning within one or multiple contexts. Challenges arise when switching between activities and issues with organization and planning hinder the ability to function independently
Level 2 (requires substantial support)	Significant deficiencies are observed in both verbal and nonverbal social communication skills. These social challenges persist even when suitable assistance is provided. Individuals might display limited initiation of social interactions and show decreased or atypical reactions to social gestures from others. For example, a person who communicates using basic sentences, showcases a restricted scope of interests, and presents highly distinctive nonverbal communication	The rigid nature of behavior, struggles with adjusting to changes, and other restricted or repetitive behaviors are conspicuous enough to be noticeable by casual observers. These behaviors create substantial disruptions in functioning across different situations, and individuals might encounter distress and face challenges in redirecting their focus or altering their actions
Level 3 (requires very substantial support)	Profound shortcomings are evident in both verbal and nonverbal social communication skills, leading to notable hindrances in functioning. There is minimal initiation of social interactions and limited response to social gestures from others. As an example, an individual with only a handful of understandable words in their speech, who seldom initiates interaction, and when they do, adopts unconventional methods to satisfy their needs. They might only respond to very direct social approaches	The inflexibility of behavior, extreme difficulty in adapting to change, and other restricted/repetitive behaviors significantly disrupt functioning in all areas of life. There is a notable level of distress and significant difficulty in shifting focus or changing actions

TABLE 2: Various autism screening tools.			
Tool	*Age*	*Format*	*Psychometric properties*
Infant-toddler checklist (ITC)	6–24 months	24-item questionnaire	Sensitivity and specificity of 88.9%[37]
Parent's Observations of Social Interactions (POSI)	16–35 months	The seven-item assessment completed by parents and includes five out of the six critical items from the M-CHAT, along with two additional questions pertaining to behavior	Sensitivity of 83% and specificity of 75%[38]
Screening Tool for Autism in Toddlers and Young Children (STAT)	24–36 months	12 activities across four domains are observed. Two activities related to play, two activities involving requesting, four activities focused on directing attention, and four activities centered around motor imitation	A cut-off score of 2.75 had sensitivity of 95% and specificity of 73%[39]
Social Communication Questionnaire (SCQ)	4 years and older	Parent-reported, 40 yes/no questions	A cut-off score of 15 has sensitivity of 71% and specificity of 79%[40]
Autism Spectrum Screening Questionnaire (ASSQ)	7–16 years	27-item checklist rated on a 3-point scale by parents or teachers	A cut-off score of 17 or more has sensitivity of 91% and specificity of 86%[41]
AQ child	4–11 year	Parent reported 50 questions	A cut-off score of 76 has sensitivity 95% and specificity of 95%[42]
Chandigarh Autism Screening Instrument	1.5–10 years	A 37-item instrument, reported by parents in Hindi, requires yes/no responses	A cut-off score of 10 has sensitivity and specificity of 89%[43]
Indian Autism Screening Questionnaire (IASQ)	3–18 years	Parent-reported, 10-item scale, available in Hindi and English	At a cut-off of 1 has sensitivity of 99% and specificity of 62%[44]

20 questions that caregivers respond to with either a yes or no. Subsequently, in the second stage, the same questions are posed, but in greater detail, exploring the symptoms further. This stage is conducted by a healthcare professional.[34] The positive predictive value of M-CHAT-RF is 57.7% and has sensitivity of 82.6% and specificity of 45.7%.[35] After the completion of the initial stage of the questionnaire, the interpretation is as follows:

- *0-2 (low risk):* If no other risk factors are present, no further evaluation is required.
- *3-7 (medium risk):* The second stage of the screening should be administered. If the second stage results in a score of 2 or higher, immediate referral for diagnostic evaluation and early intervention is recommended.
- *8-20 (high risk):* Scores falling within this range indicate a high risk for ASD. Urgent referral for diagnostic assessment and early intervention is necessary, with no requirement for a subsequent follow-up interview.

The M-CHAT-RF is available in English and other Indian languages such as Hindi, Marathi, Bangla, Tamil, Telugu, and Urdu.[36] Other screening tools for autism used worldwide and in India are briefly summarized in **Table 2**.

DIAGNOSTIC TOOLS

Autism spectrum disorder is clinically diagnosed according to the criteria outlined in DSM-5. However, in addition to clinical observations, various validated tools are utilized to complement the diagnostic process. The diagnostic tools require training for administration. The various commonly used autism diagnostic tools are briefly summarized in **Table 3**.

EVALUATION OF COMORBIDITIES

Autism spectrum disorder is associated with various comorbidities and three-fourths have at least one associated comorbidity.[50] Screening for and addressing these accompanying conditions are essential to provide comprehensive care for individuals with ASD. The prevalence of common comorbidities is discussed here:

- *Epilepsy:* Around 10% prevalence overall and higher prevalence rate among adults with ASD.[51]
- *Attention-deficit/hyperactivity disorder:* It is the most common comorbidity associated with ASD.[50] Lifetime prevalence rate of around 40% in children with ASD.[52]

TABLE 3: Autism diagnostic tools.		
Tool	*Description*	*Psychometric properties*
Autism Diagnostic Observation Schedule, Second Edition (ADOS-2)	The assessment is administered by trained examiners and consists of five modules with the selection of modules based on the individual's level of expressive language	Widely recognized as "gold standard". (ADI-R) and ADOS have highest sensitivity and specificity for diagnosis of ASD[45]
Autism Diagnostic Interview, Revised (ADI-R)	The assessment comprises a total of 93 items designed to assess three areas of functioning: language, reciprocal social interactions, and restricted, repetitive, and stereotyped behaviors, and interests. Trained examiners administer an interview to caregivers. Depending on the age, a diagnostic algorithm is employed to methodically select a subset of questions. The determination of autism spectrum disorder (ASD) versus non-ASD is made using specific thresholds for each domain[46,47]	
Childhood Autism Rating Scale, Second Edition (CARS-2)	15 questions are rated on a scale of 1–4, based on severity. There are two versions of scale: (1) CARS2-ST (standard version) and (2) CARS2-HF (high functioning). The CARS2-ST scale is utilized for individuals under the age of 6 with communication difficulties or an estimated IQ below average. CARS2-HF scale is used for verbally fluent individuals who are 6 years old and above and have an IQ higher than 80	Sensitivity 81–100% and specificity 70–100% for both versions and varying cut-off values[48]
AIIMS-modified-INCLEN Diagnostic Tool for Autism Spectrum Disorder (INDT-ASD) Tool	Two sections and total of 37 questions and physician administered. Validated for 1–14 years of age	A score of 14 or higher suggests severe ASD, with a corresponding CARS score of >36.5. The sensitivity and specificity of the tool are 80 and 80.7%, respectively[49]

- *Anxiety disorder:* Anxiety in autistic children can be specific, social, or a generalized anxiety disorder. Prevalence rates vary from 1.6 to 62%.[53]
- *Obsessive-compulsive disorder:* Much higher prevalence in comparison to the general population and estimated around 17% in children with autism.[54]
- *Intellectual disability:* Around 70% of individuals diagnosed with ASD experience varying degrees of ID and the two entities share varied genetic etiologies with many candidate genes.[55]
- *Learning disability (LD):* Prevalence rates range between 60 and 70%.
- *Sleep disorders:* Around 75% of children with ASD encounter sleep disturbances. Typical sleep problems in autistic children encompass diminished sleep efficiency, shorter periods of rapid eye movement, and slow-wave sleep as well as an elevated desaturation index.[56]
- Other common related disorders in children with autism include depression, motor delay, tic disorder, bowel and bladder symptoms, and oppositional defiant disorder.[50]

ROLE OF INVESTIGATIONS IN ASD

Neuroimaging

Magnetic resonance imaging (MRI) brain has low yield in absence of epilepsy, focal neurological deficits, microcephaly, macrocephaly, or atypical regression. The yield of a pathological finding on MRI in autism without these associated features is very low.[57] The American Academy of Pediatrics advises against performing routine MRI scans in typical cases, emphasizing that the decision to undergo neuroimaging should be based on the patient's medical history and physical examination.[58]

Electroencephalogram

Children with autism exhibit epileptiform discharges on their electroencephalogram (EEG) without experiencing distinct clinical seizures. The clinical relevance of such epileptiform activity in autism patients remains a subject of controversy.[59] During the routine baseline evaluation, an EEG is not recommended unless there are seizures, atypical regression, or other abnormalities observed during history-taking and examination.[58]

Metabolic Testing

Metabolic testing should be routinely avoided in children with autism in view of low yield and cost-effectiveness.[60] Clinical indications are unusual regression, premature childhood fatalities within the family, pronounced hypotonia or weakness, visual impairment, auditory dysfunction, and dysmorphism. When necessary and indicated clinically, a targeted approach to metabolic testing should be adopted which may include blood glucose, pH and bicarbonate, urine ketone, fasting ammonia, plasma amino acid levels, urine organic acid levels, and acylcarnitine metabolite levels.[58]

Genetic Testing

Genetic evaluation in autistic children is guided clinically. Severe ID and dysmorphism are more likely to be associated with a genetic etiology.[61] Children who exhibit motor delay should undergo evaluations to screen for cerebral creatine deficiency and thyroid insufficiency. After conducting a comprehensive history and examination, if there is suspicion of a particular genetic etiology such as Rett syndrome, fragile X syndrome, or tuberous sclerosis, it is advisable to perform a targeted test to confirm the same. In cases where the underlying cause remains unknown, it is recommended to offer clinical microarray testing, which has a yield of 5–15%. If the results from the clinical microarray are inconclusive, the next step would be next-generation sequencing, which has a yield of 8–20%.[58] **Flowchart 1** summarizes the diagnostic approach to a child with ASD.

CONCLUSION

The risk factors for ASD are vast and varied and definitive single causative factors are still unclear. Genetic-environment interaction plays a vital role in the pathogenesis of ASD. Early features of autism may be subtle and high-risk children should undergo a formal screening/diagnostic evaluation. Investigations for the genetic etiology of autism should be personalized based on the clinical features.

REFERENCES

1. Parenti I, Rabaneda LG, Schoen H, Novarino G. Neurodevelopmental Disorders: From Genetics to Functional Pathways. Trends Neurosci. 2020;43(8):608-21.
2. American Psychiatric Association (Eds). Diagnostic and statistical manual of mental disorders: DSM-5, 5th edition. Washington, DC: American Psychiatric Association; 2013. p. 947.
3. Salari N, Rasoulpoor S, Rasoulpoor S, Shohaimi S, Jafarpour S, Abdoli N, et al. The global prevalence of autism spectrum disorder: a comprehensive systematic review and meta-analysis. Ital J Pediatr. 2022;48(1):112.
4. Li YA, Chen ZJ, Li XD, Gu MH, Xia N, Gong C, et al. Epidemiology of autism spectrum disorders: Global burden of disease 2019 and bibliometric analysis of risk factors. Front Pediatr. 2022;10:972809.
5. Maenner MJ. Prevalence and Characteristics of Autism Spectrum Disorder Among Children Aged 8 Years—Autism and Developmental Disabilities Monitoring Network, 11 Sites, United States, 2020. MMWR Surveill Summ. 2023;72(2):1-14.
6. Gulati S, Kaushik JS, Saini L, Sondhi V, Madaan P, Arora NK, et al. Development and validation of DSM-5 based diagnostic tool for children with Autism Spectrum Disorder. PloS One. 2019;14(3):e0213242.
7. Arora NK, Nair MKC, Gulati S, Deshmukh V, Mohapatra A, Mishra D, et al. Neurodevelopmental disorders in children aged 2-9 years: Population-based burden estimates across five regions in India. PLoS Med. 2018;15(7):e1002615.
8. Modabbernia A, Velthorst E, Reichenberg A. Environmental risk factors for autism: an evidence-based review of systematic reviews and meta-analyses. Mol Autism. 2017;8(1):13.

Flowchart 1: Diagnostic approach to a child with autism spectrum disorder.

Suspicion of autism spectrum disorder
↓
- *Detailed history and examination:* Screen for seizures, family history of similar complaints, atypical regression, dysmorphism, neurocutaneous markers, etc.
- Rule out hearing impairments and screen for mimickers
- Application of DSM-5 by a trained healthcare provider
- Assess severity as per DSM-5

↓
Screen and address common comorbidities, such as ADHD, ID, anxiety, epilepsy, sleep disorders, and feeding difficulties
↓
- Neuroimaging and EEG when indicated clinically
- *Targeted genetic testing:* Fragile X syndrome, *MeCP2*, PTEN, metabolic tests, thyroid profile, clinical microarray, next-generation sequencing, etc.

↓
Disability certification and management

(ADHD: attention-deficit hyperactivity disorder; DSM-5: Diagnostic and Statistical Manual of Mental Disorders, Fifth Edition; EEG: electroencephalogram; ID: intellectual disability)

9. Bölte S, Girdler S, Marschik PB. The contribution of environmental exposure to the etiology of autism spectrum disorder. Cell Mol Life Sci. 2019;76(7):1275-97.
10. Wu S, Wu F, Ding Y, Hou J, Bi J, Zhang Z. Advanced parental age and autism risk in children: a systematic review and meta-analysis. Acta Psychiatr Scand. 2017;135(1):29-41.
11. Lam J, Sutton P, Kalkbrenner A, Windham G, Halladay A, Koustas E, et al. A Systematic Review and Meta-Analysis of Multiple Airborne Pollutants and Autism Spectrum Disorder. PLoS One. 2016;11(9):e0161851.
12. Rossignol DA, Genuis SJ, Frye RE. Environmental toxicants and autism spectrum disorders: a systematic review. Transl Psychiatry. 2014;4(2):e360.
13. King S, Kildea S, Austin MP, Brunet A, Cobham VE, Dawson PA, et al. QF2011: a protocol to study the effects of the Queensland flood on pregnant women, their pregnancies, and their children's early development. BMC Pregnancy Childbirth. 2015;15(1):109.
14. Halladay AK, Bishop S, Constantino JN, Daniels AM, Koenig K, Palmer K, et al. Sex and gender differences in autism spectrum disorder: summarizing evidence gaps and identifying emerging areas of priority. Mol Autism. 2015;6(1):36.
15. Hansen SN, Schendel DE, Francis RW, Windham GC, Bresnahan M, Levine SZ, et al. Recurrence Risk of Autism in Siblings and Cousins: A Multinational, Population-Based Study. J Am Acad Child Adolesc Psychiatry. 2019;58(9):866-75.
16. Yenkoyan K, Grigoryan A, Fereshetyan K, Yepremyan D. Advances in understanding the pathophysiology of autism spectrum disorders. Behav Brain Res. 2017;331:92-101.
17. Beopoulos A, Géa M, Fasano A, Iris F. Autism spectrum disorders pathogenesis: Toward a comprehensive model based on neuroanatomic and neurodevelopment considerations. Front Neurosci. 2022;16:988735.
18. Wang Z, Hong Y, Zou L, Zhong R, Zhu B, Shen N, et al. Reelin gene variants and risk of autism spectrum disorders: An integrated meta-analysis. Am J Med Genet B Neuropsychiatr Genet. 2014;165(2):192-200.
19. Xu X, Miller EC, Pozzo-Miller L. Dendritic spine dysgenesis in Rett syndrome. Front Neuroanat. 2014;8:97.
20. El-Ansary A, Al-Ayadhi L. GABAergic/glutamatergic imbalance relative to excessive neuroinflammation in autism spectrum disorders. J Neuroinflammation. 2014;11(1):189.
21. Peterson C. Theory of mind understanding and empathic behavior in children with autism spectrum disorders. Int J Dev Neurosci. 2014;39(1):16-21.
22. Pardo CA, Vargas DL, Zimmerman AW. Immunity, neuroglia and neuroinflammation in autism. Int Rev Psychiatry. 2005;17(6):485-95.
23. Sarovic D. A Unifying Theory for Autism: The Pathogenetic Triad as a Theoretical Framework. Front Psychiatry. 2021;12:767075.
24. Yoon SH, Choi J, Lee WJ, Do JT. Genetic and Epigenetic Etiology Underlying Autism Spectrum Disorder. J Clin Med. 2020;9(4):966.
25. Rylaarsdam L, Guemez-Gamboa A. Genetic Causes and Modifiers of Autism Spectrum Disorder. Front Cell Neurosci. 2019;13:385.
26. Leblond CS, Cliquet F, Carton C, Huguet G, Mathieu A, Kergrohen T, et al. Both rare and common genetic variants contribute to autism in the Faroe Islands. NPJ Genomic Med. 2019;4(1):1-10.
27. Citrigno L, Muglia M, Qualtieri A, Spadafora P, Cavalcanti F, Pioggia G, et al. The Mitochondrial Dysfunction Hypothesis in Autism Spectrum Disorders: Current Status and Future Perspectives. Int J Mol Sci. 2020;21(16):5785.
28. Iwata K, Matsuzaki H, Takei N, Manabe T, Mori N. Animal Models of Autism: An Epigenetic and Environmental Viewpoint. J Cent Nerv Syst Dis. 2010;2:37-44.
29. Wolterink G, Daenen LE, Dubbeldam S, Gerrits MA, van Rijn R, Kruse CG, et al. Early amygdala damage in the rat as a model for neurodevelopmental psychopathological disorders. Eur Neuropsychopharmacol. 2001;11(1):51-9.
30. Parmeggiani A, Corinaldesi A, Posar A. Early features of autism spectrum disorder: a cross-sectional study. Ital J Pediatr. 2019;45(1):144.
31. Landa RJ, Gross AL, Stuart EA, Faherty A. Developmental trajectories in children with and without autism spectrum disorders: the first 3 years. Child Dev. 2013;84(2):429-42.
32. DSM Library. [2013]. Diagnostic and Statistical Manual of Mental Disorders: DSM-5, Fifth edition. [online] Available from: https://dsm.psychiatryonline.org/doi/book/10.1176/appi.books.9780890425787 [Last accessed September, 2023].
33. Lipkin PH, Macias MM; Council on Children with Disabilities, Section on Developmental and Behavioral Pediatrics. Promoting Optimal Development: Identifying Infants and Young Children with Developmental Disorders Through Developmental Surveillance and Screening. Pediatrics. 2020;145(1):e20193449.
34. M-CHAT™. [2009]. M-CHAT™—Autism Screening. [online] Available from https://mchatscreen.com/ [Last accessed September, 2023].
35. Aishworiya R, Ma VK, Stewart S, Hagerman R, Feldman HM. Meta-analysis of the Modified Checklist for Autism in Toddlers, Revised/Follow-up for Screening. Pediatrics. 2023;151(6):e2022059393.
36. M-CHAT™. (2023). MCHAT R/F Translations. [online] Available from https://mchatscreen.com/mchat-rf/translations/ [Last accessed September, 2023].
37. Wetherby AM, Brosnan-Maddox S, Peace V, Newton L. Validation of the Infant-Toddler Checklist as a broadband screener for autism spectrum disorders from 9 to 24 months of age. Autism Int J Res Pract. 2008;12(5):487-511.
38. Smith NJ, Sheldrick RC, Perrin EC. An Abbreviated Screening Instrument for Autism Spectrum Disorders. Infant Ment Health J. 2013;34(2):149-55.

39. Stone WL, McMahon CR, Henderson LM. Use of the Screening Tool for Autism in Two-Year-Olds (STAT) for children under 24 months: an exploratory study. Autism Int J Res Pract. 2008;12(5):557-73.
40. Eaves LC, Wingert HD, Ho HH, Mickelson ECR. Screening for autism spectrum disorders with the social communication questionnaire. J Dev Behav Pediatr. 2006;27(Suppl 2):S95-S103.
41. Posserud MB, Lundervold AJ, Gillberg C. Validation of the autism spectrum screening questionnaire in a total population sample. J Autism Dev Disord. 2009;39(1):126-34.
42. Auyeung B, Baron-Cohen S, Wheelwright S, Allison C. The Autism Spectrum Quotient: Children's Version (AQ-Child). J Autism Dev Disord. 2008;38(7):1230-40.
43. Arun P, Chavan BS. Development of a screening instrument for autism spectrum disorder: Chandigarh Autism Screening Instrument. Indian J Med Res. 2018;147(4):369-75.
44. Chakraborty S, Bhatia T, Sharma V, Antony N, Das D, Sahu S, et al. Psychometric properties of a screening tool for autism in the community—The Indian Autism Screening Questionnaire (IASQ). PLoS One. 2021;16(4):e0249970.
45. Falkmer T, Anderson K, Falkmer M, Horlin C. Diagnostic procedures in autism spectrum disorders: a systematic literature review. Eur Child Adolesc Psychiatry. 2013;22(6):329-40.
46. Oh M, Song DY, Bong G, Yoon NH, Kim SY, Kim JH, et al. Validating the Autism Diagnostic Interview-Revised in the Korean Population. Psychiatry Investig. 2021;18(3):196-204.
47. Kim SH, Lord C. Autism Diagnostic Interview, Revised. In: Kreutzer JS, DeLuca J, Caplan B (Eds). Encyclopedia of Clinical Neuropsychology. New York, NY: Springer; 2011. pp. 313-5.
48. Dawkins T, Meyer AT, Van Bourgondien ME. The Relationship Between the Childhood Autism Rating Scale: Second Edition and Clinical Diagnosis Utilizing the DSM-IV-TR and the DSM-5. J Autism Dev Disord. 2016;46(10):3361-8.
49. Gulati S, Patel H, Chakrabarty B, Dubey R, Arora NK, Pandey RM, et al. Development and validation of AIIMS modified INCLEN diagnostic instrument for epilepsy in children aged 1 month-18 years. Epilepsy Res. 2017;130:64-8.
50. Khachadourian V, Mahjani B, Sandin S, Kolevzon A, Buxbaum JD, Reichenberg A, et al. Comorbidities in autism spectrum disorder and their etiologies. Transl Psychiatry. 2023;13(1):71.
51. Liu X, Sun X, Sun C, Zou M, Chen Y, Huang J, et al. Prevalence of epilepsy in autism spectrum disorders: A systematic review and meta-analysis. Autism. 2022;26(1):33-50.
52. Rong Y, Yang CJ, Jin Y, Wang Y. Prevalence of attention-deficit/hyperactivity disorder in individuals with autism spectrum disorder: A meta-analysis. Res Autism Spectr Disord. 2021;83:101759.
53. Vasa RA, Keefer A, McDonald RG, Hunsche MC, Kerns CM. A Scoping Review of Anxiety in Young Children with Autism Spectrum Disorder. Autism Res. 2020;13(12):2038-57.
54. Meier SM, Petersen L, Schendel DE, Mattheisen M, Mortensen PB, Mors O. Obsessive-Compulsive Disorder and Autism Spectrum Disorders: Longitudinal and Offspring Risk. PLoS One. 2015;10(11):e0141703.
55. Srivastava AK, Schwartz CE. Intellectual Disability and Autism Spectrum Disorders: Causal Genes and Molecular Mechanisms. Neurosci Biobehav Rev. 2014;46(Pt 2):161-74.
56. Aathira R, Gulati S, Tripathi M, Shukla G, Chakrabarty B, Sapra S, et al. Prevalence of Sleep Abnormalities in Indian Children With Autism Spectrum Disorder: A Cross-Sectional Study. Pediatr Neurol. 2017;74:62-7.
57. Cooper AS, Friedlaender E, Levy SE, Shekdar KV, Bradford AB, Wells KE, et al. The Implications of Brain MRI in Autism Spectrum Disorder. J Child Neurol. 2016;31(14):1611-6.
58. Hyman SL, Levy SE, Myers SM; Council on Children with Disabilities, Section on Developmental and Behavioral Pediatrics. Identification, Evaluation, and Management of Children with Autism Spectrum Disorder. Pediatrics. 2020;145(1):e20193447.
59. Ghacibeh GA, Fields C. Interictal epileptiform activity and autism. Epilepsy Behav. 2015;47:158-62.
60. Campistol J, Díez-Juan M, Callejón L, Fernandez-De Miguel A, Casado M, Garcia Cazorla A, et al. Inborn error metabolic screening in individuals with nonsyndromic autism spectrum disorders. Dev Med Child Neurol. 2016;58(8):842-7.
61. Tammimies K, Marshall CR, Walker S, Kaur G, Thiruvahindrapuram B, Lionel AC, et al. Molecular Diagnostic Yield of Chromosomal Microarray Analysis and Whole-Exome Sequencing in Children with Autism Spectrum Disorder. JAMA. 2015;314(9):895-903.

Chapter 3

Management of Autism Spectrum Disorder

Kaushik Ragunathan, Richa Tiwari, Gautam Kamila, Sheffali Gulati

INTRODUCTION

Autism spectrum disorder (ASD) is a multifaceted neurodevelopmental condition characterized by difficulties in social communication and behavioral patterns. Emerging in early childhood, ASD affects individuals differently, ranging from mild difficulties to profound impairments in cognitive and emotional processing. Core deficits include repetitive behaviors, restricted interests, and impairments in social communication and interaction.[1] Early diagnosis and intervention are crucial in promoting positive outcomes and fostering a supportive environment for those living with ASD.

Presently, there is no known cure for ASD, but timely intervention can help. The goal of treatment is to maximize the child's functioning and improve their social, communication, functional, and behavioral skills. Nonpharmacological interventions continue to be the mainstay of therapy. Pharmacological agents are not curative but when used with nonpharmacological approaches improve core symptoms and may also help to reduce few associated comorbidities.

Role of complementary and alternative medicine (CAM), newer technologies, such as augmentative and alternative communication (AAC), artificial intelligence (AI) including deep learning models, virtual reality, and robotics, noninvasive neuromodulation, such as direct current stimulation (DCS) and transcranial magnetic stimulation (TMS) in management of ASD seems promising but needs further exploration.

NONPHARMACOLOGICAL MANAGEMENT IN AUTISM SPECTRUM DISORDER

Autism spectrum disorder management is not a one-size-fits-all approach and each person presents with unique strengths, weaknesses, and challenges. By acknowledging the distinct characteristics of each child, interventions can be tailored to optimize their potential and result in the most favorable functional outcomes **(Fig. 1)**. Families and caregivers should work closely with specialists and educators to adapt interventions to specific needs of the child.[2,3]

Autism spectrum disorder necessitates a personalized, multidisciplinary management strategy, targeting

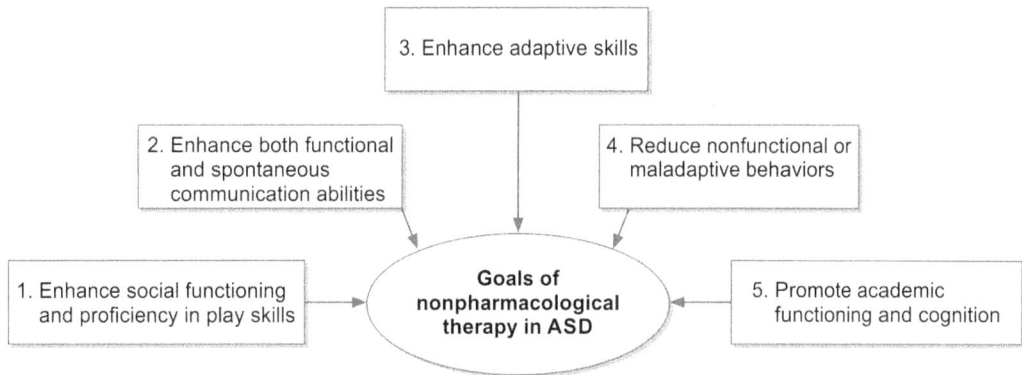

Fig. 1: Goals of nonpharmacological therapy in autism spectrum disorder (ASD).

social, communication, and adaptive skill enhancement while reducing negative behaviors. Early intervention, capitalizing on individual strengths, and engaging caregivers are crucial for success. Tailored evidence-based therapies, such as applied behavior analysis (ABA) and speech therapy, ensure optimal progress. Regular assessments monitor development and guide necessary adjustments, aiming to maximize functioning and foster independence for each child. Collaboration among professionals, educators, and parents ensures a comprehensive approach to child's specific needs, ultimately improving their quality of life **(Table 1)**.[4]

Prompt diagnosis and immediate and intensive treatment have the capacity to significantly influence outcomes, especially in terms of behavior, functional abilities, and communication. While a cure remains elusive, over time, symptoms have the potential to ameliorate, and in a few instances, may reduce to the extent that they no longer result in impairment. The body of evidence supporting effectiveness of early intervention is growing, highlighting the importance of initiating interventions as soon as possible. Therapies can be administered through early intervention programs. As the child becomes older, school-based special education programs have a more prominent role in providing therapy.[4]

Treatment modalities that are used are summarized in **Figure 2** and include:[5]

Behavioral Approaches

Behavioral strategies have the most evidence in improving ASD symptoms. They center on modifying behaviors by comprehending antecedents and consequences of a particular behavior. These include ABA. ABA promotes favorable behaviors while discouraging undesirable ones, aiming to enhance a range of skills. The process involves monitoring and assessing progress. Various types of ABA can be used as per problem at hand. Most prominently used approaches are described here:

- *Discrete trial training (DTT):* Utilizes incremental instructions to teach desired behavior or response. Lessons are deconstructed into their fundamental components, with positive reinforcement for desired outcomes and behaviors, while undesired responses are discouraged.
- *Pivotal response training (PRT):* It takes place in a natural setting rather than a clinic setting. The goal of

TABLE 1: Key points to consider in planning individualized management of autism spectrum disorder (ASD).	
Comprehensive assessment	To identify the individual's strengths, weaknesses, and specific needs, involving input from diverse professionals—psychologists, speech/occupational therapists, educators
Person-centered goals	Treatment plans must revolve around the individual's goals and aspirations, maximizing functional abilities and overall quality of life
Strength-based approach	Acknowledging and leveraging an individual's strengths enhances active engagement and motivation in therapy by capitalizing on their interests and abilities
Early intervention	Identifying and addressing challenges as early as possible for better progress and increased independence in the long run
Multidisciplinary collaboration	Holistic ASD management involves a multidisciplinary team of professionals including educators, therapists, physicians, and psychologists
Tailored therapies	Diverse evidence-based therapies including applied behavior analysis (ABA), speech therapy, occupational therapy, and social skills training tailored to the individual's unique needs and objectives
Communication support	Individuals with ASD benefit from augmentative and alternative communication (AAC) systems, aiding communication, and overcoming challenges in expression
Parent and caregiver involvement	Caregivers play a crucial role in implementing strategies at home and supporting the individual's progress beyond therapy sessions
Ongoing monitoring and adjustments	Consistent evaluation and progress monitoring are essential to ensure the ongoing effectiveness and relevance of the treatment plan, adapting it to the individual's evolving needs
Emphasis on independence	Integral to ASD management is fostering independence through life skills, empowering individuals for autonomy and confidence

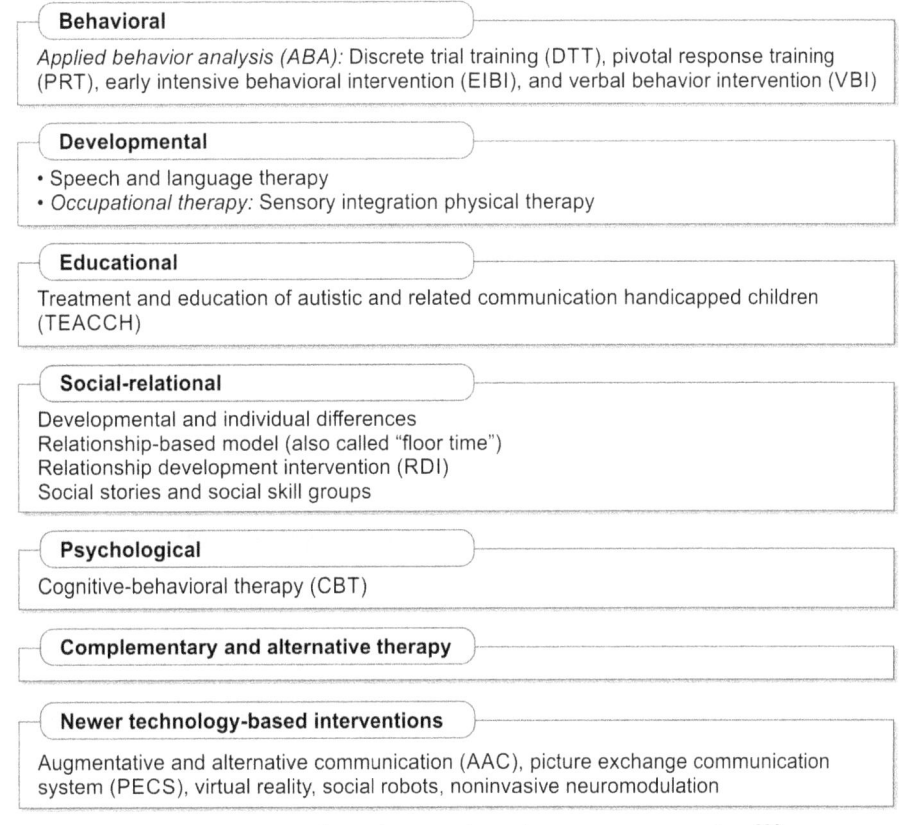

Fig. 2: Summary of nonpharmacological treatment approaches.[6,8,9]

PRT is to improve a few "pivotal skills" that will help the person learn many other skills. One example of a pivotal skill is to initiate communication with others.
- *Early intensive behavioral intervention (EIBI):* For children under age 5 years
- *Verbal behavior intervention (VBI)* focuses on language skills
- *Others:* Language paradigms and incidental teaching (teaching as events occur in the context of the natural environment).

Developmental Approaches

Developmental approaches aim to enhance distinct developmental skills like language or physical abilities as well as interconnected developmental capacities, and are often complemented by behavioral strategies. Common developmental therapies used in ASD are:
- *Speech and language therapy:* To enhance speech, language, and communication skills accommodating verbal, nonverbal, and alternative forms of expression in ASD such as signs/gestures/technology-assisted communication.
- *Occupational therapy:* It fosters independence by teaching skills, such as dressing, eating, bathing, and social interaction. It includes:
  • *Sensory integration therapy:* To address sensory challenges that may be restrictive or overwhelming.
  • *Physical therapy:* For enhancing motor skills. It includes motor training (including fine skills such as handwriting as well as gross motor training involving balance and posture).

The Early Start Denver Model (ESDM) is a broad developmental approach based on the principles of ABA. It is used with children 12–48 months of age.

Other developmental models are Social Communication, Emotional Regulation, and Transactional Support (SCERTS) program, and Joint Attention, Symbolic Play, Engagement and Regulation (JASPER). Parents and therapists employ play, social interactions, and shared focus within authentic environments to enhance language, social, and learning abilities.

Educational Approaches

Structured educational programs with a team are given in a classroom setting. Intensive and individualized interventions during preschool years have shown positive results in many studies. These school curricula-based education programs with high staff-to-student ratio and specialized teachers create supportive and structured environments utilizing functional behavior analysis. Family involvement and close monitoring and transition planning are integral to the child's progress. These comprehensive interventions empower and optimize learning experiences and overall development of children with ASD. They help foster independence and social integration while addressing their unique challenges and strengths.

A notable type of educational approach is *Treatment and Education of Autistic and Related Communication Handicapped Children (TEACCH)*. It harnesses the consistency and visual learning capability of children with ASD, e.g., written/drawn daily routines in clear sight, boundaries around learning stations, and verbal instructions supplemented with visual instructions such as picture cards or physical demonstrations to aid learning objectives. Lessons are broken down into small steps, so they are easier.

Social-relational Approaches

Interventions center on enhancing social abilities and fostering emotional connections, often involving parental or peer mentor involvement.
- *Developmental, individual differences, and relationship-based model (also called "floor time")*: It promotes aligning with individual interests to broaden communication possibilities and nurturing emotional and intellectual development through skill acquisition.
- *Relationship development intervention (RDI)*: It involves activities that increase motivation, interest, and abilities to participate in shared social interactions.
- *Social stories* provide simple descriptions of what to expect in a social situation.
- *Social skills groups* provide opportunities for people with ASD to practice social skills in a structured environment.

Psychological Approaches

Assist individuals with ASD in managing anxiety, depression, and mental health challenges. *Cognitive-behavioral therapy (CBT)* targets thought-behavior-emotion links. CBT enables collaborative goal setting and cognitive reframing for adaptive responses.

Complementary and Alternative Therapy

They comprise diverse practices beyond conventional medicine. Alternative therapies replace standard treatments, while complementary therapies supplement them. Integrative medicine combines both approaches with supportive evidence. CAM may merge into conventional practice with time as new and better evidence is generated. Families often explore CAM options alongside conventional therapies such as behavioral analysis in search for improvement. While CAM's allure in pursuit of a cure is strong, its efficacy varies **(Fig. 3)**. When discussing about CAM with family of child with ASD, maintain an open-minded and nonjudgmental stance. Inquire without presumptions understanding motivations behind choices suggested by them. Acknowledge and handle concerns about mainstream treatments and side effects, aim to be an ally and offer relevant resources.[6]

Technology-based Interventions and Supports

Augmentative and alternative communication, computer applications and software, and picture exchange communication system (PECS)—visual-based treatment that uses symbols instead of picture cards to enable communication, social robots, teleconferencing, video modeling, virtual reality [including virtual and three-dimensional (3D) environments to mimic social situations], and wearable sensors are all examples of the types of technology in this subcategory of publications.[7]

Increasing awareness of autism calls for essential interventions for toddlers, yet optimal strategies remain unclear. Limited ASD-specific interventions exist for those under 2 years old outside research settings. Integrative developmental behavioral models show effectiveness. Early intervention services, including speech and language interventions, are strongly recommended for toddlers with ASD. Emphasizing natural learning, sensorimotor exploration, communication development, and enriched environments is crucial. Limited research evaluates comprehensive programs for older ASD individuals, but ABA-based strategies show promise. Educational interventions for adolescents target social competence, emotional regulation, education, and independence skills.

No benefits demonstrated or may be detrimental	Possible benefits (can be tried after discussion with parents)	Unknown benefits (can be tried after discussion with parents)
No benefit - Secretin - Facilitated communication **Unknown benefit, potential risk** - Intravenous immunoglobulin - Chelation - Hyperbaric oxygen therapy - Antimicrobial agents - Vitamin B_6, vitamin A, vitamin D (tolerable upper intake level) - Magnesium - Homeopathy - Vagus nerve stimulation - Stem cell therapy	**Possible benefit, low risk** - Music therapy - Melatonin, oxytocin, and sulforaphane - Therapeutic horseback riding - Animal/pet therapy - Transcranial magnetic stimulation - Biofeedback/neurofeedback - Yoga, massage, Reiki - Hypnotherapy - Vitamin C, vitamin B_{12} **Possible benefit, potential risk if taken unsupervised** - Gluten-free casein-free diet	**Unknown benefit, low risk** - Auditory integration therapy - Omega 3 fatty acids, probiotics - Oxidative therapies other than vitamin C (methylcobalamin, folate, N-acetyl cysteine) - Zinc - Herbal products - Amino acids (taurine, dimethylglycine) - Mindfulness therapy - Acupuncture and chiropractic

Fig. 3: Complementary and alternative therapy in autism spectrum disorder (ASD).
Source: Autism spectrum disorder in children and adolescents: Pharmacologic interventions. (2021) Available from: URL: https://www.uptodate.com/contents/autism-spectrum-disorder-in-children-and-adolescents-pharmacologic-interventions.

Transition care of a child with ASD needs utmost sensitivity and must be started early but gradually to allow time for adequate adjustments. Commencing transition planning at age 10 necessitates a collaborative approach with a multidisciplinary team responsible for the child's care, emphasizing the development of self-advocacy skills and ensuring parental comfort as key priorities.

ADDRESSING ASD RELATED COMORBIDITIES USING NONPHARMACOLOGICAL APPROACHES

Autism spectrum disorder is frequently associated with various comorbidities, often presenting unique challenges for affected individuals. Understanding these coexisting conditions are vital for providing comprehensive support.

Among these, comorbid conditions are intellectual disabilities, with approximately 40-50% of individuals with ASD experiencing coexisting cognitive impairments.

Additionally, attention-deficit/hyperactivity disorder (ADHD) is commonly observed, affecting about 30-60% of those with ASD.

Anxiety and depression are prevalent, affecting around 30-50% of individuals, as are motor coordination difficulties and language disorders.

Gastrointestinal (GI) issues, epilepsy, and sleep disturbances are also known comorbidities. Attending to these concerns can enhance focus, learning, and improve associated behaviors as well.

Sleep disturbances represent a common comorbidity in children with ASD, with prevalence ranging from 50 to 80%. A stepwise approach to sleep disturbances in children has been practiced even conventionally. This includes sleep education and implementation of healthy sleep practices followed by specific behavioral strategies. If nonsuccessful, medications can be cautiously titrated to the lowest effective dose for optimal treatment. The same principle applies to ASD. Parent-based sleep education has shown effectiveness in the general pediatric population and some children with ASD. Behavioral interventions, such as complete extinction (removing reinforcement to decrease a behavior) or graduated extinction and scheduled awakenings, are commonly used and have positive effects on various sleep problems. Other interventions, such as weighted blankets and aromatherapy, have limited evidence. Physical activity and yoga may also impact sleep in ASD children, but the findings are mixed. Massage has been found to induce improvements in sleep quality, diurnal behavior, and attention in children. Further research is needed for a comprehensive understanding of sleep interventions in this population.[9,10]

In conclusion, nonpharmacological therapies play a crucial role in the comprehensive management of ASD. These therapies offer a range of benefits, addressing core symptoms and improving the overall quality of life for individuals on the spectrum. Behavioral interventions, such as ABA, help enhance social skills, communication, and adaptive behaviors. Speech and language therapy aids in improving communication abilities, while occupational therapy supports the development of essential life skills and sensory integration. Additionally, social skill training fosters meaningful interactions and relationships. Sensory-based therapies promote coping mechanisms for sensory sensitivities. It is essential to recognize the individuality of each person with ASD, tailoring interventions to their unique needs and strengths. By embracing a holistic approach that incorporates these nonpharmacological therapies, we can create a more inclusive and supportive environment for individuals on the autism spectrum, empowering them to reach their fullest potential.

PHARMACOLOGICAL MANAGEMENT OF AUTISM SPECTRUM DISORDER

Principles of Pharmacotherapy in Autism Spectrum Disorder

The primary modality of treatment of ASD is nonpharmacological. There is no single medication that directly addresses the cognitive impairment in Autism. There are three approaches to plan pharmacotherapy in patients with ASD. The first and foremost measure is to target the core symptoms. Second is to address the comorbidities related to ASD. Third is still in its primitive stages of evidence which targets the basic underlying neurobiological processes related to syndromic autism (as in fragile X syndrome).[11]

However, over the last decade, there has been increasing evidence of polypharmacy in ASD ranging from 35 to 65%. It has been observed that the use of medications in autism increases with increasing age, associated intellectual disability (ID), and other psychological comorbidities.[4]

The initial assessment should include history and examination to rule out correctable medical factors that can cause/worsen the problem behavior in autistic children (e.g. gastroesophageal reflux and constipation that can worsen irritability and epilepsy that can add onto hyperactivity). The principles of initiating psychotropic medications in ASD are similar to that of any other typically developing child. However, the treating clinician should carefully weigh the risk-benefit ratio before doing so *because children with ASD are slightly more sensitive to adverse effects of these medications.* Hence, it should be started at a lower dose, gradually titrated to response at a very slower rate. The medication may be gradually tapered off when symptoms have been adequately controlled and have been taken care of by the non-pharmacological behavioral interventions.

PHARMACOLOGICAL TREATMENT OF CORE SYMPTOMS IN ASD

Repetitive Behaviors

Pharmacotherapy when used alone will not act on repetitive behaviors, which includes motor stereotypes, behavioral rigidity, and compulsions. But, it may be utilized as a part of comprehensive behavioral intervention for better results. Dopamine receptor blockers (atypical antipsychotics) may have some effect on repetitive behaviors. Studies suggest that short-term courses of aripiprazole or risperidone may show benefits in aggression and tantrum related to repetitive behaviors.[11]

The other medications that have been tried include antiseizure drugs (divalproex sodium and topiramate) and selective serotonin reuptake inhibitor (SSRI) (fluoxetine and fluvoxamine).

Impaired Communication and Reciprocal Social Interaction

There are no medications targeting social communication in ASD. However, treating comorbidities can result in some improvement in this domain.

PHARMACOLOGICAL TREATMENT OF COMORBIDITIES RELATED TO ASD

Hyperactivity, Impulsivity, and Inattention

Hyperactivity and inattention are one of the most common presenting core symptoms in ASD. Stepwise management has been suggested in children. During the first visit, a thorough baseline behavioral assessment is done and targeted interventions are advised. After a period of 3–6 months, the child is again assessed for the same and if there is no response, a trial of pharmacotherapy can be initiated. This is undertaken on the basis that children with ASD are more sensitive to psychostimulant doses and especially those with ID and other comorbidities may not respond well to medicines.[4]

The first-line medication is usually a stimulant medication (dextroamphetamine salts or methylphenidate) initiated in a low dose. The dose is gradually titrated for response. In case of adverse effects or no response to the first-line medications, a trial of selective norepinephrine reuptake inhibitor (SNRI) (atomoxetine) may be given. The other options include α-adrenergic agonists (guanfacine and clonidine) and atypical antipsychotics (aripiprazole and risperidone).

Irritability and Disruptive Behaviors

The United States Food and Drug Administration (USFDA) has approved two medications for irritability in autism. *Risperidone*, a second-generation atypical antipsychotic (D2 receptor antagonist), was approved in 2006 for irritability, aggression, tantrums, and deliberate self-injury in patients >5 years of age. *Aripiprazole* was approved in 2009 by FDA for children and adolescents of age 6–17 years. These two medications have an affinity for dopamine, serotonin, histaminergic, and α-adrenergic receptors in the brain. The treating clinician should keep a watch for weight gain and sedation. The other medicines of this family, olanzapine and quetiapine, are not FDA approved and lack sufficient evidence for routine use in children.[11]

Few other medications for irritability include α-2 adrenergic agonists (clonidine and guanfacine), SSRIs (fluvoxamine and citalopram), antiseizure medications (ASMs) (valproic acid and divalproex sodium), and SNRI (venlafaxine). These drugs are commonly used off-label for irritability but lack sufficient evidence to be used as the first-line agent.

Minocycline has been tried in ASD with fragile X syndrome. Arbaclofen has been studied in smaller patient groups. Amantadine [noncompetitive N-methyl-D-aspartate (NMDA) antagonist] has yielded positive effects in irritability and hyperactivity. However, we need blinded randomized controlled trials (RCTs) with large sample size before a recommendation can be made for these three drugs.

Anxiety and Depression

The anxiety disorders amenable to pharmacotherapy include social phobias, generalized anxiety disorder, and separation anxiety. The first-line treatment option for anxiety related to ASD is always CBT. Pharmacotherapy includes SSRI (fluoxetine, sertraline, escitalopram, and citalopram), α-agonists (guanfacine and clonidine), atypical antipsychotics, and β-blockers (propranolol). Short-acting benzodiazepine (lorazepam) has been tried for event-related anxiety. For mood-related disorders, starting on a mood stabilizer and/or a second-generation antipsychotic drug is recommended.

For depression, SSRIs are widely used in children. However, it has been noted that ASD children are more sensitive to adverse effects. Hence, it is recommended that they are started in a lower dose and very gradual titration to response may be tried. Particularly in adults, fluoxetine seems to be best tolerated among serotonergic agents.

Obsessive-Compulsive Disorder Related Disorders (OCD Related Disorders)

First-line therapy in obsessive-compulsive disorder (OCD) related disorders is CBT, although it may be less effective in children with ASD. A trial of SSRI may be given particularly if associated with anxiety or depression. Risperidone and clomipramine are alternative options.

Sleep Disorder

Children with ASD are well known to have sleep issues such as decreased sleep duration, increased sleep latency, and disturbed sleep. Studies suggest that low melatonin level in children with ASD is related to altered circadian rhythm. A low dose of oral melatonin supplement can be added along with behavioral intervention and sleep hygiene measures. The usual dose ranges from 1 to 6 mg. α-adrenergic agents (clonidine) and antihistamines (diphenhydramine) are being used off-label for insomnia, but there is insufficient evidence to support the same. Melatonin, when used along with CBT, shows better results.

Gastrointestinal and Feeding Issues

Common GI symptoms in children with ASD include constipation, vomiting, gastroesophageal reflux, abdominal pain, feeding issues, and diarrhea. The medical management is the same as that of any other typically developing child. But autistic children may benefit from consistent behaviorally informed interventions for encopresis and constipation.

Autistic children have feeding issues in the form of food selectivity, rumination, pica, and compulsive eating. This is usually related to their repetitive behavior. Feeding problems affect nutrition and can cause micro-/macronutrient deficiencies. The management is same as in any other typically developing child, but in addition targeted behavioral interventions on a case-to-case basis should be designed. If they fail, gastrostomy-tube placement and nonoral feeding should be tried.

Pica may be associated with the risk of iron deficiency, lead poisoning, ingestion of nonedible substances including bezoars leading to obstruction or intestinal perforation.

Seizures, Epilepsy, and EEG Abnormalities in ASD

In the following description, we have tried to arrive at a reasonable strategy to approach an autistic child with seizure and an autistic child with no seizure but with electroencephalogram (EEG) abnormalities.

Child with ASD and clinical seizure: Incidence of epilepsy is high in autistic patients as compared to typically developing children. The risk is even greater if there is an associated ID. The challenge is to rightly identify the clinical seizure, especially in those with complex motor stereotypes. Focal seizures with impaired awareness are the most common semiology, but generalized tonic, or tonic-clonic seizures may also occur. Autistic kids may have some complex stereotypes such as staring episodes or gaze deviation which may be mistaken as seizure. Video documentation of events and EEG documentation may help in deciding regarding initiation of ASM. The term, *interictal spike discharges,* is used to denote the occurrence of EEG abnormalities between seizures.

In syndromic causes of autism such as fragile X and tuberous sclerosis complex (TSC), there is a need for ASM therapy and dosage is optimized till clinical response. There are even specific choices of ASM like that in management of spasms in TSC with vigabatrin.

Subclinical electroencephalographic abnormalities (SEAs) or isolated epileptiform discharges (IEDs) are at times used interchangeably to indicate epileptiform discharges on EEG but complete absence of identifiable clinical seizures. Several studies have reported SEAs in the range of 4–86% in ASD even if no clinical seizures have been noted. The discharges were most frequently noted from the right temporal lobe or bilateral temporal region, which is usually implicated in social deficits and language dysfunction respectively. The presence of EEG abnormalities has been associated with lower IQ, impaired adaptive skills, marked increase in stereotypies and aggression.[12]

EEG Abnormalities in ASD: To Treat or Not to Treat?

The *first step* in approaching SEAs in autistic children is to look for the contributory role of these discharges in cognitive and behavioral abnormalities. In conditions such as electrical status epilepticus in sleep (ESES), where there may not be ongoing clinical seizures but high incidence of electrical discharges during sleep may contribute to cognitive regression and significant behavioral problems (hyperactivity, aggression, and irritability). The management differs from the rest of the epileptic conditions. Steroids (pulse methylprednisolone) and benzodiazepines are proven successful modalities in ESES. A similar condition is Landau–Kleffner syndrome where steroids are the first-line therapy. Lennox-Gastaut syndrome is distinct from the two above-mentioned conditions since it presents with multiple semiology of seizures and characteristic EEG findings.

After ruling out the above-mentioned conditions or direct contributory role of the EEG discharges to ASD, *the next step* is to make an individualized approach on a case-to-case basis. At present, there is insufficient evidence to support initiating ASM for treating epileptiform discharges in ASD even in autistic regression. However, it has been noted that there can be some tangential benefit in behavioral problems due to the mood stabilizing action of a few ASM.[13]

Choice of ASM: The most frequently used medications include valproate, levetiracetam, and lamotrigine. Valproate has a broad spectrum of action when used as an ASM and in addition has been well known for its mood stabilizing action. It has some role in improving aggression, irritability, and repetitive behavior in autistic cohorts. Lamotrigine has a very similar neuropsychiatric profile to valproate. These two medications (and carbamazepine) are used in instances where there are associated mood disorders or depression.[13]

The following medications are to be used with caution in those with cognitive impairment: phenobarbitone, topiramate, zonisamide, and phenytoin.[13]

The following medications should be used with caution in those with psychiatric/behavioral concerns: levetiracetam, phenobarbitone, zonisamide, phenytoin, topiramate, and perampanel.

TABLE 2: Summary of common medications used in ASD.

Pharmacotherapy	Symptoms targeted	Adverse effects	Comments

Atypical antipsychotics:
• Risperidone—D$_2$ receptor antagonist
  – Dose range (0.25–3.5 mg/day)
  – Doses up to 10 mg/day have been reported in literature for children >45 kg
• Aripiprazole—D$_2$ receptor antagonist with partial agonist properties
  – Dose range (2.5 mg/day to a maximum of 15 mg/day has been tried)[14]
	• Irritability
	• Disruptive traits
		• Increased appetite, weight gain, sedation, fatigue, and drooling
		• Elevated prolactin levels and tremors
		• Start at a lower dose, very gradual titration, monitor for sedation, and extrapyramidal adverse effects
		• *Serious adverse effects:* Metabolic syndrome, dyslipidemia and hyperglycemia
		• Sedation (after risperidone) is likely to reduce after 8 weeks of therapy
		• As compared to risperidone, aripiprazole is noted to have less sedation and lower incidence of extrapyramidal symptoms
			Risperidone and aripiprazole are *FDA-approved medications* targeting irritability in ASD[4]

α-2 adrenergic agonists: Clonidine and guanfacine	• Irritability • Hyperactivity	• Sedation and drowsiness • Fatigue • Constipation • Worsening of irritability and aggression • Appetite suppression, hypotension, and bradycardia	α-2 agonists can be considered in: • Children <5 years with ADHD symptoms, and hyperarousal • Failed response/intolerance to stimulant medications/SNRIs • Coexisting sleep issues[4]
Serotonergic medications: This category includes the SSRIs, SNRIs (serotonin-norepinephrine reuptake inhibitors), and tricyclic antidepressants	• Anxiety • OCD • Disruptive behaviors • Irritability • Mood disorders • Repetitive behaviors	Autistic children may be more sensitive to behavioral activation with SSRIs	Serotonin dysregulation has been reported in autism in relation to anxiety, depression symptoms, and repetitive behaviors
SSRIs: • Fluvoxamine • Clomipramine (5–10 mg/day) • Fluoxetine (5–20 mg/day) • Buspirone (2.5–5 mg/day) • Citalopram (2.5–20 mg/day)		These medications may cause activation, sedation, insomnia, diarrhea, dry skin, pruritus, and rarely worsening of stereotypies	• There is insufficient evidence to support SSRIs for core symptoms but may help in anxiety and depression symptoms • FDA has mentioned caution in children with ASD taking SSRI (especially fluoxetine) due to concerns regarding suicidal ideation in depressed children with ASD. So, these children should be carefully monitored
SNRIs (atomoxetine): Inhibit the presynaptic norepinephrine transporter	Hyperactivity (nonstimulant medication)		• Atomoxetine may be considered if failure/intolerance/no response to first-line stimulant medications • It is preferred in coexisting anxiety

Contd…

Pharmacotherapy	Symptoms targeted	Adverse effects	Comments
Psychostimulant medications: Methylphenidate, dexmethylphenidate, lisdexamfetamine, and dextroamphetamine	• Inattention • Hyperactivity • Impulsivity	• Insomnia and appetite suppression are well-known adverse effects • Worsening of irritability and depressive symptoms	In case of inattention/hyperactivity, a stepwise approach is usually implemented with regard to pharmacotherapy, as children may be more sensitive to adverse effects (as explained in the text)
Antiseizure medications: • Levetiracetam • Lamotrigine • Divalproex sodium • Bumetanide	• For indications, other than management of seizures • Mood stabilizing effects • Irritability • Repetitive behaviors		There have been constant discussions over the role of levetiracetam in worsening of behavioral problems, but till date there is no conclusive evidence to support the use as first-line ASM or to avoid levetiracetam in those with ASD

(ADHD: attention-deficit hyperactivity disorder; ASD: autism spectrum disorder; FDA: Food and Drug Administration; OCD: obsessive-compulsive disorder; SSRIs: selective serotonin reuptake inhibitors)

DRUGS TARGETING NEUROBIOLOGICAL PROCESSES RELATED TO SYNDROMIC AUTISM (ROLE OF PRECISION MEDICINE)

The functional effect of tuberous sclerosis is related to activation of the mammalian target of rapamycin (mTOR) complex. There are several ongoing trials utilizing everolimus (mTOR inhibitor) as an adjunctive therapy in drug refractory epilepsy in TSC. The initial results are assuring.

SCN2A mutations have been related to ID and autism with or without epilepsy. There is a role for sodium channel blockers (phenytoin). PCDH19 (protocadherin-19)-related disorders are associated with drug refractory epilepsy with or without behavioral problems. PCDH19 is suspected to have a role in gamma-aminobutyric acid type A (GABA$_A$) function. Ganaxolone plays a role in GABA$_A$ function. Its role in epilepsy and neuropsychiatric problems is yet to be investigated.[13]

The other two common genetic associations in ASD are *SCN1A* and *MECP2*. Mutations in *SCN1A* are related to Dravet syndrome. Nonepilepsy phenotypes are associated with autistic traits. In *MECP2*-related Rett syndrome, hand stereotypies are a common autistic feature although these kids may have good social interaction.

NEWER TREATMENT STRATEGIES

After extensive review of the newer drugs/ongoing trials on pharmacotherapy in ASD, the authors felt that the following drugs are worth mentioning. The other treatment options have been listed in **Table 3**.

Oxytocin is a neurohypophyseal peptide synthesized in the hypothalamus and is actively related to the receptors in nucleus accumbens, amygdala and hippocampus that play a role in social behaviors. Several trials have shown benefit with intranasal/intravenous oxytocin in terms of short-term improvement in social communication. But, there is insufficient evidence to support its long-term use. Intranasal oxytocin has adverse effects such as nasal irritation, skin irritation, fatigue, and diarrhea.

Till date, there is no robust evidence to support probiotics for GI symptoms or behavioral problems in ASD. The existing blinded RCTs have found no significant difference in terms of GI symptoms/behavior. However, the studies regarding prebiotics are assuring. Especially the combination of prebiotics and exclusion diet (casein and gluten-free diet) has reduced GI symptoms and antisociability scores.

Cannabidiol is the nonpsychotropic component of marijuana, and has been tried in the management of motor deficits like the tremor in Parkinson's disease and in anxiety, pain, and nausea. The possible mechanisms implicated in ASD include GABA$_A$ agonist potentiation, stimulation of 5-HT1A receptors and possible role in mitochondrial function. Large-scale studies are required to support its use in children.

A newer therapeutic option, resveratrol, a plant phytoalexin has been tried in ASD for its anti-inflammatory

TABLE 3: Newer/emerging treatment options in ASD.

Medication/supplement	Possible mechanism of action	Comment
Dietary supplements: Sulforaphane (in broccoli and many cruciferous vegetables) Omega-3 fatty acids	• Antioxidant • Anti-inflammatory • Mitochondrial protective agent	At present, the evidence to suggest the role of broccoli in improvement of core symptoms is still inconclusive
N-acetyl cysteine (NAC)	• Antioxidant action • NAC lowers glutaminergic transmission, thereby improving the imbalance between E:I (excitation:inhibition) ratio[15]	Initial studies have shown improvement in irritability and stereotypies
Metformin	• Role in specific subgroups of ASD (fragile X syndrome) • In the absence of FMRP, there is hyperactive insulin receptor, upregulation of mTORC1, MAPK/ERK pathways	• Specifically targets overeating in ASD (especially in fragile X syndrome, Prader–Willi syndrome) • Minor degrees of improvement in irritability and aggression
Oxytocin	Neuropeptide from hypothalamus with a critical role in social functioning	• Suggested role in improvement in social reciprocity, repetitive behaviors, and emotion recognition • Preliminary studies have shown some evidence of improvement in social cognition, although they require large RCTs
Phosphodiesterase-4D (PDE4D) inhibitors	cAMP level is downregulated in fragile X syndrome. PDE4D inhibitors cause inhibition of cAMP breakdown	Positive results in a small group of adult males with fragile X syndrome, in terms of cognition and behavior
Cannabidiol (CBD)	• Potentiation of $GABA_A$ agonist action • Stimulation of 5-HT1A receptors • Improves mitochondrial function	• Trials of oral and topical cannabidiol in ASD are ongoing • Role of CBD in drug refractory epilepsy such as Dravet and Lennox–Gastaut syndrome has been well established • However, there is no sufficient evidence at present to support its role in behavioral problems
Probiotics and prebiotics	Commonly tested options are: • *Bifidobacterium, Lactobacillus*, and *Lacticaseibacillus*-based probiotic preparations • They increase the production of microbial metabolites, such as short-chain fatty acids (SCFA) and many other anti-inflammatory cytokines	• Benefits of probiotics on core behavioral symptoms of ASD are not satisfactory based on the existing trials • However, prebiotic and symbiotic combinations have shown assuring results on trials. But at present there is no sufficient quality of evidence to provide recommendations for the same

(ASD: autism spectrum disorder; cAMP: cyclic adenosine monophosphate; ERK: extracellular signal-regulated kinase; FMRP: fragile X mental retardation protein; MAPK: mitogen-activated protein kinase; mTORC1: mTOR complex 1; RCTs: blinded randomized controlled trials)

and antioxidant properties. However, the existing RCTs have shown conflicting results between studies and hence require large-scale studies.

There are several ongoing studies worldwide with focus on newer neurobiological pathways and with a scope for precision medicine which may be the future of pharmacotherapy in autism.

CONCLUSION

The primary modality of treatment in ASD is nonpharmacological; drug therapy can be used as a bridge or on a short-term basis as a support to the behavioral interventions. Nonpharmacological approaches must be highly individualized. The choice of therapy approach and its delivery is a team effort with a common goal in view.

Therapies must always be given by a well-trained professional in collaboration with other team members. Behavior, developmental, and integrative models of therapy should never be ignored while the child is started on medications. None of the existing medications target cognitive improvement in ASD; the medications are targeted predominantly toward comorbidities of ASD. Risperidone and Aripiprazole are FDA-approved medications targeting irritability (disruptive behaviors) in ASD. When pharmacotherapy is planned for an autistic patient, a detailed baseline cognitive and behavioral assessment should be documented by a qualified psychologist and should be repeated frequently to document response to the medication. At present, there definitely is no sufficient evidence for initiating ASM in a child with ASD with subclinical EEG abnormalities. The decision has to be taken on a case-to-case basis if the contributory role of the SEAs to the behavioral problems is proven.

REFERENCES

1. American Psychiatric Association (Eds). Diagnostic and statistical manual of mental disorders: DSM-5, 5th edition. Washington, DC: American Psychiatric Association; 2013. p. 947.
2. Narzisi A, Costanza C, Umberto B, Filippo M. Non-Pharmacological Treatments in Autism Spectrum Disorders: An Overview on Early Interventions for Pre-Schoolers. Curr Clin Pharmacol. 2014;9(1):17-26.
3. Myers SM. Management of autism spectrum disorders in primary care. Pediatr Ann. 2009;38(1):42-9.
4. Hyman SL, Levy SE, Myers SM; Council on Children with Disabilities, Section on Developmental and Behavioral Pediatrics. Identification, Evaluation, and Management of Children With Autism Spectrum Disorder. Pediatrics. 2020;145(1):e20193447.
5. Nash K, Carter KJ. Treatment options for the management of pervasive developmental disorders. Int J Psychiatry Med. 2016;51(2):201-10.
6. Cheng A. (2019). Benefits of Nonpharmacological and Pharmacological Treatments in Autistic Children. [online] Available from: https://scholar.dominican.edu/nursing-senior-theses/21/ [Last accessed September, 2023].
7. Lecciso F, Levante A, Fabio RA, Caprì T, Leo M, Carcagnì P, et al. Emotional Expression in Children With ASD: A Pre-Study on a Two-Group Pre-Post-Test Design Comparing Robot-Based and Computer-Based Training. Front Psychol. 2021;12:678052.
8. Linden A, Best L, Elise F, Roberts D, Branagan A, Tay YBE, et al. Benefits and harms of interventions to improve anxiety, depression, and other mental health outcomes for autistic people: A systematic review and network meta-analysis of randomised controlled trials. Autism. 2023;27(1):7-30.
9. Keogh S, Bridle C, Siriwardena NA, Nadkarni A, Laparidou D, Durrant SJ, et al. Effectiveness of non-pharmacological interventions for insomnia in children with Autism Spectrum Disorder: A systematic review and meta-analysis. PLoS OnE. 2019;14(8):e0221428.
10. Esposito D, Belli A, Ferri R, Bruni O. Sleeping without Prescription: Management of Sleep Disorders in Children with Autism with Non-Pharmacological Interventions and Over-the-Counter Treatments. Brain Sci. 2020;10(7):441.
11. Howes OD, Rogdaki M, Findon JL, Wichers RH, Charman T, King BH, et al. Autism spectrum disorder: Consensus guidelines on assessment, treatment and research from the British Association for Psychopharmacology. J Psychopharmacol. 2018;32(1):3-29.
12. Precenzano F, Parisi L, Lanzara V, Vetri L, Operto FF, Pastorino GMG, et al. Electroencephalographic Abnormalities in Autism Spectrum Disorder: Characteristics and Therapeutic Implications. Medicina (Kaunas). 2020;56(9):419.
13. Watkins LV, O'Dwyer M, Shankar R. A review of the pharmacotherapeutic considerations for managing epilepsy in people with autism. Expert Opin Pharmacother. 2022;23(7):841-51.
14. Swaiman KF, Ashwal S, Ferriero DM, Schor NF, Finkel RS, Gropman AL, et al. Swaiman's Pediatric Neurology: Principles and Practice, 6th edition. Edinburgh: Elsevier; 2018.
15. Aishworiya R, Valica T, Hagerman R, Restrepo B. An Update on Psychopharmacological Treatment of Autism Spectrum Disorder. Neurotherapeutics. 2022;19(1):248-62.

Attention-deficit Hyperactivity Disorder in Children

Monica Juneja, Smitha Sairam

INTRODUCTION

Attention-deficit hyperactivity disorder (ADHD) is one of the most common neurodevelopmental disorders of childhood characterized not only by inattention and hyperactivity, but also impulsivity. These symptoms result in significant impairment of academics and social functioning. Persistence of symptoms into adolescence, or in adulthood, may lead to difficulties with employment and relationships as well as antisocial behaviors.

EPIDEMIOLOGY

Prevalence estimates of ADHD vary with the research methodology used, type of survey (community vs. clinic sample), age group of the population surveyed, and changes in diagnostic criteria over time. Systematic reviews have estimated the global community prevalence of ADHD in children to be between 2 and 8% with an average being around 5%.[1,2] In an Indian study, the community prevalence of ADHD in children aged 6–9 years across five geographically diverse populations was found to range between 0.5 and 2.3%.[3] However, the prevalence in school and clinic-based population has been estimated to be much higher.[4] With boys outnumbering girls by a ratio of 2:1 for inattentive presentation and 3:1 for combined presentation, there is a definite male predominance in ADHD.[5] While boys are more frequently labeled with hyperactive or combined presentations, girls are more likely to have an inattentive presentation.

ETIOPATHOGENESIS OF ADHD

Attention-deficit hyperactivity disorder is a disorder with a multifactorial etiology, with a combination of genetic, epigenetic, and environmental factors contributing to the pathogenesis and heterogeneity. Structural magnetic resonance imaging (MRI) in children with ADHD is essentially normal; however, volumetric studies have shown smaller volumes of the prefrontal cortex and basal ganglia and abnormalities of the cerebellum, particularly the vermis.[6] These studies have also documented delays in achieving peak cortical thickness in ADHD. Functional MRI findings indicate low blood flow to the striatum, and deficits in dispersed functional networks in prefrontal regions, parietal lobe, and temporal lobe—areas involved in selective and sustained attention.[7]

Attention-deficit hyperactivity disorder is a highly heritable, polygenic disorder, with a heritability as high as 80%. The familial aggregation of the disorder is strong, with the relative risk of ADHD being 5–10-fold for first-degree relatives. Twin studies have found that 75% of the variance in ADHD phenotype can be attributed to genetic factors. If one identical twin has ADHD, the other twin has a >50% chance of having ADHD.[8]

At the neurochemical level, decrease in dopaminergic and noradrenergic levels mediate the core symptoms of ADHD.[9] Strong associations have been found between ADHD and multiple genes involved in dopamine and serotonin pathways, with the dopamine transporter gene (*DAT1*) and a particular form of the dopamine 4 receptor gene (*DRD4*) being most strongly implicated. Other genes that might contribute to ADHD include *COMT*, *DRD5*, *SLC6A3*, *DBH*, *SNAP25*, *SLC6A4*, and *HTR1B*.[10]

Environmental risk factors for ADHD include maternal substance use, prenatal exposure to environmental toxins, low birth weight, lead exposure, and iron deficiency. Psychosocial adversities such as poverty, exposure to violence, and undernutrition, or malnutrition can contribute to or worsen ADHD symptoms.[11]

CLINICAL FEATURES

The three core symptoms of ADHD: (1) Inattention, (2) hyperactivity, and (3) impulsivity manifest in most of the situations—at home, in school, outdoors, or in the workplace. However, the symptoms change with age.[12] In preschool children, hyperactivity is most obvious and impairing. These children run and climb excessively "are always on the go" and often act as if "driven by a motor". They may warm-up easily to strangers and talk more than other children of similar age. They usually dislike and avoid activities that require paying attention for more than few minutes, and will quickly lose interest after engaging in an activity for a short while. Preschoolers and young children with ADHD are often short-tempered and aggressive with playmates, and may sustain injuries more often due to careless and impulsive behaviors.

School-aged children with ADHD most often present with attention problems resulting in failure to complete homework, poor grades, poor organizational skills, and disruptive behaviors in the classroom such as repeatedly getting up from their seat, speaking out of turn, troubling their classmates and truancy. Interactions with peers and/or adults may be problematic because of associated hyperactivity, decreased awareness of others' space, impulsivity manifesting commonly as "butting into other people's matters and difficulty in sustaining activities or conversations." They may be easily bullied or persuaded to act in "silly" ways that often land them in trouble.

Girls generally have fewer hyperactivity symptoms, and often remain undiagnosed until later when academic demands become greater.

Adolescents with ADHD may find the increased social and academic expectations to be very challenging, even though hyperactivity decreases significantly in this age group. Without support, teenagers with ADHD tend to have lower grades, higher rates of school failure, and suspension for problem behaviors. About half of adolescents with ADHD have serious problems with peer relationships. They tend to have fewer friends, and are more likely to be ignored or rejected by peers because of their impulsive behaviors. Problems related to bullying continue into adolescence. Their impulsivity and poor emotion-regulation often leads to frustration and inability to cope with demanding situations. Adolescents with ADHD tend to indulge in smoking, alcohol use, and substance abuse earlier than their neurotypical peers. They are also more likely to indulge in risky behaviors such as rash driving, resulting in compromise of their and others' safety.

DIAGNOSIS

The diagnosis of ADHD is a clinical diagnosis using various diagnostic criteria, the most common being DSM-5.[13] It lists eighteen specific behaviors as part of the diagnostic criteria and delineates three types of presentations [(1) predominantly hyperactive-impulsive type, (2) predominantly inattentive type, and (3) combined type] based on the symptoms (**Box 1**). For establishing a diagnosis of ADHD, children should meet six of the inattentive and/or hyperactive-impulsive criteria.

BOX 1: DSM-5 diagnostic criteria for attention-deficit hyperactivity disorder (ADHD).

A. A persistent pattern of inattention and/or hyperactivity-impulsivity that interferes with functioning or development, as characterized by (1) and/or (2):
  1. *Inattention:* Six (or more) of the following symptoms have persisted for at least 6 months to a degree that is inconsistent with developmental level and that negatively impacts directly on social and academic/occupational activities:
    Note: The symptoms are not solely a manifestation of oppositional behavior, defiance, hostility, or failure to understand tasks or instructions. For older adolescents and adults (age 17 and older), at least five symptoms are required.
    a. Often fails to give close attention to details or makes careless mistakes in schoolwork, at work, or during other activities (e.g., overlooks or misses details, work is inaccurate).
    b. Often has difficulty sustaining attention in tasks or play activities (e.g., has difficulty remaining focused during lectures, conversations, or lengthy reading).
    c. Often does not seem to listen when spoken to directly (e.g., mind seems elsewhere, even in the absence of any obvious distraction).
    d. Often does not follow through on instructions and fails to finish schoolwork, chores, or duties in the workplace (e.g., starts tasks but quickly loses focus and is easily sidetracked).
    e. Often has difficulty organizing tasks and activities (e.g., difficulty managing sequential tasks; difficulty keeping materials and belongings in order; messy, disorganized work; has poor time management; fails to meet deadlines).
    f. Often avoids, dislikes, or is reluctant to engage in tasks that require sustained mental effort (e.g., schoolwork or homework; for older adolescents and adults, preparing reports, completing forms, reviewing lengthy papers).
    g. Often loses things necessary for tasks or activities (e.g., school materials, pencils, books, tools, wallets, keys, paperwork, eyeglasses, mobile telephones).

Contd...

Contd…

> h. Is often easily distracted by extraneous stimuli (for older adolescents and adults, may include unrelated thoughts).
> i. Is often forgetful in daily activities (e.g., doing chores, running errands; for older adolescents and adults, returning calls, paying bills, keeping appointments).
>
> 2. *Hyperactivity and impulsivity:* Six (or more) of the following symptoms have persisted for at least 6 months to a degree that is inconsistent with developmental level and that negatively impacts directly on social and academic/occupational activities:
> *Note:* The symptoms are not solely a manifestation of oppositional behavior, defiance, hostility, or a failure to understand tasks or instructions. For older adolescents and adults (age 17 and older), at least five symptoms are required.
>   a. Often fidgets with or taps hands or feet or squirms in seat.
>   b. Often leaves seat in situations when remaining seated is expected (e.g., leaves his or her place in the classroom, in the office or other workplace, or in other situations that require remaining in place).
>   c. Often runs about or climbs in situations where it is inappropriate. (Note: In adolescents or adults, may be limited to feeling restless).
>   d. Often unable to play or engage in leisure activities quietly.
>   e. Is often "on the go," acting as if "driven by a motor" (e.g., is unable to be or uncomfortable being still for extended time, as in restaurants, meetings; may be experienced by others as being restless or difficult to keep up with).
>   f. Often talks excessively.
>   g. Often blurts out an answer before a question has been completed (e.g., completes people's sentences; cannot wait for turn in conversation).
>   h. Often has difficulty waiting his or her turn (e.g., while waiting in line).
>   i. Often interrupts or intrudes on others (e.g., butts into conversations, games, or activities; may start using other people's things without asking or receiving permission; for adolescents and adults, may intrude into or take over what others are doing).
>
> B. Several inattentive or hyperactive-impulsive symptoms were present prior to age 12 years.
> C. Several inattentive or hyperactive-impulsive symptoms are present in two or more settings (e.g., at home, school, or work; with friends or relatives; in other activities).
> D. There is clear evidence that the symptoms interfere with, or reduce the quality of social, academic, or occupational functioning.
> E. The symptoms do not occur exclusively during the course of schizophrenia or another psychotic disorder and are not better explained by another mental disorder (e.g., mood disorder, anxiety disorder, dissociative disorder, personality disorder, substance intoxication or withdrawal).
>
> *Specify whether:*
> - 314.01 (F90.2) Combined presentation: If both criteria A1 (inattention) and A2 (hyperactivity-impulsivity) are met for the past 6 months.
> - 314.00 (F90.0) Predominantly inattentive presentation: If criterion A1 (inattention) is met but criterion A2 (hyperactivity-impulsivity) is not met for the past 6 months.
> - 314.01 (F90.1) Predominantly hyperactive-impulsive presentation: If criterion A2 (hyperactivity-impulsivity) is met and criterion A1 (inattention) is not met for the past 6 months.
>
> *Specify if:*
> *In partial remission:* When full criteria were previously met, fewer than the full criteria have been met for the past 6 months, and the symptoms still result in impairment in social, academic, or occupational functioning.
>
> *Specify current severity:*
> *Mild:* Few, if any, symptoms in excess of those required to make the diagnosis are present, and symptoms result in no more than minor impairments in social or occupational functioning.
> *Moderate:* Symptoms or functional impairment between "mild" and "severe" are present.
> *Severe:* Many symptoms in excess of those required to make the diagnosis, or several symptoms that are particularly severe, are present, or the symptoms result in marked impairment in social or occupational functioning.

Source: DSM-Diagnostic and Statistical Manual of Mental Disorders.

However, for adolescents, the number of criteria has been decreased to five in either/both domains. In addition, diagnostic criteria for ADHD include ascertaining the presence of several symptoms before the age of 12 years, presence of the symptoms in two or more major settings, which lead to significant difficulties in learning, and/or social interactions. DSM-5 also classifies the symptoms as mild, moderate, or severe. Further, the symptoms should not be attributable to any other mental health condition. Children who do not meet full criteria for ADHD, but have significant difficulties in functioning, are said to be in partial remission if they had met the full criteria earlier (*see* **Box 1**).

A thorough history is required to elucidate the symptoms specified in DSM-5, including their impact and manifestations in various settings, and assess commonly associated conditions and comorbidities. Important components of history and examination are given in **Table 1**. A review of collateral information, such as school performance and testing results from other observers, helps to understand and assesses the degree of functional impairment. It is also important to identify treatable conditions and other disorders that may present with symptoms of inattention, hyperactivity, and/or impulsivity **(Table 2)**.

BEHAVIOR RATING SCALES FOR ADHD

A number of behavior rating scales for ADHD are available. These are useful in establishing the severity of symptoms and monitoring response to intervention, but should not be solely used to establish a diagnosis of ADHD, as symptoms may be under or overreported. These measures include, but are not limited to, the Vanderbilt ADHD Diagnostic Rating Scale, the Conners Rating Scales (parent and teacher), ADHD Rating Scale-5, the Swanson, Nolan, and Pelham Checklist (SNAP), and the ADD-H-Comprehensive Teacher's Rating Scale (ACTeRS).

COMORBIDITIES AND ASSOCIATED CONDITIONS

More than two-thirds of children with ADHD have a comorbid neurodevelopmental or psychiatric disorder.[15] Common comorbidities include oppositional defiant disorder (25-75%), conduct disorder (35%), major depression (6-30%), anxiety disorders (25%), bipolar disorder (20%), intellectual disability (15%), tic disorder (10%), autism spectrum disorder (10%), and epilepsy and specific learning disability (20-60%). ADHD criteria

TABLE 1: Comprehensive history and examination components for children with possible attention-deficit hyperactivity disorder (ADHD).

Essential components of history

Prenatal and birth history:
- Prenatal exposure to substances associated with symptoms of ADHD (tobacco, cocaine, and alcohol)
- Gestational age, birth weight
- History of adverse perinatal events

Developmental and behavioral history:
- Motor development
- Language development
- *Early regulatory behaviors:* Feeding problems, sleep problems in infancy
- History of onset of behavioral concerns
- Temperament
- Sleep habits
- Fears, worries, and routines
- *Social relationships:* Family, friends, and history of bullying

Third generation family history:
- Diagnosis of ADHD, anxiety, mood, language, or learning disorders
- Difficulty with school completion, poor job performance, and substance abuse

Psychosocial history:
- Socioeconomic class
- Frequent changing of home and school
- Exposure to domestic violence
- History of abuse and neglect

Medical history (child and family):
Tics, epilepsy, cardiac symptoms, vision, and hearing, drug history, and family medical history, especially cardiac*, such as sudden death below 40 years or death associated with exercise

Examination
- Anthropometry including height, weight and body mass index (BMI)
- Pulse and blood pressure
- Pallor
- *Dysmorphology assessment for associated syndromes:* Fragile X syndrome, Williams syndrome, DiGeorge syndrome, Klinefelter's syndrome, Turner syndrome, etc.
- *Neurocutaneous markers:* Tuberous sclerosis complex
- Cardiac examination*
- Neurological examination
- Assessment of vision and hearing

*Cardiac history of patient and family members and cardiac examination are essential before initiating stimulant medications.

TABLE 2: Alternate conditions that may mimic attention-deficit hyperactivity disorder (ADHD) symptomatology.[14]

Symptoms consistent with ADHD	Alternative conditions/diagnosis to be ruled out	Red flags suggestive of a non-ADHD diagnosis	Other clinical considerations
Inattention	• Hearing impairment • Visual impairment • Seizure disorder • Autism spectrum disorder • Sleep apnea and narcolepsy • Anxiety disorders • Thyroid disorders • Drugs (antiepileptics, benzodiazepines, antihistaminics, etc.) and toxins such as lead	• Excessive worries • Fearfulness • Stereotypic behaviors	Cognitive level of child (not able to comprehend/excessively bored)
Talks excessively	• Anxiety disorders • Bipolar disorder	• Excessive worries • Fearfulness • Grandiosity	
School failure or underachievement	• Learning disorders • Adjustment disorder • Psychosocial stressors	ADHD symptoms only in setting requiring academics (school; homework)	Consider behaviors during vacations versus school year
Fidgety	• Anxiety disorders • Tic disorder • Stereotypical movement	Repetitive motor or vocal movements	High level of activity but not affecting performance

Source: Adapted and modified from Prock LA, Rappaprt L. Attention and Deficits of Attention. In: Carey WB (Ed). Developmental-Behavioral Pediatrics, 4th edition. Philadelphia, PA: Saunders/Elsevier; 2009. pp. 524-34.

can also be met as part of the presentations of fragile X syndrome, fetal alcohol spectrum disorder, and Tourette disorder. The presence of comorbidities complicates the diagnostic process, affects the course, prognosis, and management. Assessment and management of comorbid disorders are as important as the assessment and treatment of ADHD symptoms and often warrant referral to specialists.

MANAGEMENT OF ADHD

The treatment of ADHD includes behavioral management and pharmacotherapy. Psychoeducating the child and important others about the diagnosis is the first step to ensuring a good outcome. The discussion should include an understanding that ADHD is a neurodevelopmental disorder, and is not caused because of poor parenting or intentional misbehavior. Its propensity to improve through medication and behavioral therapy should be emphasized. Family preferences should be considered while deciding the intervention plan, as this can increase adherence to treatment. Also, many parents who have ADHD themselves, may need extra support to help them follow a consistent schedule for medications and behavioral programs.

Prior to starting intervention, the clinician should preferably document the baseline severity of symptoms in the child using ADHD parent and teacher rating scales.

Behavioral Interventions

For preschool children (younger than 6 years) with ADHD and those with ADHD-like behaviors without a verified diagnosis, evidence-based behavioral interventions constitute the first line of management.[16] Recommendations for behavioral interventions should be individualized, based on specific treatment goals, be age-appropriate, and acceptable and feasible for the child, family, and teachers. Parent training in behavior management (PTBM) helps parents to understand age-appropriate behaviors, achieve consistent and positive interactions with their children, and teaches parents to provide appropriate consequences for their child's behaviors. It also helps children to improve their abilities to manage their own behaviors. Behavioral interventions are most effective if caregivers understand the principles of behavior therapy (i.e., identification of antecedents and altering the consequences of behavior) and the techniques are consistently implemented. Some strategies for managing behaviors at home are given in **Box 2**.

Medications may be considered in preschoolers if behavioral interventions do not provide significant improvement or if evidence-based behavioral interventions are not available, or cannot be implemented. In such cases, the clinician should weigh the risks of starting medication against the harm of delaying treatment.

Pharmacotherapy

Medications are the first line of treatment in children older than 6 years of age, and adolescents with ADHD, preferably in combination with behavioral and educational intervention.[16] The recommended first-line and most widely prescribed drugs for ADHD are psychostimulants, which act as dopamine and norepinephrine reuptake inhibitors thereby increasing the available dopamine and norepinephrine in the caudate nucleus and prefrontal cortex. Of the two stimulant medications, methylphenidate (MPH) and amphetamine, only MPH is available in India. The other class of drugs is nonstimulants, which act as norepinephrine reuptake inhibitors and block the presynaptic norepinephrine transporter in the prefrontal cortex. Atomoxetine (ATX) is a nonstimulant drug, and is generally prescribed when stimulants are not effective or cause significant adverse effects. Second-line or adjuvant medications for ADHD include central-acting α-2 adrenergic agonists, such as clonidine and guanfacine. The drugs used for treatment of ADHD along with dosing and titration have been given in **Table 3**.

Stimulant medications have an early onset of action with behavioral effects seen within 30–45 minutes. With short-acting preparations, a peak and trough effect may occur, wherein rebound symptoms of hyperactivity are seen as effect of medication wears off. This can be countered by using long-acting preparations of the drug. It is estimated that at least 80% of children respond to the stimulants, if used in correct doses.

Initial response to nonstimulants (ATX) can occur between 1 week and 23 days, the response may continue to increase incrementally beyond 6–9 weeks. The efficacy of ATX is lower than that of stimulants.

After obtaining an adequate treatment response, medications should be continued for as long as they

BOX 2: Strategies for parents to manage behaviors in attention-deficit hyperactivity disorder (ADHD).

- Give clear and brief instructions or commands
- Set reasonable but consistent rules and boundaries
- Reward positive behaviors
- Create a calm and nondistracting environment for activities that require attention (e.g., homework)
- Schedule in-between breaks for activities that may be complicated or rigorous for the child
- Maintain a daily schedule or routine, and encourage child to follow the schedule
- Break difficult tasks into smaller, simpler, and achievable tasks
- Provide specific places where child can put away his items
- Establish a consistent sleep routine
- Be vigilant about dangerous activities that child may indulge in
- Involve child in activities or sports that he/she is good at

TABLE 3: Medications for attention-deficit hyperactivity disorder (ADHD).

Name of drug	Dosage forms	Dosing	Maximum dose/day	Duration of effects
Stimulants				
Methylphenidate short-acting	5 mg, 10 mg, 20 mg tablets	Start with 2.5–5 mg twice daily, titrate over the first 4 weeks till desired effect/maximum dose/or, side effects appear	60 mg/day	3–5 hours
Methylphenidate intermediate-acting (sustained release)	10 mg, 20 mg tablets	Start with 10–20 mg/day in single dose, increase slowly by 10 mg weekly	60 mg/day	6–8 hours
Methylphenidate OROS	18 mg, 36 mg capsule	Start with 18 mg/day	• *6–12 years:* 54 mg • *13–17 years:* 72 mg	10–12 hours
Nonstimulant				
Atomoxetine	10 mg, 18 mg, 25 mg	Start with 0.3 mg/kg/day in two divided doses. Titrate over 1–3 weeks to 1.2–1.4 mg/kg/day	1.4 mg/kg/day or 100 mg, whichever is lower	Up to 24 hours

(OROS: osmotic-release oral system)

remain effective. Drugs should ideally not be stopped during times of stress or transitions (changing schools, examinations, etc.). Dose reduction or drug holidays may be considered during vacations or school breaks after a minimum of 1–2 years of symptom resolution, when functional burden and expectations from the child are not high. Signs that ADHD has remitted include lack of need to adjust dose despite robust growth, lack of deterioration when a dose is missed, and ability to concentrate during drug holidays. However, any recurrence or worsening of symptoms that may occur on reducing or stopping medication warrants restarting the medication or increasing dose appropriately.

ADVERSE EFFECTS OF MEDICATIONS

Common short-term adverse effects associated with stimulants include appetite loss, abdominal pain, headaches, and sleep disturbance. Appetite loss with MPH is often bothersome to parents, and hence, it is recommended to give the medications after meals. Stimulant medications may increase the heart rate by an average of 1–2 beats/min and blood pressure by 1–4 mm Hg (systolic and diastolic). Though the changes are insignificant in most patients, a small subset may experience substantial increases of 5–15%, and hence, monitoring of these signs is important.

Stimulants do not increase risk of sudden cardiac death, contrary to earlier beliefs. Nevertheless, relevant cardiac history in child and family should be obtained before initiating treatment, and risk factors should prompt safety concerns regarding use of the stimulant medication. Stimulants may have a long-term effect on growth velocity with diminished growth being 1–2 cm from predicted adult height.

Adverse effects associated with ATX include increases in heart rate and blood pressure, somnolence, abdominal pain, and decreased appetite. Hepatitis and increase in suicidal thoughts are rare adverse effects.

Combined Intervention

Studies indicate that a combination of medication and behavioral therapies have positive effect, especially in preadolescent children. Parents and teachers expressed more satisfaction with the treatment plan in combined intervention. Additionally, combined therapy may allow use of lower stimulant dosages, potentially reducing adverse effects.

BOX 3: Classroom accommodations for children with attention-deficit hyperactivity disorder (ADHD).
- Preferential seating in an area with fewer distractions
- Breaking long assignments into smaller parts
- Providing clear instructions and ensuring that child has understood them
- Providing more time to complete tasks and assignments
- Using a timer or alarm to help with time management
- Providing breaks in-between long or monotonous tasks
- Assigning a peer or a shadow teacher who can support in organizing, planning, and completion of classwork, homework, and assignments
- Providing positive reinforcement

School Interventions

Effective communication with teachers regarding the diagnosis and management goes a long way in improving behaviors as well as classroom learning. Some classroom accommodations that can help the child with ADHD learn effectively are given in **Box 3**.

PROGNOSIS

Even though ADHD is a chronic disorder, effective treatments are available that ameliorate the symptoms and improve functioning in individuals with the disorder. The long-term outcome for children with ADHD depends on the type and severity and type of symptoms, associated comorbidities, cognitive abilities, family environment, and response to treatment. Almost 60–80% of children with ADHD retain the diagnosis in adolescence and 40–60% of adolescents have symptoms persisting into adulthood. Initial symptom severity, parental mental health, and childhood comorbidity may contribute to persistence of ADHD symptoms. Studies of adults with ADHD show that they are likely to have fewer years of education, unstable jobs, more work difficulties, and lower rates of employment. In addition, they also have lower self-esteem, poor interpersonal relationships, substance abuse, and increased risk for accidents. However, regular treatment may lower the risk of substance abuse disorders and other adverse outcomes.

CONCLUSION

Even though ADHD is a chronic disorder, effective treatments are available that ameliorate the symptoms and improve functioning in individuals with the disorder. The long-term outcome for children with ADHD depends on the type and severity and type of symptoms, associated comorbidities, cognitive abilities, family environment, and response to treatment. Almost 60–80% of children with ADHD retain the diagnosis in adolescence, and 40–60% of adolescents have symptoms persisting into adulthood. Initial symptom severity, parental mental health, and childhood comorbidity may contribute to persistence of ADHD symptoms. Studies of adults with ADHD show that they are likely to have fewer years of education, unstable jobs, more work difficulties, and lower rates of employment. In addition, they also have lower self-esteem, poor interpersonal relationships, substance abuse, and increased risk for accidents. However, regular treatment may lower the risk of substance abuse disorders and other adverse outcomes.

REFERENCES

1. Salari N, Ghasemi H, Abdoli N, Rahmani A, Shiri MH, Hashemian AH, et al. The global prevalence of ADHD in children and adolescents: a systematic review and meta-analysis. Ital J Pediatr. 2023;49(1):48.
2. Sayal K, Prasad V, Daley D, Ford T, Coghill D. ADHD in children and young people: prevalence, care pathways, and service provision. Lancet Psychiatry. 2018;5(2):175-86.
3. Arora NK, Nair MKC, Gulati S, Deshmukh V, Mohapatra A, Mishra D, et al. Neurodevelopmental disorders in children aged 2-9 years: Population-based burden estimates across five regions in India. PLoS Med. 2018;15(7):e1002615.
4. Kuppili PP, Manohar H, Pattanayak RD, Sagar R, Bharadwaj B, Kandasamy P. ADHD research in India: A narrative review. Asian J Psychiatr. 2017;30:11-25.
5. Ramtekkar UP, Reiersen AM, Todorov AA, Todd RD. Sex and age differences in attention-deficit/hyperactivity disorder symptoms and diagnoses: implications for DSM-V and ICD-11. J Am Acad Child Adolesc Psychiatry. 2010;49(3): 217-28. e1-3.
6. Firouzabadi FD, Ramezanpour S, Firouzabadi MD, Yousem IJ, Puts NAJ, Yousem DM. Neuroimaging in Attention-Deficit/Hyperactivity Disorder: Recent Advances. AJR Am J Roentgenol. 2022;218(2):321-32.
7. Dickstein SG, Bannon K, Castellanos FX, Milham MP. The neural correlates of attention deficit hyperactivity disorder: an ALE meta-analysis. J Child Psychol Psychiatry. 2006;47(10):1051-62.
8. Larsson H, Chang Z, D'Onofrio BM, Lichtenstein P. The heritability of clinically diagnosed attention deficit hyperactivity disorder across the lifespan. Psychol Med. 2014;44(10):2223-9.
9. Mehta TR, Monegro A, Nene YR, Fayyaz M, Bollu PC. Neurobiology of ADHD: A Review. Curr Dev Disord Rep. 2019;6:235-40.
10. Thapar A, Stergiakouli E. An Overview on the Genetics of ADHD. Xin Li Xue Bao. 2008;40(10):1088-98.
11. Froehlich TE, Anixt JS, Loe IM, Chirdkiatgumchai V, Kuan L, Gilman RC. Update on environmental risk factors for attention-deficit/hyperactivity disorder. Curr Psychiatry Rep. 2011;13(5):333-44.
12. Kumperščak HG. ADHD Through Different Developmental Stages. In: Banerjee S (Ed). Attention Deficit Hyperactivity Disorder in Children and Adolescents. Rijeka, Croatia: InTech; 2013.
13. American Psychiatric Association. Diagnostic and statistical manual of mental disorders, 5th edition. Arlington: American Psychiatric Association; 2013.
14. Prock LA, Rappaprt L. Attention and Deficits of Attention. In: Carey WB (Ed). Developmental-Behavioral Pediatrics, 4th edition. Philadelphia, PA: Saunders/Elsevier; 2009. pp. 524-34.
15. Radmanović MB, Burgić SS. Comorbidity in Children and Adolescents with ADHD. In: Kumperščak HG (Ed). ADHD: From Etiology to Comorbidity. United Kingdom: IntechOpen; 2021.
16. Winner JD, Zurhellen W; Subcommittee on Children and Adolescents with Attention-Deficit/Hyperactive Disorder. Clinical Practice Guideline for the Diagnosis, Evaluation, and Treatment of Attention-Deficit/Hyperactivity Disorder in Children and Adolescents. Pediatrics. 2019;144(4):e20192528.

Anxiety Disorders in Children and Adolescents

Prahbhjot Malhi

INTRODUCTION

Anxiety disorders are among the most frequently diagnosed mental health disorders in children and adolescents. Rational worries and fears play an adaptive role and are generally present in early childhood, however, disproportionate, and excessive fearful responses to otherwise benign situations are considered as anxiety responses. When these responses routinely start to interfere with the school and daily activities and persist over time (generally 6 months) then the child is diagnosed with an anxiety disorder. Anxiety disorders are characterized by avoidance behaviors, social difficulties, performance uncertainties, and physical symptoms, such as palpitations, difficulty in breathing, and dizziness. Anxiety is therefore a multidimensional construct that comprises somatic, emotional, cognitive, and behavioral components.[1] Several biological, environmental (parenting and stressful events), cognitive (intolerance for uncertainty), and developmental (fear conditioning and abnormal safety learning in childhood) risk factors have been identified for developing anxiety disorders although their interactional mechanisms remain debatable.[2] Anxiety has strong genetic underpinnings and carries a 2–7 times increased risk for children of parents with anxiety disorders.[3] Anxiety disorders are also characterized by neuroendocrine, neurotransmitter, and neuroanatomical disruptions that originate from either decreased inhibitory or increased excitatory transmission.[4]

The Diagnostic and Statistical Manual of Mental Disorders, Fifth Edition (DSM-5) includes a range of anxiety conditions, such as specific phobias, social anxiety, panic, separation anxiety, and selective mutism (SM).[1] Anxiety may have diverse presentations and some common signs to look out for in children are presented in **Box 1**. Anxiety disorders often co-occur with chronic medical conditions,

BOX 1: Some common signs to look out for in children with anxiety.
- Difficulty in concentrating
- Clingy, tearful, extreme shyness, withdrawn, and regressive behaviors
- Avoids social situations (school refusal) and social activities
- Difficulty sleeping, frequent waking in the night, and bad dreams
- Frequent worrying, imaging the worst, and negative thinking
- Looks nervous
- Tense and restless
- Irritable, easily frustrated, angry outbursts, and mood swings
- Frequent headaches, stomach aches, flushed face, and trouble breathing

such as the presence of asthma, diabetes, epilepsy, or gastrointestinal illness and the relationship may be bidirectional.[5] It is therefore important that pediatricians recognize and treat comorbid mental health conditions along with the physical illness of young people.

PREVALENCE

Anxiety disorders are common psychiatric disorders among children and adolescents and research documents prevalence rates between 10 and 20%.[6-9] Anxiety disorders contribute considerably to the global burden of disease among the youth.[10] Separation anxiety disorder (SAD) is the most frequently diagnosed and the earliest presentation and accounts for nearly half of the referrals for anxiety-related conditions. Overall, girls are twice as likely to be diagnosed with an anxiety disorder relative to boys.[11]

Anxiety disorders tend to have an earlier age of onset as compared to other internalizing psychiatric problems. Indeed, evidence indicates that nearly three-fourths of adult anxiety disorders start in childhood years.[12] Moreover, longitudinal studies suggest that children with anxiety disorders are at a heightened risk for developing adverse consequences and psychiatric comorbidities including depression, substance dependence, suicidal behavior, disruptive behavior, educational underachievement, sleep problems, increased healthcare utilization, and economic disadvantage in adulthood.[13,14] Despite this, very few families access services and get the treatment that their children deserve due to several barriers including stigma attached to seeking mental health services, lack of awareness, and limited confidence in physician's ability to diagnose child anxiety problems.[15]

TYPES OF ANXIETY

All children with anxiety disorders tend to overestimate their fears and underestimate their capacity to cope with the situation. Despite some common features, childhood anxiety disorders are distinguished by the focus of their fears. A brief description of various types of anxiety disorder is described here.

Separation Anxiety Disorder

Separation anxiety disorder is recurrent and excessive distress that something bad or a disaster will happen if the child is not with the attachment figure/s (parents and caregiver). Although, it is developmentally appropriate to experience some anxiety between 18 months and 3 years when a parent leaves the child, it is considered a problem when it persists beyond preschool years. The anxiety is particularly problematic as it may result in school refusal and excessive clinginess and dependence on the parents. Significant school absences can lead to decline in school work and academic underachievement. In addition, the child may refuse to sleep alone, attend a birthday party, or visit a relative. The child may also experience nightmares about actual or anticipated separation and have frequent headaches and other somatic symptoms when separation from a loved one is anticipated. At times, separation anxiety may escalate into a panic attack. Risk factors may include various types of biological, psychological, and environmental contributors (illness, divorce, death, positive family history, and difficult temperament).[16,17] Although most children with separation anxiety remit before adulthood, interventions are required to reduce impairments in functioning and improve quality of life in the childhood years.[18-20]

Panic Disorder

Panic disorder is characterized by extreme distress that may have no obvious trigger and it can come on unexpectedly and can completely overwhelm the child. Panic is associated with several somatic sensations including tachycardia, shortness of breath, tingling sensations, sweating, dizziness, nausea, and tremors. Although panic attacks do not last very long the child may experience intense fear. The parents may deem panic symptoms as a manifestation of a physical illness and this can result in increase in visits to the emergency department or specialty consultations, such as cardiology or neurology. Children may fear experiencing a panic attack and may start avoiding situations where these attacks happened and can lead to the development of agoraphobia in adulthood.[1]

Phobias

Specific phobias are excessive and irrational fears that are triggered by the anticipation or presence of an identifiable object (animals, insects, and water) or a situation (heights, closed places, and hospitals). Phobias are different from fears as they persist despite reassurance and significantly impact the child's life. Besides being fearful, children may also present with other emotional symptoms, such as crying, dependence, and acting out behaviors.[21] Evidence indicates that about 10% of persons in their lifetime will meet the criteria for a specific phobia.[12,22] Females are twice as likely than males to experience specific phobias.[23]

Social Anxiety Disorder

Social anxiety also referred to as social phobia is characterized by an intense and unreasonable fear of embarrassment in social situations. In order to meet the criteria for a diagnosis of social anxiety, the child must also respond to these social situations with distress that interferes significantly with daily functioning.[1] The overall prevalence of SAD is 2-6%.[24] SAD generally has its onset during adolescent years and is more likely to occur during school hours wherein performing social tasks (talking to peers, athletics, reading aloud in class, and called upon by the teacher to answer questions) can trigger intense social discomfort.[25] Social anxiety, if left unaddressed, can be associated with several adverse consequences, such as difficulties with social competence, poorer functioning at school, peer and friendship problems, greater risk for school dropout, and an overall reduction in quality of life.[26,27]

Generalized Anxiety Disorders

Children who experience disproportionate and irrepressible worry across several domains that is expressed on most days for at least 6 months are more likely to meet the criteria for generalized anxiety disorder (GAD). The symptoms are not a response to recent stressful event/s or any specific situation/s. Besides anxiety, patients may also experience tiredness, irritability, sleep difficulties, and concentration problems.[1] GAD occurs in about 10% of children and adolescents and is more prevalent in girls.[28] A high proportion of GAD patients display physical complaints and other psychiatric comorbidities particularly other anxiety disorders and depressive disorders.[29] GAD is more likely to respond to relaxation training rather than behavioral therapy as the focus of symptoms is diffuse.

Selective Mutism

Selective mutism is a rare disorder (1–2%) and typically emerges in early years (2–5 years) but symptoms become apparent when children enter school for the first time.[30] It is characterized by the child being mute in specific situations or with certain people, for at least a month, while he/she may communicate normally at places where they feel comfortable. This can result in substantial social and academic deficits over time. Communication delays, bilingualism, temperamental, environmental, and neurodevelopmental factors contribute to the development of this disorder. Assessment involves audio/video recordings, behavioral observations, and the use of questionnaires, such as the selective mutism questionnaire for children, parents, and teachers.[31] School-based assessments are also critical to understand the child's interactions with classmates and teachers. Psychosocial interventions, such as gradual exposure to social situations, parent-based contingency management, social skills training, and modeling play an important role in the management of SM.[32,33]

EVALUATING A CHILD WITH AN ANXIETY DISORDER

Generally, anxiety assessment involves a detailed clinical interview, behavioral observation in the clinic, and administration of assessment tools. While evaluating, clinicians need to differentiate anxiety disorders from developmentally appropriate fears, worries, and responses to environmental and traumatic stressors such as starting school, parental divorce, abuse, and death in the family. Assessing a child for an anxiety disorder is challenging for the pediatrician as symptoms of anxiety (changes in eating, sleeping, and school function; problems with social interaction; and avoidance of situations) often mimic features that are present in other mental health diagnoses among the pediatric age population such as externalizing problems and mood disorders. For example, there is considerable overlap between symptoms of anxiety and depression among youth and distinguishing these two conditions can at times be difficult.[20] Obtaining a family history is essential as a positive family history besides highlighting the genetic factors for the development of anxiety may also be a source of behavioral modeling for the child.

Since anxiety includes several components including physiological, emotional, cognitive, and behavioral, it is important to gather objective information about how a child feels, thinks, does, and how his body reacts in an anxiety-provoking situation. Garnering information from multiple informants including school-teachers and parents is usually helpful and the clinician needs to use his/her clinical judgment to integrate all the information collected.[34] It is important to recognize that the level of agreement among informants about the presence and severity of symptoms tends to be low at times given the diverse settings that the various informants observe the child and the inherent difficulty in assessing internal emotional experiences of children.[35] The mental health of parents can lead to bias as evidence indicates that negative affect can lead to overestimation of the child's anxiety symptoms.[36] While evaluating, the clinician should also review the protective factors that are present in the child's environment to identify sources of available support.

Screening Tools for Anxiety

A detailed, in-depth, multi-method, and multi-informant assessment is recommended before initiating empirical treatments in clinical practice. Several diagnostic interviews have been developed to establish diagnoses according to the DSM classification, such as the Anxiety Disorders Interview Schedule (ADIS), the Diagnostic Interview for Children and Adolescents (DICA), and the Diagnostic Interview Schedule for Children, Version IV (DISC-IV).[37-39] The ADIS is a semistructured interview and the parent and child are interviewed separately and information from both the interviews is combined into a composite diagnostic status. These diagnostic tools require training and may be too time-consuming to administer in a busy office practice.

Using brief, easy-to-administer, and score screening tools to assess various symptoms of anxiety is a useful strategy to gather objective information from various sources. Several measures are available for screening and assessing emotional problems and anxiety among children.[40] **Table 1** summarizes some of the commonly used screening tools. Many of the scales have not specifically been adapted for the Indian population nevertheless they have been used in clinical settings as they provide useful information that may not be available otherwise. In addition, several authors have used them in India to measure anxiety and reported their utility in providing valid information.[41-52] However, there is a need to develop culturally appropriate screening tools for Indian children.

TABLE 1: Screening tools for anxiety disorders in children and adolescents.

Screening tool	Brief description	Format	Strengths
Broad-based screens			
Strengths and Difficulties Questionnaire (SDQ)[41]	Five subscales with five items each (emotional symptoms, conduct problems, hyperactivity/inattention, peer relationship problems, and prosocial behavior). Scores on subscales can be combined into externalizing (hyperactivity/inattention and conduct problems), internalizing (emotional problems and peer relationship problems), and a total score (all four subscales)	Parent, teacher, youth, and child forms are available for children (2–17 years), 25 items	Well-established tool. Brief, easy to administer and score, cutoff scores categorize scores in normal, borderline, and abnormal range. Hindi translation is available. Can be accessed at https://www.sdqinfo.org/a0.html
Vanderbilt Assessment Scales[42]	Primary focus is on ADHD but also has items to assess anxiety and impairment across school, peers, and home	Child, parent, and teacher forms are available	Wide age range, easy to administer and score; can also be used to assess impact of treatment
Anxiety-specific screening tools			
Social Anxiety Scale for Children-Revised (SASC-R)[43]	The SASC-R measures fear of negative evaluation, social avoidance, and distress with new or unfamiliar peers, and more generalized social avoidance and distress	22 items	
Screen for Child Anxiety Related Emotional Disorders (SCARED)[44]	Provides a total score and five subscales: Separation anxiety, generalized anxiety, social anxiety, panic/somatic, and school phobia; can be used in community and clinical settings	41 items tool, parent and child forms are available, can be used for ages 9–18 years	Cutoff scores help in distinguishing anxiety from nonanxiety conditions. Cutoff scores can also help in guiding and monitoring treatment gains. Can be assessed from https://www.pediatricbipolar.pitt.edu/clinical-services/clinical-tools
Multidimensional Anxiety Scale for Children (MASC)[45]	Provides four subscale scores (physical symptoms, social anxiety, separation/panic, and harm avoidance) and a total anxiety score	39 items; parent and child form, 8–18 years	Cost-effective screener for anxiety disorders in youth

Contd...

Contd...

Screening tool	Brief description	Format	Strengths
Spence Children's Anxiety Scale (SCAS)[46]	Measures six domains of anxiety (separation anxiety, social anxiety, obsessive-compulsive disorder, panic/agoraphobia, generalized anxiety). Yields six domain and a total anxiety score	Child (44 items) and parent (38 items) forms are available (7–17 years)	Provides cutoff scores for domain and total scores. Hindi translation is available. Can be accessed at www.scaswebsite.com
Patient health questionnaire for adolescents (PHQ-A)[47]	Assesses anxiety, mood, eating, and substance use disorders among adolescents	Brief, self-report measure	Can be used in a primary care setting; has been found to be valid for use with Indian adolescents
Children's separation anxiety scale (CSAS)[48]	Measures worry, distress, opposition about separation, and calm at separation. Differentiates anxiety symptoms from depression in children	20 items	Relatively new scale, validation studies are lacking
Pediatric Index of Emotional Distress (PI-ED)[49]	Assesses anxiety and depression that contains no somatic items	Self-report screening tool, 14 items, 8–16 years	Easy to score and interpret, cutoff scores determines the individuals who require more detailed assessment
Social Worries Anxiety Index for Young children (SWAIY)[50]	Measures social anxiety in young children	10 items, 4–8 years	Brief, easy to score and administer

(ADHD: attention-deficit hyperactivity disorder)

PSYCHOLOGICAL MANAGEMENT

Significant progress has been documented in the last decade in the treatment of anxiety disorders in children. However, there are no consensus guidelines. Some of the factors that need to be considered while selecting an intervention include the age of the child, severity, duration of symptoms, comorbidities, family preferences, and access to specialized care. It is important that clinicians also focus on improving parent-child relationship, enhancing communication skills, and reducing parental anxiety to maximize gains. Many children and adolescents use avoidant coping as a primary coping mechanism and these may be inadvertently reinforced by parents.[53] Since many children experience somatic complaints as part of their anxiety, parents can be taught simple management techniques that may be useful for managing the physical manifestation of anxiety **(Table 2)**. Some simple guidelines that parents may use at home for managing the fears and worries of their children are presented in **Box 2**.

Self-help and Mobile App-based Interventions

The most common self-help therapy is bibliotherapy. It is a popular low-intensity intervention that guides parents to help their child to overcome their anxieties through written materials, such as self-book books, storybooks, and workbooks.[54,55] There are several self-management books available for children and their parents **(Box 3)**. In a study conducted in Australia, Rappe et al. found that providing a workbook for parents was associated with recovery in one-fourth of anxious children as compared to only 7% of children who received no treatment.[56] Additionally, bibliotherapy can be augmented with alternate methods of contact with the therapist including telephone calls, particularly when traditional therapeutic services are difficult to access.[57] Indeed, research indicates that novice therapists, such as parents, can effectively deliver low-intensity therapies with good outcomes for children with subthreshold anxiety symptoms.

Mobile app-based interventions for children have been developed recently to leverage technology to improve access to treatment options for children.[58,59] Some of the popular apps for children and adolescents include positive penguins (helps 9-11 years old to understand their feelings), worry box (store and manage worries for 6-16 years old), breathe2relax (teaches deep breathing exercises), and anxiety coach (helps children to identify

TABLE 2: Managing somatic symptoms in childhood anxiety disorders.

Technique	Description
Deep breathing	Children are taught deep breathing to help their bodies to relax, to slow their heart rate, and be calm in stressful situations. Deep breathing is taught through techniques such as blowing bubbles, feathers, candles, or pieces of paper
Progressive muscle relaxation	Focuses on slowly and progressively tensing and relaxing various muscles in the body
Visualization and guided imagery techniques	Children are asked to imagine a calm and safe place, floating on a cloud, or thinking of a peaceful color. The virtual trip in mind helps the child to reduce bodily tension

BOX 2: Simple strategies that parents can use for managing anxiety at home.

- Build family routines to make daily life more predictable
- Listen to the child and take the child's fears seriously
- Be supportive but encourage the child to face their fears one step at a time
- Identify the situations that trigger child's worries
- Encourage physical activity to help reduce stress and induce relaxation
- Help the anxious child to relax by deep breathing and make relaxation a family activity
- Use guided imagery script (relaxing and happy place) to help the child feel safe
- Build self-confidence by praising the child's efforts for facing their worries
- Model healthy ways of handling anxiety
- Work on enhancing child's skills

BOX 3: Cognitive-behavioral therapy (CBT) workbooks.

- *Helping your anxious child:* A step-by-step guide (Rapee R, 2008)
- *Overcoming your child's fears and worries:* A self-help guide using cognitive-behavioral techniques (Creswell C, Willetts L, 2012)
- *Parent-led CBT for child anxiety:* Helping parents help their kids (Cathy Creswell C, Parkinson M, Thirlwall K, Willetts L, 2017)
- *CBT workbook for kids:* 40+ fun exercises and activities to help children overcome anxiety and face their fears at home, at school, and out in the world (Davidson H, 2019)
- *CBT workbook for kids:* Strategies and exercises to help children overcome their emotional disorders and fears (Miller RD, 2020)
- *Anxiety workbook for kids:* Proven tools to cure your kids paralyzing fear (Conley L, 2020)
- *The self-regulation workbook for kids:* CBT exercises and coping strategies to help children handle anxiety, stress, and other strong emotions (Berman J, 2021)
- *The resilience workbook for kids:* Fun CBT activities to help you bounce back from stress and grow from challenges (Baruch-Feldman C, Comizio R, 2022)

their worries and provides practice on exposure tasks related to their worries). Although digital platforms offer a user-friendly and innovative approach to traditional therapies, empirical evidence regarding their usefulness is still awaited. However, self-help interventions may be very useful for mild anxiety and highly motivated young persons.[59]

Cognitive Behavior Therapy

Cognitive behavior therapy (CBT) remains the treatment of choice for youth in preference to pharmacological treatment.[60] The CBT underscores that maladaptive thinking is the root cause of dysfunctional behavior and distorted cognitions need to be reframed into more positive and constructive thoughts. **Table 3** lists some cognitive distortions experienced by anxious children. The essence of CBT is cognitive restructuring and self-regulatory strategies that involves retraining the mind to think differently about anxiety-provoking situations and avoiding the pitfalls associated with thoughts that are characterized by catastrophic and all-or-nothing thinking.[61,62] The CBT involves several effective therapeutic strategies, such as psychoeducation, deep breathing, progressive muscle relaxation training, behavioral goal setting and reward, monitoring one's thoughts to become aware of connections between thoughts and behaviors, and training in coping skills **(Table 4)**. Active parental involvement in the intervention program helps in the long-term maintenance of treatment gains.[63]

Mindfulness-based Interventions

Mindfulness-based interventions (MBIs) or mindfulness-based stress reduction (MBSR) interventions have recently gained popularity as effective strategies that can be used to promote and manage the mental health of children and youth with anxiety disorders both at home and at school,

TABLE 3: Cognitive distortions experienced by anxious children.

Cognitive distortion	Description	Example
"Black and white" thinking	The child only thinks in extremes and allows for no middle ground	"If I am not successful at everything, then I am a complete failure"
Catastrophizing	Imagining the worst possible outcome of a situation	"It is raining and thundering heavily and that means my house will be flooded"
Overgeneralization	Expecting that a single poor outcome predicts what will happen in the future for similar events	Pronouncing one word wrongly while reading aloud, the child believes he is a poor reader
Disqualifying the positive	Positive experiences are ignored and the child exclusively focuses on the negatives	Even when the child gets a good grade in examination, the child attributes it to luck or an easy examination
Personalizing	Believes that the negative outcome of an event is because of him/her. Blames self when things go wrong	The child believes that because other children at a birthday party are not talking to him then they must hate him

TABLE 4: Common techniques used in cognitive-behavioral therapy (CBT).

Technique	Description
Psychoeducation	Educates parents and the child about the nature and etiology of anxiety disorders, the interrelationship between anxiety-related thoughts, feelings, and behaviors; and the steps involved in the treatment in an easy-to-understand language
Relaxation training	Focuses on teaching children to develop awareness and control over their physiological responses to anxiety and then trains them in progressive muscle relaxation through systematic tension-releasing exercise
Cognitive restructuring	Emphasis is identifying anxiety-related thoughts, teaching skills that teach reframing negative talk and replacing it with positive self-statements (this does not look hard, I can do it), challenging unrealistic beliefs, and making concrete plans to realistically cope with the feared situation
Graduated exposure	To face fears in a graded and manageable manner. Developing a worry/fear hierarchy and helping the child to start with the least intense fear and moving up the hierarchy
Contingency management	Uses behavioral contingency management procedures to motivate the child to stick to the plan by using behavioral contracts and reward

particularly trauma victims.[64-67] Mindfulness involves focusing one's attention on one's emotions and thoughts in the present moment. Since MBIs are simple, sharing child-friendly books with parents may be an effective way for families to teach mindfulness to their children. For example, Mindfulness Activities for Kids (And Their Grown-ups): Learn Calm, Focus, and Gratitude for a Lifetime workbook authored by Sally Arnold can be used with as young as 3–7 years old and is a cost-effective way to teach children simple strategies to navigate big feelings.

School-based Programs

In addition to family-based counseling, guidelines for school teachers should also be considered as part of the overall management plan. School-based treatments for anxiety disorders are very useful as many young people display significant anxiety symptoms in the social and academic settings at school. Peers and teachers can greatly help socially anxious children in facing their worries in the classroom, such as fears related to public speaking, taking a school test, and facing negative feedback.[68] Several manualized anxiety school-based treatment programs have documented significant success in managing anxieties at school. Some of the school programs include the skills for academic and social success,[69] Cool Kids Program: School Version,[70] Baltimore Child Anxiety Treatment Study in the Schools,[71] and the Fun FRIENDS programs[72] for youth with social anxiety disorder. In India,

> **BOX 4:** Simple strategies that teachers can use for managing anxiety in the classroom.
>
> - Preferential seating where the student feels safe (near a door, teacher, or a friend)
> - Provide social support (assign a "buddy")
> - Manage work output by providing additional time to complete assignments
> - Normalize "mistakes", teach students that mistakes provide opportunities to learn
> - Do not call upon child to present before class unexpectedly
> - Give advance notice for planned social situations and school tests
> - Give seat breaks when child feels overwhelmed
> - Allow the child to call home at specified time and keep a self-calming object (parents picture)
> - Avoid reprimanding and pointing mistakes in front of classmates
> - Praise and encourage child's efforts to stay calm
> - Be patient and allow the student time to calm down
> - Start with what a child can do comfortably and gradually build from there

school-based anxiety prevention studies are not available, nevertheless, school teachers can be guided to implement simple strategies in the classroom for anxious school children **(Box 4)**.

PROGNOSIS AND OUTCOME

Childhood anxiety disorders have an early onset and a chronic and progressive course, especially if left untreated. Untreated anxiety can have an unremitting and persistent course and may persist into adolescent and adulthood years.[73] Remission rates range from 20 to 85%.[74,75] Prognosis depends on the severity of symptoms, type of treatment, and the family's resilience and follow through with treatment. For example, a study from South India reported that adolescents with greater severity and comorbidities required increased levels of intervention and longer follow-up.[74] In the Child/Adolescent Anxiety Multimodal Extended Long-term Study (CAMELS), younger age, male sex, higher youth functioning, and higher family functioning were found to predict stable remission.[75,76] Improvements in family functioning and reductions in caregiver strain is also related to better outcomes for anxious youth.[77]

PREVENTION

Parents can be coached to help prevent anxiety and foster their child's competence in managing their fears. Since anxiety runs in families several anxiety promoting behaviors, such as parental modeling, overprotective, and overcautious parenting are targeted in prevention programs. A recently developed parental program successfully targeted three risk factors that were thought to be responsible for parent-child transmission of anxiety, such as criticism/low warmth, overprotection, and modeling of anxiety.[78] Family-based and school-based programs have also been documented to be moderately successful in preventing anxiety in children.[78,79]

PHARMACOTHERAPY

Pharmacologic interventions are believed to confer clinical benefit by reducing the degree of anxious reactivity, thereby increasing the range of opportunities for children to relearn more adaptive responses to stressful stimuli responsible for anxiety.

TREATMENT OF ANXIETY DISORDERS

A multimodal approach to clinical treatment of youth with anxiety disorder is optimal, as studies not only show benefit of both therapeutic and pharmacologic interventions but also suggest that they work in tandem to confer greater improvement in symptoms. When functional impairments are mild, initial intervention with CBT is preferred over starting a medication, but for moderate to severe symptoms of anxiety disorder combination of medication and CBT is recommended. Consistent evidence, including randomized controlled trials (RCTs), supports the benefit of selective serotonin reuptake inhibitors (SSRIs), both alone or in combination with therapy for treatment of anxiety disorder in children and adolescents. Medication intervention may be started concurrently with psychotherapy which might be needed to reduce the impairing nature of severe symptoms before psychotherapy can proceed in an effective manner. It may also be used as an augmentation strategy if initial psychotherapy does not provide relief of symptoms.

Following medications have been tried for the treatment of anxiety disorders:[80]

- *Selective serotonin reuptake inhibitors and selective norepinephrine reuptake inhibitors:* Three of four medications approved by US Food and Drug Administration (FDA) specifically for treatment of obsessive-compulsive disorder (OCD) in children and adolescents are SSRIs: sertraline (6 years and older), fluoxetine (7 years and older), and fluvoxamine

(8 years and older). No medication has yet been approved for treatment of non-OCD anxiety in youth. RCTs of SSRIs have shown efficacy in treatment of GAD, SAD, and social anxiety disorder, often in mixed populations that include children and adolescents with any one or combination of these disorders. When pharmacologic treatments in RCTs are segregated by anxiety subtype (OCD vs. non-OCD), treatment response for non-OCD seems slightly greater than OCD. These findings suggest that although monotherapy with either medication or psychotherapy can be effective for treating anxiety disorders, a multimodal approach is more likely to be successful. The recommendation of a combination of medication and therapy for anxiety disorders also mirrors recommendations for pediatric depression and complex forms of attention-deficit/hyperactivity disorder (ADHD).

Adverse effects: Common side effects include nausea, stomachaches, headaches, insomnia, and restlessness. These may emerge intermittently as per dosage adjustments and may resolve spontaneously. Adolescents should also be cautioned regarding potential sexual side effects. Furthermore, these drugs may potentiate suicidal thinking, a low frequency event that warrants informed consent.

- *Tricyclic antidepressants:* Tricyclic antidepressants including imipramine and clomipramine have shown efficacy in several RCTs of social or school refusal. Clomipramine has an FDA indication for treatment of OCD, but is less preferred because of the potential for problematic side effects including cardiac abnormalities, constipation, sedation, etc.
- *Other agents:*
  - Buspirone, a partial agonist of serotonin receptors with some evidence for generalized anxiety in adults, but there is no data regarding use in youth.
  - Similarly, bupropion, an inhibitor of dopamine and norepinephrine has not been studied.
  - Clonidine, α-2 agonist, was shown to decrease arousal and anxiety.
  - Controlled trials do not support the use of benzodiazepines in children, but there has been history of clinical use for anxious children and considerable evidence of effectiveness in adults.

A treatment algorithm is summarized in **Table 5**.

TABLE 5: Pharmacological agents used for treatment of anxiety disorders.

Medication	Starting dose	Total therapeutic dose range	Common side effect profile	Special warning/ monitoring	Specific indications	FDA approval
Sertraline (SSRI)	12.5–25 mg	50–100 mg	Nausea, sedation, and headache	Suicidality, activation (restlessness and impulsivity), and serotonin syndrome*	GAD	For OCD; ≥6
Fluoxetine (SSRI)	5–10 mg	10–60 mg	Activation, nausea, and insomnia	___do___	Long half-life	For OCD; ≥7
Fluvoxamine (SSRI)	12.5–25 mg	50–200 mg (prescribe twice a day more than 50 mg)	Hyperactivity and abdominal discomfort	___do___	___	For OCD; ≥8
Citalopram (SSRI)	5–10 mg	10–40 mg	Somnolence, insomnia, and diaphoresis	___do___	No RCTs, few interactions	For adults
Paroxetine (SSRI)	5–10 mg	10–40 mg	Sedation, nausea, and dry mouth	___do___	Social phobia; nondepressed	For adults
Venlafaxine XR (VFX) (SNRI)	37.5 mg	75–225 mg (prescribe every night or twice a day)	Nausea, sedation, and dizziness	HTN, tachycardia, and suicidality	GAD; nondepressed	For adults

Contd...

Contd...

Medication	Starting dose	Total therapeutic dose range	Common side effect profile	Special warning/ monitoring	Specific indications	FDA approval
Clomipramine (tricyclic)	25 mg	100–150 mg	Dry mouth, constipation, and diaphoresis	HTN, rebound HTN, lethal in OCD; level ≤400	OCD; EKG, BP monitoring to minimize overdose risk	For OCD; ≥10
Buspirone (5-HTa PA)	5 mg three times a day	15–60 mg (prescribe three times a day)	Sedation, disinhibition, and headache	Safe with benzodiazepines	Augmentation; sexual side effects	For adults
Mirtazapine (tetracyclic)	7.5–15 mg	7.5–30 mg (prescribe every night)	Hunger, sedation, and dizziness	Weight gain	Appetite stimulation, insomnia; few interactions	For adults
Clonazepam (benzodiazepine)	0.25–0.5 mg	0.25–3 mg (prescribe every day three times a day)	Sedation and confusion	Disinhibition, tolerance, and seizure from discontinuation	Short-term relief of acute anxiety; longer acting	For adults
Lorazepam (benzodiazepine)	0.5–1 mg	0.5–6 mg (Prescribe every day 4 times a day)	Sedation and confusion	Disinhibition, tolerance, and seizure from discontinuation	Short-term relief of acute anxiety; shorter acting; liver impaired	For adults

Note: *Develop safety plan and means to assess early side effects, which may resolve in 1–2 weeks. Avoid abrupt discontinuation with paroxetine, sertraline, fluvoxamine, and citalopram.

(BP: blood pressure; EKG: electrocardiogram; FDA: Food and Drug Administration; GAD: generalized anxiety disorder; HTN: hypertension; OCD: obsessive-compulsive disorder; RCTs: randomized controlled trials; SNRI: norepinephrine reuptake inhibitor; SSRI: selective serotonin reuptake inhibitor)

Source: Adapted and modified from Kodish I, Rockhill C, Ryan S, Varley C. Pharmacotherapy for anxiety disorders in children and adolescents. Pediatr Clin N Am. 2011;58:55-72.

CONCLUSION

The public health burden of anxiety disorders and the associated long-term adverse consequences underscores the need for concerted preventive measures, timely diagnosis, and effective interventions. Although considerable progress in the assessment and treatment of children and adolescents with anxiety disorders have been made in the recent past, culturally specific valid tools for Indian children are still unavailable. In the case of mild or subthreshold anxiety symptoms, psychoeducation, a list of workbooks, encouragement, and mobile app-based interventions may alone be sufficient, however, for debilitating symptoms specific evidence-based face-to-face therapies are more useful. For severe anxiety, the need to use medications along with psychological therapies may be warranted. There is an imperative need to build clinical expertise among pediatricians to address the mental health needs of the children and youth in the country.

REFERENCES

1. American Psychiatric Association. Diagnostic and statistical manual of mentaldisorders, 4th edition. Washington, DC: American Psychiatric Association; 1994.
2. Varela RE, Sanchez-Sosa JJ, Biggs BK, Luis TM. Parenting strategies and socio-cultural influences in childhood anxiety: Mexican, Latin American descent, and European American families. J Anxiety Disord. 2009;23(5):609-16.
3. Bögels SM, Brechman-Toussaint ML. Family issues in child anxiety: Attachment, family functioning, parental rearing and beliefs. Clin Psychol Rev. 2006;26(7):834-56.
4. Martin EI, Ressler KJ, Binder E, Nemeroff CB. The neurobiology of anxiety disorders: brain imaging, genetics, and psychoneuroendocrinology. Psychiatr Clin North Am. 2009;32(3):549-75.
5. Cobham VE, Hickling A, Kimball H, Thomas HJ, Scott JG, Middeldorp CM. Systematic review: Anxiety in children and adolescents with chronic medical conditions. J Am Acad Child Adolesc Psychiatry. 2020;59(5):595-618.
6. Sagar R, Pattanayak RD, Chandrasekaran R, Chaudhury PK, Deswal BS, Lenin Singh RK, et al. Twelve-month prevalence

and treatment gap for common mental disorders: Findings from a large-scale epidemiological survey in India. Indian J Psychiatry. 2017;59(1):46-55.
7. Polanczyk GV, Salum GA, Sugaya LS, Caye A, Rohde LA. Annual research review: A meta-analysis of the worldwide prevalence of mental disorders in children and adolescents. J Child Psychol Psychiatry. 2015;56(3):345-65.
8. Canals J, Voltas N, Hernández-Martínez C, Cosi S, Arija V. Prevalence of DSM-5 anxiety disorders, comorbidity, and persistence of symptoms in Spanish early adolescents. Eur Child Adolesc Psychiatry. 2019;28(1):131-43.
9. Ghandour RM, Sherman LJ, Vladutiu CJ, Ali MM, Lynch SE, Bitsko RH, et al. Prevalence and treatment of depression, anxiety, and conduct problems in US children. J Pediatr. 2019;206:256-67.e3.
10. Global Burden of Disease Pediatrics Collaboration; Kyu HH, Pinho C, Wagner JA, Brown JC, Bertozzi-Villa A, et al. Global and national burden of diseases and injuries among children and adolescents between 1990 and 2013: Findings from the Global Burden of Disease 2013 Study. JAMA Pediatr. 2016;170(3):267-87.
11. Ohannessian CM, Milan S, Vannucci A. Gender differences in anxiety trajectories from middle to late adolescence. J Youth Adolesc. 2017;46(4):826-39.
12. Kessler RC, Berglund P, Demler O, Jin R, Merikangas KR, Walters EE. Lifetime prevalence and age-of-onset distributions of DSM-IV disorders in the National Comorbidity Survey Replication. Arch Gen Psychiatry. 2005;62:593-602.
13. Woodward LJ, Fergusson DM. Life course outcomes of young people with anxiety disorders in adolescence. J Am Acad Child Adolesc Psychiatry. 2001;40(9):1086-93.
14. Asselmann E, Wittchen HU, Lieb R, Beesdo-Baum K. Sociodemographic, clinical, and functional long-term outcomes in adolescents and young adults with mental disorders. Acta Psychiatr Scand. 2018;137(1):6-17.
15. Reardon T, Harvey K, Baranowska M, O'Brien D, Smith L, Creswell C. What do parents perceive are the barriers and facilitators to accessing psychological treatment for mental health problems in children and adolescents? A systematic review of qualitative and quantitative studies. Eur Child Adolesc Psychiatry. 2017;26:623-47.
16. Masi G, Mucci M, Millepiedi S. Separation anxiety disorder in children and adolescents: epidemiology, diagnosis and management. CNS Drugs. 2001;15(2):93-104.
17. Suveg C, Aschenbrand SG, Kendall PC. Separation anxiety disorder, panic disorder, and school refusal. Child Adolesc Psychiatr Clin N Am. 2005;14(4):773-95.
18. Foley DL, Pickles A, Maes HM, Silberg JL, Eaves LJ. Course and short-term outcomes of separation anxiety disorder in a community sample of twins. J Am Acad Child Adolesc Psychiatry. 2004;43(9):1107-14.
19. Foley DL, Rowe R, Maes H, Silberg J, Eaves L, Pickles A. The relationship between separation anxiety and impairment. J Anxiety Disord. 2008;22(4):635-41.
20. Cummings CM, Caporino NE, Kendall PC. Comorbidity of anxiety and depression in children and adolescents: 20 years after. Psychol Bull. 2014;140(3):816-45.
21. Davis TE III, Ollendick TH. Empirically supported treatments for specific phobia in children: Do efficacious treatments address the components of a phobic response? Clin Psychol Sci Pract. 2005;12(2):144-60.
22. Becker E, Rinck M, Türke V, Kause P, Goodwin R, Neumer S, et al. Epidemiology of specific phobia subtypes: findings from the Dresden Mental Health Study. Eur Psychiatry. 2007;22(2):69-74.
23. Bekker MH, van Mens-Verhulst J. Anxiety disorders: sex differences in prevalence, degree, and background, but gender-neutral treatment. Gend Med. 2007;4 Suppl B:S178-93.
24. Aune T, Nordahl HM, Beidel DC. Social anxiety disorder in adolescents: Prevalence and subtypes in the Young-HUNT3 study. J Anxiety Disord. 2022;87:102546.
25. Alves F, Figueiredo DV, Vagos P. The prevalence of adolescent social fears and social anxiety disorder in school contexts. Int J Environ Res Public Health. 2022;19(19):12458.
26. Hebert KR, Fales J, Nangle DW, Papadakis AA, Grover RL. Linking social anxiety and adolescent romantic relationship functioning: indirect effects and the importance of peers. J Youth Adolesc. 2013;42(11):1708-20.
27. Jystad I, Bjerkeset O, Haugan T, Sund ER, Vaag J. Sociodemographic correlates and mental health comorbidities in adolescents with social anxiety: The Young-HUNT3 study, Norway. Front Psychol. 2021;12:663161.
28. Keeton CP, Kolos AC, Walkup JT. Pediatric generalized anxiety disorder: epidemiology, diagnosis, and management. Paediatr Drugs. 2009;11(3):171-83.
29. Masi G, Millepiedi S, Mucci M, Poli P, Bertini N, Milantoni L. Generalized anxiety disorder in referred children and adolescents. J Am Acad Child Adolesc Psychiatry. 2004;43(6):752-60.
30. Bergman RL, Keller ML, Piacentini J, Bergman AJ. The development and psychometric properties of the selective mutism questionnaire. J Clin Child Adolesc Psychol. 2008;37(2):456-64.
31. Kearney CA, Rede M. The heterogeneity of selective mutism: a primer for a more refined approach. Front Psychol. 2021;12:700745.
32. Hua A, Major N. Selective mutism. Curr Opin Pediatr. 2016;28(1):114-20.
33. Klein ER, Armstrong SL, Skira K, Gordon J. Social Communication Anxiety Treatment (S-CAT) for children and families with selective mutism: a pilot study. Clin Child Psychol Psychiatry. 2017;22(1):90-108.
34. De Los Reyes A, Epkins CC. Introduction to the special issue. A dozen years of demonstrating that informant discrepancies are more than measurement error: Toward guidelines for integrating data from multi-informant assessments of youth mental health. J Clin Child Adolesc Psychol. 2023;52(1):1-18.

35. Becker EM, Jensen-Doss A, Kendall PC, Birmaher B, Ginsburg GS. All anxiety is not created equal: Correlates of parent/youth agreement vary across subtypes of anxiety. J Psychopathol Behav Assess. 2016;38(4):528-37.
36. Fjermestad KW, Nilsen W, Johannessen TD, Karevold EB. Mothers' and fathers' internalizing symptoms influence parental ratings of adolescent anxiety symptoms. J Fam Psychol. 2017;31(7):939-44.
37. Silverman WK, Albano AM. Anxiety disorders interview schedule for children for DSM-IV: Child and parent versions. San Antonio, TX: The Psychological Corporation-Harcourt, Brace & Company; 1996.
38. Herjanic B, Reich W. Development of a structured psychiatric interview for children: agreement between child and parent on individual symptoms. J Abnorm Child Psychol. 1982;10(3):307-24.
39. Shaffer D, Fisher P, Lucas CP, Dulcan MK, Schwab-Stone ME. NIMH Diagnostic Interview Schedule for Children Version IV (NIMH DISC-IV): description, differences from previous versions, and reliability of some common diagnoses. J Am Acad Child Adolesc Psychiatry. 2000;39(1):28-38.
40. Viswanathan M, Wallace IF, Cook Middleton J, Kennedy SM, McKeeman J, Hudson K, et al. Screening for anxiety in children and adolescents: Evidence report and systematic review for the US Preventive Services Task Force. JAMA. 2022;328(14):1445-55.
41. Goodman R. The strengths and difficulties questionnaire: a research note. J Child Psychol Psychiatry. 1997;38:581-6.
42. Wolraich ML, Lambert W, Doffing MA, Bickman L, Simmons T, Worley K. Psychometric properties of the Vanderbilt ADHD diagnostic parent rating scale in a referred population. J Pediatr Psychol. 2003;28(8):559-67.
43. La Greca AM, Stone WL. Social anxiety scale for children-revised: Factor structure and con-current validity. J Clin Child Psychol. 1993;22:17-27.
44. Birmaher B, Khetarpal S, Brent D, Cully M, Balach L, Kaufman J, et al. The Screen for Child Anxiety Related Emotional Disorders (SCARED): scale construction and psychometric characteristics. J Am Acad Child Adolesc Psychiatry. 1997;36(4):545-53.
45. March JS, Parker JD, Sullivan K, Stallings P, Conners CK. The Multidimensional Anxiety Scale for Children (MASC): factor structure, reliability, and validity. J Am Acad Child Adolesc Psychiatry. 1997;36(4):554-65.
46. Spence SH. A measure of anxiety symptoms among children. Behav Res Ther. 1998;36(5):545-66.
47. Johnson JG, Harris ES, Spitzer RL, Williams JB. The patient health questionnaire for adolescents: validation of an instrument for the assessment of mental disorders among adolescent primary care patients. J Adolesc Health. 2002;30(3):196-204.
48. Méndez X, Espada JP, Orgilés M, Llavona LM, García-Fernández JM. Children's separation anxiety scale (CSAS): psychometric properties. PLoS One. 2014;9(7):e103212.
49. O'Connor S, Ferguson E, Carney T, House E, O'Connor RC. The development and evaluation of the paediatric index of emotional distress (PI-ED). Soc Psychiatry Psychiatr Epidemiol. 2016;51(1):15-26.
50. Stuijfzand S, Dodd HF. Young children have social worries too: Validation of a brief parent report measure of social worries in children aged 4-8 years. J Anxiety Disord. 2017;50:87-93.
51. Malhi P, Bharti B, Sidhu M. Aggression in schools: psychosocial outcomes of bullying among Indian adolescents. Indian J Pediatr. 2014;81(11):1171-6.
52. Madasu S, Malhotra S, Kant S, Sagar R, Mishra AK, Misra P, et al. Anxiety disorders among adolescents in a rural area of Northern India using Screen for Child Anxiety-Related Emotional Disorders Tool: A community-based study. Indian J Community Med. 2019;44(4):317-21.
53. Walter HJ, Bukstein OG, Abright AR, Keable H, Ramtekkar U, Ripperger-Suhler J, et al. Clinical practice guideline for the assessment and treatment of children and adolescents with anxiety disorders. J Am Acad Child Adolesc Psychiatry. 2020;59(10):1107-24.
54. Kopcsó K, Láng A, Coffman MF. Reducing the nighttime fears of young children through a brief parent-delivered treatment-effectiveness of the Hungarian version of Uncle Lightfoot. Child Psychiatry Hum Dev. 2022;53(2):256-67.
55. Malhi P, Bharti B. Healing with storybooks: Using bibliotherapy to help children cope with death. Indian J Soc Psychiatry; 2023;(3):198-300.
56. Rapee RM, Abbott MJ, Lyneham HJ. Bibliotherapy for children with anxiety disorders using written materials for parents: a randomized controlled trial. J Cons Clin Psychol. 2006;74:436-44.
57. Lyneham HJ, Rapee RM. Evaluation of therapist-supported parent-implemented CBT for anxiety disorders in rural children. Behav Res Ther. 2006;44(9):1287-300.
58. Bry LJ, Chou T, Miguel E, Comer JS. Consumer smartphone apps marketed for child and adolescent anxiety: a systematic review and content analysis. Behav Ther. 2018;49(2):249-61.
59. Williams JE, Pykett J. Mental health monitoring apps for depression and anxiety in children and young people: a scoping review and critical ecological analysis. Soc Sci Med. 2022;297:114802.
60. World Health Organization. Psychosocial interventions, treatment of emotional disorders. Geneva: World Health Organization; 2015.
61. Higa-McMillan CK, Francis SE, Rith-Najarian L, Chorpita BF. Evidence base update: 50 years of research on treatment for child and adolescent anxiety. J Clin Child Adolesc Psychol. 2016;45(2):91-113.
62. Peris TS, Caporino NE, O'Rourke S, Kendall PC, Walkup JT, Albano AM, et al. Therapist-reported features of exposure tasks that predict differential treatment outcomes for youth with anxiety. J Am Acad Child Adolesc Psychiatry. 2017;56(12):1043-52.

63. Cardy JL, Waite P, Cocks F, Creswell C. A systematic review of parental involvement in cognitive behavioural therapy for adolescent anxiety disorders. Clin Child Fam Psychol Rev. 2020;23(4):483-509.
64. Burke CA. Mindfulness-based approaches with children and adolescents: A preliminary review of current research in an emergent field. J Child Fam Stud. 2010;19:133-44.
65. Dunning DL, Griffiths K, Kuyken W, Crane C, Foulkes L, Parker J, et al. Research review: The effects of mindfulness-based interventions on cognition and mental health in children and adolescents—a meta-analysis of randomized controlled trials. J Child Psychol Psychiatry. 2019;60(3):244-58.
66. Monsillion J, Zebdi R, Romo-Desprez L. School mindfulness-based interventions for youth, and considerations for anxiety, depression, and a positive school climate—a systematic literature review. Children (Basel). 2023;10(5):861.
67. Catani C, Kohiladevy M, Ruf M, Schauer E, Elbert T, Neuner F. Treating children traumatized by war and Tsunami: a comparison between exposure therapy and meditation-relaxation in North-East Sri Lanka. BMC Psychiatry. 2009;9:22.
68. Herzig-Anderson K, Colognori D, Fox JK, Stewart CE, Masia Warner C. School-based anxiety treatments for children and adolescents. Child Adolesc Psychiatr Clin N Am. 2012;21(3):655-68.
69. Masia C, Beidel DC, Albano AM, Rapee RM, Turner SM, Morris TL, et al. Skills for academic and social success. New York University School of Medicine; New York: 1999.
70. Mifsud C, Rapee RM. Early intervention for childhood anxiety in a school setting: outcomes for an economically disadvantaged population. J Am Acad Child Adolesc Psychiatry. 2005;44:996-1004.
71. Ginsburg GS, Becker KD, Drazdowski TK, Tein JY. Treating anxiety disorders in inner city schools: results from a pilot randomized controlled trial comparing CBT and usual care. Child Youth Care Forum. 2012;41:1-19.
72. Lewis KM, Barrett P, Freitag G, Ollendick TH. An ounce of prevention: Building resilience and targeting anxiety in young children. Clin Child Psychol Psychiatry. 2023;28(2):795-809.
73. Ramsawh HJ, Chavira DA, Stein MB. Burden of anxiety disorders in pediatric medical settings: prevalence, phenomenology, and a research agenda. Arch Pediatr Adolesc Med. 2010;164(10):965-72.
74. Kandasamy P, Girimaji SC, Seshadri SP, Srinath S, Kommu JVS. Favourable short-term course and outcome of pediatric anxiety spectrum disorders: a prospective study from India. Child Adolesc Psychiatry Ment Health. 2019;13:11.
75. Ginsburg GS, Becker EM, Keeton CP, Sakolsky D. Naturalistic follow-up of youths treated for pediatric anxiety disorders. JAMA Psychiatry. 2014;71(3):310-18.
76. Ginsburg GS, Becker-Haimes EM, Keeton C, Kendall PC, Iyengar S, Sakolsky D, et al. Results from the Child/Adolescent Anxiety Multimodal Extended Long-term Study (CAMELS): Primary anxiety outcomes. J Am Acad Child Adolesc Psychiatry. 2018;57(7):471-80.
77. Schleider JL, Ginsburg GS, Keeton CP, Weisz JR, Birmaher B, Kendall PC, et al. Parental psychopathology and treatment outcome for anxious youth: roles of family functioning and caregiver strain. J Consult Clin Psychol. 2015;83(1):213-24.
78. Åhlén J, Vigerland S, Lindberg M, Gunterberg O, Ghaderi A. Developing a Brief Parent Training Intervention to Prevent Anxiety in Offspring. Scand J Child Adolesc Psychiatr Psychol. 2022;10(1):123-33.
79. Teubert D, Pinquart M. A meta-analytic review on the prevention of symptoms of anxiety in children and adolescents. J Anxiety Disord. 2011;25:1046-59.
80. Kodish I, Rockhill C, Ryan S, Varley C. Pharmacotherapy for anxiety disorders in children and adolescents. Pediatr Clin N Am. 2011;58:55-72.

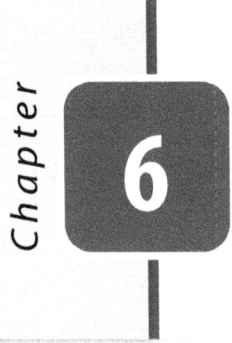

Chapter 6

Exogenous Depression in Children

GD Koolwal, Shreyance Jain

INTRODUCTION

Depression is one of the common psychiatric disorders in children.[1] Depressive disorders present with persistent sadness and/or irritability, anhedonia that is relatively unresponsive to pleasurable activities and interactions as well as lack of attention from people. Depression in children has a significant adverse effect on a child's cognitive, emotional, and social development. Early onset of major depression is associated with more depressive episodes in future, suicide attempts, greater psychiatric and medical comorbidity, and poorer quality of life.[2] Early recognition of these disorders is essential so that children may receive effective evidence-based treatments.[3]

EPIDEMIOLOGY

Prevalence studies in children with depression showed that the prevalence rate varies according to the age groups. In preschool children the prevalence rate of major depressive disorder has been reported around 1.4%. Prevalence rate of depression in infants ranges from 0.5 to 3% in clinical population sample. Community studies suggest that the prevalence of childhood depression ranges from 0.4 to 2.5%.[4] After puberty, rates of depression increase and females are affected approximately twice more commonly than males.[5] Before puberty, depressive disorders have equal prevalence in both genders.[6]

CLASSIFICATION

Term exogenous depression stems from the Latin word *"exogenous"*, which means growing by adding from outside. Exogenous depression is characterized by a reaction to external life events. The entity is often used interchangeably with other types of depression such as reactive depression or situational depression. In children, it can occur after a particular event, like the *death of parent, abuse, parental separation, inadequate social support, academic failures, presence of some personality traits, medications, chronic and debilitating medical illnesses, substance abuse,* etc.[2,7]

It is difficult to diagnose exogenous depression from endogenous depression because it becomes difficult to determine whether the external event or stress is the cause of the depression or it is because of some internal factors. As per recent classification system depressive disorders are classified on the basis of severity of illness, duration of illness and seasonal variations, and terms exogenous and endogenous are rarely used.

WHO ICD-11 CRITERIA[5]

Diagnostic Requirements

Depressive disorders are characterized by depressive mood (e.g., sad, irritable, and empty) or loss of pleasure accompanied by other cognitive, behavioral, or neurovegetative symptoms that significantly affect the individual's ability to function **(Box 1)**. A depressive disorder should not be diagnosed in individuals who have ever experienced a manic, mixed, or hypomanic episode, which would indicate the presence of a bipolar disorder.

Developmental Presentations

- Assessment of depression children is on the basis of history and report from informants, like parents, teachers, friends, etc. Episode should represent a *change from prior functioning*.
- Depressed mood may present as *somatic complaints* (e.g., headaches and stomachaches), whining, increased separation anxiety, or excessive crying.
- Depressed mood may sometimes present in children and adolescents as *pervasive irritability*.
- *Reduced ability to concentrate or sustain attention* may manifest as a decline in academic performance, increased time needed to complete school assignments, or an inability to complete assignments.

- *Hypersomnia and hyperphagia* are more common symptoms of a depressive episode in adolescents than in adults.
- Appetite disturbance in children and adolescents may manifest in *failure to gain weight* rather than weight loss.
- Increased *risk for suicidality* may manifest in passive statements (e.g., "I do not want to be here anymore") or as themes of death during play.
- *Self-injurious behaviors* that are not explicitly suicidal in terms of lethality or expressed intent may also occur in depressive episode in young children and adolescents. Examples include *head banging or scratching* in young children and *cutting or burning* in adolescents.

DSM-5 Diagnostic Criteria for Depression[8]

DSM-5 diagnostic criteria for depression have been given in **Box 2**.

> **BOX 1:** Depressive episode as per ICD-11 criteria.
>
> *Essential (required) features:*
> The concurrent presence of at least five of the following characteristic symptoms occurring most of the day, nearly every day during a period lasting at least 2 weeks. At least one symptom from the affective cluster must be present. Assessment of the presence or absence of symptoms should be made relative to typical functioning of the individual
>
> *Affective cluster:* Depressed mood as reported by the individual (e.g., feeling down and sad) or as observed (e.g., tearful and defeated appearance). In children and adolescents, depressed mood can manifest as *irritability*. Markedly diminished interest or pleasure in activities, especially those normally found to be enjoyable to the individual
>
> *Cognitive-behavioral cluster:* Reduced ability to concentrate and sustain attention to tasks, or marked indecisiveness, beliefs of low self-worth or excessive and inappropriate guilt that may be manifestly delusional, hopelessness about the future, recurrent thoughts of death (not just fear of dying), recurrent suicidal ideation (with or without a specific plan), or evidence of attempted suicide
>
> *Neurovegetative cluster:* Significantly disrupted sleep (delayed sleep onset, increased frequency of waking during the night, or early morning awakening) or excessive sleep, significant change in appetite (diminished or increased) or significant weight change (gain or loss), psychomotor agitation or retardation (observable by others, not merely subjective feelings of restlessness or being slowed down), reduced energy, fatigue, or marked tiredness following the expenditure of only a minimum of effort
>
> The symptoms are not better accounted for by bereavement, not a manifestation of another medical condition, and are not due to the effects of a substance or medication on the central nervous system including withdrawal effects. The clinical presentation does not fulfill the diagnostic requirements for a mixed episode. The mood disturbance results in significant impairment in personal, family, social, educational, occupational, or other important areas of functioning. If functioning is maintained, it is only through significant additional effort

> **BOX 2:** DSM-5 diagnostic criteria for depression.
>
> A. Five (or more) of the following symptoms have been present during the same 2-week period and represent a change from previous functioning; at least one of the symptoms is either (1) depressed mood or (2) loss of interest or pleasure
> (*Note:* Do not include symptoms that are clearly attributable to another medical condition)
> 1. Depressed mood most of the day, nearly every day, as indicated by either subjective report (e.g., feels sad, empty, and hopeless) or observation made by others (e.g., appears tearful)
> (*Note: In children and adolescents, can be irritable mood*)
> 2. Markedly diminished interest or pleasure in all, or almost all, activities most of the day, nearly every day (as indicated by either subjective account or observation)
> 3. Significant weight loss when not dieting or weight gain (e.g., a change of >5% of body weight in a month), or decrease or increase in appetite nearly every day
> (*Note: In children, consider failure to make expected weight gain*)
> 4. Insomnia or hypersomnia nearly every day
> 5. Psychomotor agitation or retardation nearly every day (observable by others, not merely subjective feelings of restlessness or being slowed down)
> 6. Fatigue or loss of energy nearly every day
> 7. Feelings of worthlessness or excessive or inappropriate guilt (which may be delusional) nearly every day (not merely self-reproach or guilt about being sick)
> 8. Diminished ability to think or concentrate, or indecisiveness, nearly every day (either by subjective account or as observed by others)
> 9. Recurrent thoughts of death (not just fear of dying), recurrent suicidal ideation without a specific plan, or a suicide attempt or a specific plan for committing suicide
> B. The symptoms cause clinically significant distress or impairment in social, occupational, or other important areas of functioning
> C. The episode is not attributable to the physiological effects of a substance or to another medical condition
> D. The occurrence of the major depressive episode is not better explained by schizoaffective disorder, schizophrenia, schizophreniform disorder, delusional disorder, or other specified and unspecified schizophrenia spectrum, and other psychotic disorders
> E. There has never been a manic episode or a hypomanic episode

Severity of Depression (DSM-5): Severity is based on the number of criterion symptoms, the severity symptoms, and the degree of functional disability.

Mild: Few, if any, symptoms in excess of those required to make the diagnosis are present, the intensity of the symptoms is distressing but manageable, and the symptoms result in minor impairment in social or occupational functioning.

Moderate: The numbers of symptoms, intensity of symptoms, and/or functional impairment are between those specified for "mild" and "severe."

Severe: The number of symptoms is substantially in excess of that required to make the diagnosis, the intensity of the symptoms is seriously distressing and unmanageable, and the symptoms markedly interfere with social and occupational functioning.

RISK OF CHILDHOOD DEPRESSION

Childhood depression has been associated with declining academic performance, poor social functioning, homicidal ideation, substance use disorders, and suicidal behavior. It can also lead increased risk of recurrent future episodes of depression.[2,9]

Comorbidity

Comorbid psychiatric illnesses are noted in 80–95% of children.[10] Anxiety disorders are commonly associated and has a common genetic underpinning.[11] Comorbidity psychiatric disorders may be because of common etiology or a consequence of depressive illness. Other common comorbidities reported are attention-deficit and hyperactivity disorder (ADHD), oppositional defiant disorder (ODD), conduct disorder (CD), and substance use disorder.[2]

ETIOLOGY

Depressive disorders in children are multifactorial and have a biopsychosocial basis of origin, since multiple factors are involved in onset and maintenance **(Table 1)**. Various theories of childhood onset of depression have been proposed, such as (1) biological theories, (2) attachment theories, (3) behavioral theories, (4) learned helplessness theory, and (5) sociocultural theories.

TABLE 1: Vulnerability factors for depression.

Genetic:	Environmental risk factors:
• Emotion regulation	• Parental depression and family discord
• Fear and anxiety	• Child maltreatment
• Behavioral disorders and irritability	• Peer victimization
• Sleep disorders	• Sexual minority status
• Comorbid medical illness	• Bereavement
	• Poor resilience

Neurotransmitters: Serotonin (5-hydroxytryptamine) is a precursor monoamine neurotransmitter of epinephrine, norepinephrine, and dopamine which plays important role, in regulation of sleep, appetite, learning, memory, temperature regulation as well as social adaptation. It is also associated with other neuropsychiatric diseases. Serotonin modulates neuroplasticity in early formative years of life and serotonergic dysregulation may contribute in pathophysiology of depression.[12]

Adverse Childhood Experiences and Stressful Life Events

In children, depression is associated with stressful life events which may also constitute potent risk factor. The onset of depressive episode not only gets triggered by major stressful life event but also by minor life events, like dropout from school, loss of friend or illness in family members, poor socioeconomic status, etc. which may precipitate the depressive episode.[13] Not all exposed to traumatic experience get depressed, but among them who had severe emotional abuse in childhood, experience higher level of depressive symptoms. Along with it *childhood temperament and critical time periods* are equally involved in onset of depression.[14]

If depressive symptoms/disorders are not explained by above factors or if family history is negative for depression/mood disorders then neurobiological factors, such as epileptic syndromes, metabolic disorders, sleep disorders, or intracranial tumors must be ruled out.[15]

Course

The episode of major depression in children lasts around 8 months and >90% of depressed children recover from it within 1–2 years. Early age of onset of depression increases the risk of anxiety disorders, substance abuse, psychiatric comorbidity, suicide attempts, psychiatric and medical hospitalization, impairment in relationships,

> **BOX 3:** Clinical assessment.
>
> - *Detail history:* Collect information from all possible sources and on multiple occasions. Different information may be obtained from discussion with school teachers, from school records, or from medical records. Clinician should interview the child and parent in separate settings so that each one can express their concerns. Children are often reluctant to disclose their feelings, thoughts, and emotions or issues related to peers in the presence of their parents. Similarly, parents may not discuss sensitive issues in presence of their children. The primary goal is to establish a good therapeutic alliance
> - *Developmental history* which includes presence of neurotic traits—thumb sucking, nail biting, and tantrums
> - *Physical examination:* Evaluate for thyroid gland swelling and nutritional disorders
> - *Mental status examination:* Signs of depression includes poor eye-to-eye contact, poor engagement/uncooperativeness, poor hygiene, downcast facies, tearfulness, psychomotor agitation or retardation, sad mood, anger outbursts, low frustration tolerance, distractibility, poverty of speech, perseverative or ruminative thought processes, guilt, or self-blame
> - *Temperament assessment:* Activity, rhythmicity, mood, adaptability, intensity of reaction, threshold of responsiveness, and attention span
> - *Comorbid psychiatric conditions:* Substance use disorders, generalized anxiety disorders, dissociative (conversion) disorder, oppositional defiant disorder, conduct disorder, and attention and deficit hyperkinetic disorder must be ruled out
> - History of suicide attempts/deliberate harm
> - *Assess for suicidal intent/behavior*
> - *Psychosocial evaluation:* It includes family discord and family functioning and psychopathology
> - *Severity and level of dysfunction:* School performance decline, school refusal/phobia, and social interaction
> - *Functionality assessment:* Social, educational, and family functioning
> - Assess the severity, subtype of depression, specifier if any, level of dysfunction, comorbid physical and psychiatric conditions, and substance use
> - *Differential diagnosis:* Rule out medication-induced depression and rule out bipolar affective disorder
> - *Diagnosis:* According to the standard ICD-11/DSM-5 diagnostic criteria

(DSM-5: Diagnostic and Statistical Manual of Mental Disorders, Fifth Edition; ICD-11: 11th Revision of the International Classification of Diseases)

more lifetime depressive episodes, nicotine dependence, educational underachievement, unemployment, early parenthood, and worse overall quality of life.[2,16]

Assessment of Children Presenting with Depression[4]

It is essential to conduct a comprehensive evaluation of a child to ensure the accuracy of the primary diagnosis as well as of comorbid diagnoses **(Box 3)**.

Additional/Optional Assessments

Rating scales: Routine clinical assessments may be supplemented by standardized rating scales to rate all aspects of depression, depending on the availability and feasibility. Children's Depression Inventory (CDI) with target age group of 7–17 years is commonly used scale to measure childhood depression. Other scale like Mood and Feelings Questionnaire (MFQ) for age group of 6–17 years can also be used. Revised Children's anxiety and depression scale for age group of 8–18 years can also be used to assess comorbid anxiety disorder, separation anxiety disorder, social phobia, and obsessive-compulsive disorder.

Neuroimaging, especially in those with suspected intracranial space-occupying lesion/tumors or other conditions such as epilepsies, metabolic disorders, and in cases of treatment-resistant depression.

Investigations: Hemogram, blood glucose levels, lipid levels, liver function tests, renal function tests, and thyroid function test (if indicated). No laboratory tests are diagnostic of depressive disorders in children,[2] only in symptomatic cases relevant investigations are indicated like if a child presents with symptom of depression and hypothyroidism then thyroid function tests should be obtained.

TREATMENT

Treatment of depression is divided into three stages:
1. Acute treatment phase (for first 2–3 months)
2. Consolidation/continuation phase (subsequent 3–6 months)
3. Maintenance phase (continuing treatment for >12 months).

In acute treatment phase target is to achieve a response (defined as minimum of 50% decrease in depressive symptoms scores on a standard rating scale and a global rating of improved to very much improve. Consolidation phase involves either continuation of treatment or dose adjustments to improve residual symptoms and to further achieve remission.[4,10]

PSYCHOTHERAPY

The two most-studied and evidence-based treatment modalities for childhood and adolescent depression are cognitive behavior therapy (CBT) and interpersonal psychotherapy (IPT).[4,17] Other psychotherapies which are used are self-management/self-control therapy, play therapy, behavior therapy/behavioral activation (BA), and problem-solving therapy.[11]

Specific Psychotherapies

Cognitive behavior therapy: In CBT, patient is taught to identify faulty thoughts associated mood and behavior. Negative automatic thought identification is taught to client, along with skill testing of these thoughts and replacing them with more acceptable and adaptive thoughts. Further BA, problem-solving skills, and emotional regulation techniques with relaxation exercises are taught to children.

Interpersonal psychotherapy: It helps in identifying relationship problems, interpersonal conflicts, and role transition. It teaches problem-solving skills and improves interpersonal communication. It is very effective in dealing conflicts with family members and friends which commonly seen in childhood depressive disorders and act as risk factors for depression.

PHARMACOLOGICAL MANAGEMENT[4,10,16,17]

- Antidepressant medications are chosen on the basis of evidence, severity, chronicity, individual characteristics and previous response to treatment, family history, comorbid psychiatric and medical disorders, expectation and preferences of patient, and family members.
- Prior to administration of antidepressant drugs adequate information about risks, side effects, and benefit of these drugs should be explained to parents, caregivers, and those involve in care of the children.
- Informed consent must be obtained before initiation of drug either from parents/guardians or care givers.
- Doses, onset of effect, and the danger of drug overdose must be explained to parents and caregivers.
- Antidepressant medications are considered in the cases of moderate and severe depression with or without psychotic symptoms and in cases where psychotherapy is not feasible and if it fails to respond after adequate period of psychotherapy.
- Selective serotonin reuptake inhibitors (SSRIs), especially fluoxetine should be considered as the first choice in children aged ≥8 years unless its use is restricted by drug interactions, family nonacceptability, and lack of previous response with adequate doses and time period. There escitalopram or sertraline may be considered. Escitalopram has been studied in children with age of 12 years and above and reported to be safe and efficacious.
- In children with high risk of suicidal tendency, it is recommended that parents and caregivers should ensure to give medicines under their supervision.
- Antidepressant medicines should be started at low dosages and titrated to a level where symptom control has been achieved and side effects are minimized.
- As depression in children often has psychosocial background, there is a need to address the associated environmental and social problems with supportive measures.
- In children with first episode of depression, antidepressants can be tapered by the end of consolidation/continuation phase. Medications need to be decreased and tapered off slowly to prevent withdrawal effects.
- Before tapering of medications relapse and recurrence risk, tapering plan, and possible withdrawal symptoms which can arise during the procedure need to be discussed.
- As the risk of relapse is very high during the first 8 months after stopping treatment, patients and family must be advised to follow-up every 2–4 months during this period. If there is recurrence of symptoms, then previously effective treatment may be restarted.
- All SSRIs have a *black box warning for suicidal thinking* and behavior.
- Comprehensive treatment increases the chances of remission and also improvement in coping skills and self-esteem.
- *Medication-induced behavioral activation* presents with the symptoms of irritability, agitated and aggressive behavior, anxiety symptoms (i.e., features of panic attacks), restlessness, hostility, hypomania/

mania, and emergence of psychotic symptoms. Evidence suggests that antidepressant-associated BA is associated with the use of higher doses of medications. Hence, it is suggested that children receiving antidepressant medications must be watched closely while starting and during the period of change of doses.

- *Medication treatment algorithm:*[2] An evidence-based consensus algorithm for the treatment of major depression in children reported in which four stages of medication treatment were identified. It was recommended that if a child failed to respond to treatment in one stage, then the clinician should move to treatment in the next stage.

    Stage 1: Treatment with an SSRI
    Stage 2: Use of an alternative SSRI
    Stage 3: Selection of a different class of antidepressant medication (venlafaxine, bupropion, mirtazapine, and duloxetine) **(Table 2)**.

    If a child fails to respond to these agents, then it was recommended that there was reassessment of the diagnosis and treatment consultation.

    Consultation with psychiatrist should be done in all the cases for a better overall management and prognosis.

Neuromodulatory and brain stimulation techniques: Electroconvulsive therapy (ECT) if permitted is indicated in children who failed to respond to adequate trial of two antidepressant drugs for adequate period of time and also in situations where it is considered to be lifesaving, such as suicidality, catatonia, and refusal to accept orally.

TABLE 2: Dosing of antidepressant medicines in children.

Antidepressant drugs	Starting dose (mg/day)	Target dose (mg/day)
Selective serotonin reuptake inhibitors (SSRI)		
Fluoxetine	5–10	20–40
Escitalopram	5	10–20
Sertraline	25	100–200
Others		
Bupropion	100	100–200
Duloxetine	20	60–120
Mirtazapine	15	30–45
Venlafaxine	37.5	150–225

Inpatient Hospital Admission

Inpatient treatment should be considered for children who present with a life-threatening situation, such as risk of suicide, self-harm, or self-neglect, or when the family is not able to provide an appropriate level of supervision or follow-up with outpatient treatment recommendations, or when comprehensive assessment and diagnostic clarification is required.[16]

Psychoeducation and Supportive Management

Treatment of depressed children and adolescents should also include psychoeducation, supportive management, family involvement, and school involvement. It is important to involve parents and school in the treatment process. Psychoeducation involves educating the patient and parents about depression including causes, symptoms, course, and treatment options, including benefits and risks of treatment. Depression should be explained as an illness not a character flaw of the child or parent. The parent and child should be informed about the importance of adhering to treatment to ensure an optimal outcome.[4] Supportive management includes assisting the child with problem solving, improving coping skills, and fostering involvement in treatment. Parents can provide important information about the child's symptoms over the course of treatment. Parents may also need guidance in managing their depressed child at home. With regard to school involvement, children with depression may have academic difficulties that require school remediation or accommodation in the child's school schedule or program.

PREVENTION

The universal goal of prevention is to decrease the risk of development of depression in population including children. Targeted (selective or indicated) interventions target those children having significant risk factors for development of depression or having subclinical depressive symptoms and prevent the development of episode of major depression. Targeted interventions include *cognitive restructuring, improving coping skills and communication, and developing resilience.*[18] They have moderate effect size but more effective than universal interventions. Targeted screening of known high-risk groups having known psychosocial adversities may have a higher-yield case-finding strategy than universal screening.

CONCLUSION

Childhood depression is a debilitating and complex disorder that has a chronic and recurring course. There is need for useful biomarkers for early detection, predictors for early response, and for overall better outcome. Future research needs to study the *impact of internet and mobile use along with role of social media* in the etiology of depression. There is also need to develop *online education material for early identification* and treatment of depression in children.[3]

This is increasingly going to play a major role seeing the growth in the use of technology by healthcare providers and also effective delivery of online interventions.

REFERENCES

1. Jane Costello E, Erkanli A, Angold A. Is there an epidemic of child or adolescent depression? J Child Psychol Psychiatry. 2006;47(12):1263-71.
2. Wagner KD, Brent DA. Depressive disorders and suicide. In: Sadock BJ, Sadock VA, Ruiz P (Eds). Kaplan and Sadock's Comprehensive Textbook of Psychiatry, 10th edition. Philadelphia, PA: Lippincott Williams & Wilkins; 2017.
3. Brent D, Maalouf F. Depressive disorders in childhood and adolescence. In: Thapar A, Pine DS, Leckman JF, Scott S, Snowling MJ, Taylor EA (Eds). Rutter's Child and Adolescent Psychiatry, 6th edition. Chichester, UK: Wiley-Blackwell; 2015.
4. Grover S, Avasthi A. Clinical practice guidelines for the management of depression in children and adolescents. Indian J Psychiatry. 2019;61(8):226.
5. World Health Organisation. Mood disorders. [online]. Available from: https://icd.who.int/browse11/l-m/en#/http%3A%2F%2Fid.who.int%2Ficd%2Fentity%2F76398729 [Last accessed October, 2023].
6. Birmaher B, Ryan ND, Williamson DE, Brent DA, Kaufman J, Dahl RE, et al. Childhood and adolescent depression: a review of the past 10 years. J Am Acad Child Adolesc Psychiatry. 1996;35(11):1427-39.
7. Schimelpfenin N. (2022). Endogenous vs. Exogenous Depression: What Are the Differences? [online] Available from: https://www.verywellmind.com/what-is-endogenous-depression-1067283 [Last accessed October, 2023].
8. American Psychiatric Association. Diagnostic and statistical manual of mental disorders, 5th edition. Washington, DC: American Psychiatric Association; 2013.
9. Thapar A, Pine DS, Leckman JF, Scott S, Snowling MJ, Taylor E. Rutter's Child and Adolescent Psychiatry, 6th edition. Chichester, UK: John Wiley & Sons, Ltd; 2015.
10. Patra S. Assessment and management of pediatric depression. Indian J Psychiatry. 2019;61(3):300-6.
11. Middeldorp CM, Cath DC, Van Dyck R, Boomsma DI. The co-morbidity of anxiety and depression in the perspective of genetic epidemiology. A review of twin and family studies. Psychol Med. 2005;35(5):611-24.
12. Kraus C, Castrén E, Kasper S, Lanzenberger R. Serotonin and neuroplasticity—Links between molecular, functional and structural pathophysiology in depression. Neurosci Biobehav Rev. 2017;77:317-26.
13. Shapero BG, Black SK, Liu RT, Klugman J, Bender RE, Abramson LY, et al. Stressful Life Events and Depression Symptoms: The Effect of Childhood Emotional Abuse on Stress Reactivity. J Clin Psychol. 2014;70(3):209-23.
14. Caspi A, Sugden K, Moffitt TE, Taylor A, Craig IW, Harrington H, et al. Influence of Life Stress on Depression: Moderation by a Polymorphism in the 5-HTT Gene. Science. 2003;301(5631):386-9.
15. Bernaras E, Jaureguizar J, Garaigordobil M. Child and Adolescent Depression: A Review of Theories, Evaluation Instruments, Prevention Programs, and Treatments. Front Psychol. 2019;10:543.
16. Walter HJ, DeMaso DR. Mood disorders. In: Kliegman RM, III JWSG, Blum NJ, Shah SS, Tasker RC, Wilson KM, et al. (Eds). Nelson Textbook of Pediatrics, 21st edition. Canada: Elsevier Inc.; 2020.
17. Walter HJ, Abright AR, Bukstein OG, Diamond J, Keable H, Ripperger-Suhler J, et al. Clinical Practice Guideline for the Assessment and Treatment of Children and Adolescents with Major and Persistent Depressive Disorders. J Am Acad Child Adolesc Psychiatry. 2023;62(5):479-502.
18. Rey JM, Bella-Awusah TT, Jing L. Depression in children and adolescents. In: Rey JM (Ed). International Association for Child and Adolescent Psychiatry and Allied Professions (IACAPAP) e-Textbook of Child and Adolescent Mental Health. International Association for Child and Adolescent Psychiatry and Allied Professions; Geneva: 2015.

Chapter 7

Nonsuicidal Self-injury and Suicide in Adolescence

RK Maheshwari, Shivji Ram Choudhary

NONSUICIDAL SELF-INJURY

INTRODUCTION

Adolescence is a most challenging period of life. It is a period of dependence to independence. While this period is associated with onset of maturity but at the same time due to varied reasons it is also a time when young individuals may grapple with an array of challenges and instead of facing them properly they resort to cause harm to themselves. This may be with or without suicidal intent nonsuicidal self-injury (NSSI). The intricate relationship between NSSI and suicide, sharing common risk factors and emotional struggles, underscores the urgency of addressing these issues comprehensively. Early intervention can prevent many youth to take extreme steps.

DEFINITION

Nonsuicidal self-injury or self-mutilation is defined as the deliberate, direct, self-inflicted destruction of body tissue, done to relieve emotional pain or stress but without suicidal intent and for purposes not socially sanctioned.[1-3] Common examples include cutting, burning, scratching, and banging or hitting, embedding objects under the skin, punching hard objects, preventing wounds from healing, and other forms of external injury. Cutting by far is said to be the most common method employed.[4] It may also include internal or emotional harm, e.g., consuming toxic amounts of alcohol or drugs or even deliberately participating in unsafe sex.[5]

Arms, legs, and torso are the most common areas where injury is inflicted. Razors, broken glass, knives/scissors, or other sharp objects are commonly used for the purpose.[4]

The behavior often becomes habitual and may persist in adult life.[6] Most people who self-injure use multiple methods. It is typically associated with emotional and psychiatric distress and increases risk for suicide.[1,2]

PREVALENCE

It is prevalent all across the globe. The statistical incidence varies from study to study (15-20%).[7] It is most common among adolescents and young adults. Onset typically occurs around 13-14 years of age, more commonly in person with emotional distress, such as negative emotionality, depression, anxiety, and in people prone to self-directed negative emotions and self-criticism.[1]

Incidence is either equal in both sexes or more in females though methods adopted are different. While females mostly resort to cutting, males commonly adopt hitting or burning. Incidence is also more in people with nonheterosexual orientations (for example, homosexual and bisexuals).[1]

CAUSES[1,5,8]

- This is done most often as a temporary, albeit maladaptive coping strategy to manage the distress. Body injury is said to result in release of endorphins or raise dopamine (serotonin) levels in brain leading to an elevated mood thus taking the person out of depressed states of mind.
- Also done to express self-directed anger or self-punishment (self-criticism).
- Sometimes done to influence others or to produce a physical sign of emotional distress or letting others know how I feel!

RISK FACTORS[4,9,10]

There are many risk factors or factors which precipitate NSSI such as:
- Childhood sexual abuse or family violence or childhood trauma. There is high correlation between cutting and childhood sexual abuse.
- Familial factors, e.g., parental divorce, poor harmony between parents, loss of a parent or caregiver, especially

in early age, highly punitive parental practice, or breakup with boyfriend/girlfriend.
- In ability to express strong negative emotions (e.g., pain, hurt, and anger)
- Persons who experience dissociation
- Persons suffering from psychological disorders, e.g., depression, poor impulse control, eating disorders, anxiety, and impulsivity
- Alcohol or drug abuse
- *Socioeconomic factors:* Poor economic status increases the incidence
- Personality disorder and delinquency
- Poor scholastic performance
- Chronic illness
- *Social media:* Persons indulging in NSSI may post their stories on social media and this sometimes promotes others to follow.

Nonsuicidal Self-injury Versus Suicide Versus Bipolar Personality Disorder

Nonsuicidal self-injury and suicidal behaviors are both forms of suicidal ideation and behaviors (SIBs) and have been found to coexist in both community and psychiatric populations yet they differ in several important ways as shown in **Table 1,** hence both of them have been included in the Diagnostic and Statistical Manual of Mental Disorders, Fifth Edition (DSM-5) as a separate entities.

Many individuals engage in both behaviors. Hence, it is better to put both of them on a continuum line.[11]

Nonsuicidal self-injury and bipolar personality disorder (BPD) are also separate entities and must be differentiated. BPD primarily manifests as extreme irritability, aggressive outbursts, and violent behavior. This is basically a mood or manic disorder.

DIAGNOSTIC CRITERIA

The diagnostic criteria for nonsuicidal self-injury disorder (NSSID) in the DSM-5 (American Psychiatric Association, 2013) include the following:
1. Engagement in NSSI on five or more days in the past year (Criterion A)
2. The expectation that NSSI will solve an interpersonal problem, provide relief from unpleasant thoughts and/or emotions, or induce a positive emotional state (Criterion B)
3. The experience of one or more of the following: (a) Interpersonal problems or negative thoughts or emotions immediately prior to NSSI, (b) preoccupation with NSSI that is difficult to manage, or (c) frequent thoughts about NSSI (Criterion C)
4. The NSSI is not socially sanctioned or restricted to minor self-injurious behaviors (Criterion D)
5. The presence of NSSI-related clinically significant distress or interference across different domains of functioning (e.g., work, relationships; Criterion E)
6. The NSSI does not occur only in the context of psychosis, delirium, or substance use/withdrawal and is not better accounted for by another psychiatric disorder or medical condition (Criterion F).

TABLE 1: Differences between suicide and nonsuicidal self-injury (NSSI).

	Suicide	*NSSI*
Prevalence	Less common than NSSI	More common than suicide
Intent	To end life	No intention to die (nonlethal) but done for diversion of negative thoughts
Modus operandi	Hanging, drowning, gunshot injuries, etc.	Cutting, self-burning, drug overdose, etc.
Repeat attempts	Usually employ same method to get the desired goal	Usually change the method to self-inflict
Suicidal ideation	Present	Usually absent
Precipitating disorder (e.g., psychiatric disorders)	Moderate to severe	Mild
Cognition and affect	Hopelessness and helplessness predominate even if the attempt fail	Usually relieved of negative effect
Inter-relationship	Does not increases incidence of NSSI	Increases suicidal rates
Biological cause	• Serotonergic and dopaminergic dysfunction • Immature prefrontal cortex, especially in adolescents	Endogenous opioid system is said to be involved

OUTCOME OF NONSUICIDAL SELF-INJURY

Many patients are reported to feel better but nearly 15–20% repeat within 1 year and nearly 25% repeat within 4 years.[10,11] Repeated attacks are associated with enhancement of suicidal tendencies. NSSI is one of the strongest predictors of suicide attempts, above and beyond previous suicidal behavior. Usually, the person does not share this with others and tries to hide scar, etc. but many behave just in opposite way and even publicize it on social media.

Factors which indicate recurrence: Following factors, if present, are indicative of high incidence of recurrence:
- Planned attacks
- Attacks undertaken with precaution that it remains hidden or undiscovered
- Patient does not seek help.
- Writing a suicidal type of note
- Patient undertaking the act fully knowing that it is dangerous.
- Communicating intent to others.

MANAGEMENT

Management of a case of NSSI must be done by a team consisting of family persons, social workers, pediatricians, and psychologists/psychiatrists.
- First of all a detailed history must be taken and the cause behind must be pinpointed.
- Patients must be assured of confidentiality.
- Underlying cause (e.g., depression, alcoholism, etc.) must be treated.
- All these patients must be closely monitored for a long period.
- Support group consisting of family, friends, and nongovernmental organization (NGOs) must be made available to him/her.
- He/she must be encouraged to express emotions and values of hope must be affirmed.
- Medications have a little role; however, antipsychotic agents such as risperidone or olanzapine have been tried in low doses. Mood elevators have also been used.

General Advice for Families[12]
- Parents must keep an eye on social media used by their wards and also they must monitor their peers. They must communicate in a healthy way with their child and try to address their issues.
- Parents must talk to their children about use of drugs, alcohol, etc. and they must warn them about their ill effects.
  - No firearms in home
  - Limit access to medication including over-the-counter medicines
  - Remove access to parent's medications
  - Remove sharp objects such as razors from bathroom
  - Increase supervision (e.g., keep doors open)
  - Advise them to seek help if suicidal thoughts develop or worsen.

SUICIDE IN ADOLESCENCE

INTRODUCTION

Suicide is the act of intentionally causing one's own death. The act is initiated and performed with the knowledge/expectation of its fatal outcome. In majority of cases, it is well planned with precautions taken against discovery and is preceded by a stressful precipitating event. Usually, the person gives sufficient hints to his friends/relatives about his/her intent.[11] The act is committed mostly out of despair/frustration.[13] The Government of India classifies a death as suicide if it meets the following three criteria:[14]
1. It is an unnatural death.
2. The intent to die originated within the person
3. There is a reason for the person to end his/her own life. The reason may have been specified in the suicide note or unspecified.

Though suicide is a serious issue affecting all age groups, but teenagers and young adults have the highest rates of suicide compared to other ages.[15] However, completed suicide is rare below 12 years of age. Suicide in adolescence is a major issue because death of a teen leads to an enormous toll due to significant years of potential life lost.[16] Every suicide is a tragedy affecting families, communities vis-à-vis the entire country and has long-lasting effects on the people left behind.[17] The issue becomes more grave as many suicidal deaths (especially young age suicidal deaths) can be prevented by timely intervention. There is an urgent need to educate not only the affected group but also their caretakers (parents as well as school/college authorities), social as well as political leaders and rather all those who come in their contact.

INCIDENCE

Suicidal deaths are global. The world witnesses >800,000 suicidal deaths every year or one suicidal death every 40 seconds. Social stigma, accompanying legal consequences and the fact that many suicidal deaths are labeled as accidental deaths contributes to underreporting. The reported figures also do not include failed suicidal attempts or cases who have suicidal thoughts/ideation.[18] Suicide rates are higher in persons involved in NSSI.

It is one of the leading causes of death among 15–29 years old.[18] Youth suicidal ideation, attempt, and completion are on rise.[15,16,19]

Across the globe suicide is more common in male than in females (ratio could be 2:1 or more). Success rate is higher in males whereas attempt rate is higher in females.

Adolescence Suicide Versus Old Age Suicide

Adolescence period is best defined as transition from dependence to independence. It is associated with biological, cognitive, psychological, sexual, and social development. Adolescents or young adults are more vulnerable to suicides as developmentally, their judgment and decision-making abilities are still not mature as the prefrontal cortex—the brain's executive control center—does not fully develop until one's mid-20s. This makes adolescents more emotional as well as impulsive. This can also explain their high susceptibility to peer pressure. Thus, they cannot weigh risks and consequences or values in quite the same way that their older counterparts will. In contrast to married persons who many a times are in a better position to handle the crisis as they can expect support from each other and they also get a proper second opinion, the young adults/students are mostly single and hence, many a times they fail to handle the crisis situation and resort to ulterior path.[15]

Among the adolescents and young adult suicidal deaths, a high proportion is of student suicide which is fast increasing. This situation must alert the sociologists, politicians, academicians, etc.

CAUSES OF SUICIDE

In India (all age groups), following were the causes of suicide in the year 2021:[20]
- Family problems (33.2%)
- Illness (18.6%)
- Drug abuse/alcoholic addiction (6.4%). Suicide by drug overdose is fast increasing.
- Marriage-related issues (4.8%)
- Love affairs (4.6%)
- Bankruptcy or indebtedness (3.9%)
- Unemployment (2.2%)
- Professional/career problem (1.6%)
- Death of dear person (1.2%)
- Poverty (1.1%)
- Property dispute (1.1%)
- Failure in examination (1.0%)
- Fall in social reputation (0.5%)
- Suspected/illicit relationships (0.4%)
- Impotency/infertility (0.2%)
- Causes not known (9.7%)
- Other causes (9.2%).

PRECIPITATING FACTORS

- Prior attempts of suicide/NSSI
- Family history of suicide
- Suicide of close friend/love interest
- Suicide rates are always higher in persons with psychiatric comorbidity (depression, anxiety, post-traumatic stress disorder, schizophrenia, bipolar disorders, conduct disorders, and personality disorders). Depression is most common entity among this group.
- *Poor harmony:* Young adults especially those who are aggressive and defy family norms often feel less supported by family and friends. Rather, sometimes less familial support is cause of aggressiveness. This makes them hopeless and blunts their positive coping/problem-solving skills. Bullying in educational institutions/workplace or otherwise always adds fuel to fire. Bullied teens and socially challenged teens have twice the suicide rate than their counterparts.
- *Substance use/abuse:* Influence of alcohol/drugs increases suicide rate by at least three times in females and 17 times in males. They tend to increase underlying problems while providing initial relief (masking effect). Besides they make the person more impulsive and increase their risk-taking behaviors. They also increase the feeling of guilt and self-loathing, compound existing problems, and interferes neurologically with healthy decision making and problem saving. They also increase the habit of feeling sorry for themselves and create a sneaky and secretive culture.
- Gay and bisexual male adolescents have higher rate of suicide than their heterosexual counterparts since they

are associated with high rates of parental rejection, peer rejection, social stigma, and victimization.
- Low self-concept, low self-esteem, low social self-concept, and poor social skills.[21,22] These causes are more common in female adolescents as they feel isolated or rejected.
- *Internet/mass media:* Their role is increasing day by day. The person gets information on how to commit suicide, from where to get drugs/poison, etc.
- Certain video/computer games (gaming addiction) and programs on TV showing suicide also increase the suicidal rates. Some websites are loaded with self-harm or suicide concept. False stories can also lead to depression and anxiety. Sometimes young person's imitate highly publicized suicides (Werther syndrome).
- Loss of a parent to death or divorce
- Physical and sexual abuse
- Lack of a support network
- Feeling of social isolation, inferiority or rejection, and unemployment
- Chronic diseases, e.g., malignancy, acquired immunodeficiency syndrome (AIDS)
- *Biological factors:* Suicidal tendencies have been linked to decreased activity of 5-hydroxytryptamine (5-HT) pathways in brain.
- Availability of firearms in house or easy access to them
- Incarceration
- Sibling rivalry.

Means Adopted for Committing Suicide[20-23]

As depicted in **Table 2** hanging and poisoning are by far the most common means adopted for suicide in our country.

High Risk Occupational Groups

Doctors: Doctors especially female doctors have been observed to have a higher rate of suicide than in general population.[11] This could be because of easy availability of drugs, addiction to alcohol/drugs, stressful work, and reluctance to undertake treatment for depression, etc.

Farmers: Increased suicidal rate in this group is said to be due to easy availability of poison and firearms, stressful work, and financial constraints.

Suicide Pacts

In suicide pacts, two or more people, usually having a close relationship, agree to commit the act simultaneously.

TABLE 2: Means adopted for committing suicide in India (2020–21).

Means/mode adopted	%cases in 2021
By hanging	57.0
By poison	25.1
Drowning	5.1
Fire/self-immolation	2.6
By coming under running vehicles/trains, etc.	2.4
By jumping	1.1
Consuming sleeping pills	0.4
By touching electric wire	0.4
By self-inflicting injuries	0.3
Firearms	0.2
By other means	5.3

PREVENTION

Unfortunately, suicide prevention is too often a low priority for governments and policy-makers. Suicide prevention needs to be prioritized on the global public health and public policy agendas. The Mental Health Action Plan adopted by WHO (2013) includes suicide prevention as a priority and fixed a target of reducing suicide rate by 10% by 2020. Suicide prevention is also included in the Sustainable Development Goals for 2030.

It is duty of Government, Society, and all those who are in touch with the teen to make available to him/her professional/psychological help. He/she must be assured that there are many well-wishers and they must be told that there is solution to every issue.

To prevent adolescent suicides, a multidimensional approach must be made and all concerned must feel their responsibility and act as suggested here:
- *Knowing the signs:*[24] Roughly 80% suicidal deaths are preceded by warning signals. Following points, if observed, must alert the observer:
  • Depressed mood, extreme anxiety, or changes in personality
  • Increase in drug/alcohol use, prescription medicine abuse
  • Feeling of being a burden, disappointment, or "not measuring up"
  • Wanting to die or kill him/herself
  • Increase in mental health symptoms, medications/therapy "not working"

- Acting angry, agitated, and anxious (conflicted psyche)
- Isolating from friends, quitting activities, giving things of value away
- Sleeping too little or too much
- Goodbye or "last time" conversation with friends or families
- Significant behavioral change, friends, and dark interests
- Preoccupation with firearms
- Helpless, hopeless, or avoidants
- Withdrawal from family/peers
- Loss of interest in previously pleasurable activities
- Difficulty in concentration
- Neglect of personal appearance
- Change in eating patterns—either too little or too much
- Talking about or making plans for suicide

- *Making it more difficult to die in an act of deliberate self-harm:* Interventions include building barriers on bridges, removing guns or firearms from homes, and reducing the medication load available and making drug availability difficult.
- *Improving access to mental health resources:* Wide publicity to online websites/phone numbers that provides suggestions/motivation or counseling services, especially when one is in distress. The Suicide Prevention India Foundation maintains a list of telephone numbers they can call to speak in confidence. iCALL, a counseling service run by TISS, has maintained a crowd sourced list of therapists across the country. You could also take them to the nearest hospital. Social media must be used as a weapon to distract the youth from taking extreme steps and help centers must be given a wide publicity. Government should open psychological counseling centers at multiple sites, especially near coaching centers, etc.
- *Religion:* Religion sometimes can infuse hope and confidence in some cases. Leaving the problem to almighty GOD can be game-changer in some cases.[25]
- *Role of teachers:* Teachers have a very big role to play. They must be trained to detect students who might be at risk for suicide. They can note change in behavior or mood and change in class attendance. They should be alert if a student who was otherwise active suddenly dissociates from the group.[26] They must interact with students in positive ways and help them to engage with peers and other adults in the school community during the school/college day and extracurricular activities. Connectedness is an important factor in improving academic achievement and healthy behaviors, and it is related to reductions in suicidal thoughts and attempts.[27] Teachers should see that these children are not left alone and they must seek appointment with the counselors. Every school/college must have a crisis team.
- *Role of parents/families:* The typical Indian families are not as supportive as they appear to be. Parents in fact at times behave as a dictator and force the goals on their wards. Family pressure is a common cause of student suicide. Parents must play a supportive role. They must keep talking to their children regularly (especially fathers). If possible have a video talk so that you can read their faces. Do not jump on their failures. Never compare them with peers. Talk to them on nonacademic issues too. See that they consider you friends and not dictator. Ask them to pursue their goals of their own choice. Make an environment in which he/she can share with you his/her failures, choices.
- *Role of friends:* Friends are many times in a important position to detect presuicidal states. Any change in behavior/mood, etc. must alert them. In such cases, they must inform appropriate authorities and take precautionary actions. They must motivate their friend in trouble. They must never keep it a secret.
- *Role of policymakers:* Policymakers must frame the policies so that the students do not feel the exploitation, gender differences, caste inequalities, unemployment, and peer pressure. Menace of coaching classes and the pressure that they create over the students must also be taken care of. Course curriculum should be less theoretical and more practical and job oriented.
- *Role of community:* In India, the phenomenon of suicide is constantly individualized or personalized, allowing society to escape accountability. Communities can play a crucial role in suicide prevention.[19] They must not take it as a problem of a particular family. They must keep a watch over the teenagers and must always be helpful to them. They must never make a joke of their failures, etc. on community platforms.
- *Role of NGOs:* They also can play a vital role. They can constitute teen clubs and provide psychological help services. They can also take lead to educate people about the ill effects of social media. They must publicize centers which can help the youth in crisis.

- *Role of drugs:* Lithium prophylaxis and clozapine have been used to reduce suicidal rates especially in patients with schizophrenia.
- *Role of media:* Visual media must be made more responsible in reporting or displaying suicides.
- *Socioeconomic factors:* Social policies to provide better employment as well-adopting policies not to isolate anybody from society could be very helpful.

TREATMENT

- Treat underlying psychiatric disorder
- Person must be kept under supervision of a multidisciplinary team consisting of pediatricians/physicians, sociologists, psychiatrists, etc.

CONCLUSION[27]

The increasing rate of adolescent's suicide (student suicide in particular) must awake all concerned. We must recognize it as a grave crisis. The fact that over 82% who fail expressed remorse and regret for attempting suicide show failure of the system and warrant urgent proper action.

REFERENCES

1. Klonsky ED, Victor SE, Saffer BY. Nonsuicidal self-injury: what we know, and what we need to know. Can J Psychiatry. 2014;59(11):565-8.
2. Gratz KL, Dixon-Gordon KL, Chapman AL, Tull MT. Diagnosis and Characterization of DSM-5 Nonsuicidal Self-Injury Disorder using the Clinician-Administered Nonsuicidal Self-Injury Disorder Index. Assessment. 2015;22(5):527-39.
3. Yang SY, Lee D, Jeong H, Cho Y, Ahn JE, Hong KS, et al. Comparison of patterns of non-suicidal self-injury and emotion dysregulation across mood disorder subtypes. front psychiatry. 2022;13:757933.
4. Moseley LR, Sinclair-McBride K, DeMaso DR, Walter HJ. Self-injurious behavior. In: Kliegman RM, III JWSG, Blum NJ, Shah SS, Tasker RC, Wilson KM, et al. (Eds). Nelson Textbook of Pediatrics, 21st edition. Canada: Elsevier Inc.; 2020, pp. 243-4.
5. Prasad M. (2022). Non-suicidal self-Injury. [online] Available from: https://www.slideshare.net/ColMukteshwarPrasad/non-suicidal-selfinjurynssipptx [Last accessed October, 2023].
6. Stanley B, Sher L, Wilson S, Ekman R, Huang YY, Mann JJ. Non-suicidal self-injurious behavior, endogenous opioids and monoamine neurotransmitters. J Affect Disord. 2010;124(1-2):134-40.
7. Burke TA, Ammerman BA, Hamilton JL, Alloy LB. Impact of Non-Suicidal Self-Injury Scale: Initial Psychometric Validation. Cognit Ther Res. 2017;41(1):130-42.
8. Boland RJ, Verduin ML, Ruiz P (Eds). Kaplan and Sadock's Synopsis of Psychiatry, 12th edition. Philadelphia, PA: Wolters Kluwer; 2022. p. 333.
9. Slideshare. (2013). Non-suicidal self-injury. [online] Available from: https://www.slideshare.net/sagedayschool/non-suicidal-selfinjury-webinar-slides-27334035 [Last accessed October, 2023].
10. Harrison P, Cowen P, Burns T, Fazel M. Suicide and deliberate self-harm. In: Harrison P, Cowen P, Burns T, Fazel M (Eds). Shorter Oxford Textbook of Psychiatry, 7th edition. United Kingdom: Oxford University Press; 2022. pp. 609-30.
11. Masi G, Lupetti I, D'Acunto G, Milone A, Fabiani D, Madonia U, et al. A comparison between severe suicidality and nonsuicidal self-injury behaviors in bipolar adolescents referred to a psychiatric emergency unit. Brain Sci. 2021;11(6):790.
12. Brown RC, Plener PL. Non-suicidal self-injury in adolescence. Curr Psychiatry Rep. 2017;19(3):20.
13. Slideshare. (2012). Adolescent suicide. [online] Available from: https://www.slideshare.net/ranjanir123/adolescent-suicide [Last accessed October, 2023].
14. Kumari P, Masih P. Suicide in adolescence: a review of the literature. IAHRW Int J Soc Sci Rev. 2019;7(2):269-72.
15. Cohen S. (2022). Suicide rates among young people continue to rise, but there are ways to help. [online] Available from: https://connect.uclahealth.org/2022/03/15/suicide-rate-highest-among-teens-and-young-adults/ [Last accessed October, 2023].
16. Americashealthranking's. (2019). Teen suicide in United States. [online] Available from: https://www.americashealthrankings.org/explore/health-of-women-and-children/measure/teen_suicide [Last accessed October, 2023].
17. World Health Organization. (2023). Suicide. [online] Available from: https://www.who.int/news-room/fact-sheets/detail/suicide [Last accessed October, 2023].
18. Dattani S, Rodés-Guirao L, Ritchie H, Roser M, Ortiz-Ospina E. (2023). Suicide. [online] Available from https://ourworldindata.org/suicide#:~:text=Globally%2C%20close%20to%20800%2C000%20people,being%20classified%20as%20unintentional%20injuries [Last accessed October, 2023].
19. World Health Organization. (2018). Suicide prevention: the role of communities. [online] Available from: https://apps.who.int/iris/bitstream/handle/10665/272860/9789241513791-eng.pdf?sequence=1&isAllowed=y [Last accessed October, 2023].
20. Scroll.in. (2022). Deaths by suicide highest ever in India in 2021, domestic problems biggest reason, shows NCRB data. [online] https://scroll.in/latest/1031595/deaths-by-suicide-highest-ever-in-india-in-2021-ncrb-data-shows [Last accessed October, 2023].
21. Ncrb.gov. (2020). Academic Distress' and Student Suicides in India: A Crisis That Needs to be Acknowledged. [online] Available from: https://thewire.in/rights/

academic-distress-and-student-suicides-in-india [Last accessed October, 2023].

22. Suicide in India. [online] Available from: https://ncrb.gov.in/accidental-deaths-suicides-in-india-adsi.html.

23. Medbroadcast. Adolescent suicide. [online] Available from: https://medbroadcast.com/condition/getcondition/adolescent-suicide [Last accessed October, 2023].

24. Wasserman D. (2021). Oxford Textbook of Suicidology and Suicide Prevention. [online] Available from: https://academic.oup.com/book/31744 [Last accessed October, 2023].

25. Nadeem E, Kataoka SH, Chang VY, Vona P, Wong M, Stein BD. The role of teachers in school-based suicide prevention: a qualitative study of school staff perspectives. School Ment Health. 2011;3(4):209-21.

26. Suicide Prevention Resource Center. (2019). Preventing Suicide. Role of High School Teachers. [online] Available from: https://sprc.org/sites/default/files/resource-program/Role%20of%20High%20School%20Teachers%209_22.pdf [Last accessed October, 2023].

27. Runcan R. (2020). Suicide in Adolescence: A Review of Literature. [online] Available from: https://www.researchgate.net/profile/Remus-Runcan/publication/343125743_Suicide_in_Adolescence_A_Review_of_Literature/links/5f32b7d6458515b7291693c6/Suicide-in-Adolescence-A-Review-of-Literature.pdf [Last accessed October, 2023].

Obsessive-Compulsive Disorder

Sanjay Gehlot, Indraja Sharma

INTRODUCTION

It has long been assumed and observed that people can have obsessions and compulsions whether or not they have obsessive-compulsive disorder (OCD). This has had a significant impact on human history and religion, with some referring to it as "religious scrupulosity". Morality-focused scrupulosity was recognized as a symptom of obsessive-compulsive personality disorder in the Diagnostic and Statistical Manual of Mental Disorders, Fourth Edition, Text Revision (DSM-IV-TR) published by the American Psychiatric Association. Obsessive-compulsive traits and disorders in children and adolescents have received more medical attention in the 20th and 21st centuries, with a focus on epidemiology, etiology, diagnosis, differential diagnosis, comorbidities, and management. The purpose of this discussion is to examine how pediatric OCD is currently understood.[1]

EPIDEMIOLOGY

According to studies done over the past few decades, OCD affects anywhere between 1 and 4% of people worldwide including kids, teenagers, and adults. About 4 out of 10 OCD sufferers experience this condition as a chronic one, which can have a significant negative impact on their lives. OCD is also frequently kept a secret from others by its sufferers. OCD has been ranked among the top 10 most incapacitating disorders by the World Health Organization (WHO). OCD can begin in childhood, and about 8 in 10 people experience it before turning 18 years of age. Based on the conditions' underlying causes, researchers are attempting to categorize OCD into various subtypes. For instance, early onset OCD, a subtype of OCD in children, is connected to a neurodevelopmental viewpoint.[1]

ETIOLOGY

Research reveals a variety of underlying etiologic factors in the development of OCD in humans of various ages. These include interconnecting issues based on:

- *Behavioral etiology:* Various psychological and neuropsychological models of etiology describe a complex process in which the OCD person learns or is driven to determine what are perceived as errors in their thinking patterns in order to cope with deep-seated anxiety. People with OCD often pinpoint what they believe to be flaws in their thought processes as a way to manage their intense anxiety. Particularly in light of recent advances for studying the central nervous system, the effects of overly protective parenting styles with strict rules, a conviction that one actions are never acceptable to others, and other adverse childhood experiences are still up for debate.[1]
- *Neurological causes:* Neurological dysfunctions can result from changes in the cortico-striato-thalamo-cortical circuits and white matter of the brain, which have been identified by brain scans, such as magnetic resonance imaging (MRI), functional magnetic resonance imaging (fMRI), whole-brain voxel-based morphometry (VBM), and diffusion tensor imaging (DTI). The frontal-striatal-thalamic model of neurological dysfunction has been the focus of this research, which has demonstrated that it can lead to a variety of problems including frontoparietal-limbic dysfunction, orbitofrontal dysfunction, decreased brain volume, basal ganglia dysfunction, and error-related brain activity. Additional research has discovered changes in the serotonergic-dopaminergic, glutamatergic, and hippocampus.[1]
- *Immunological etiology:* According to research connecting this condition with proinflammatory

cytokines, such as tumor necrosis factor α (TNF-α), interleukin 12 (IL-12), and immunological mechanisms are postulated to be involved in pediatric OCD. When proinflammatory cytokines are measured, it is possible to observe inflammatory damage to monocytes in OCD patients that is altered by the effects of OCD medication.[1]

- *Pediatric autoimmune neuropsychiatric disorders associated with streptococcal infections/pediatric acute-onset neuropsychiatric syndrome (PANDAS/PANS):* There are intriguing relationships between childhood OCD and immune-infectious factors including the relationship between OCD symptoms (1–10%) and the hypothesized PANDAS with positive antistreptolysin O and antideoxyribonuclease B (anti-DNase B) antibody levels, as well as PANS.[1]
- *The etiology of the gastrointestinal (GI) microbiome:* The presence of different GI microbes, as influenced by different internal and external factors (stressors), can cause or influence conditions, such as depression, OCD, PANS, PANDAS, and others. Group A β-hemolytic *Streptococcus* and Bacteroidetes (i.e., *Bacteroides*, *Odoribacter*, and *Oscillospira*) are among the bacteria being researched.[1]
- *Genetic etiology:* First-degree relatives of an OCD sufferer are twice as likely to also have the condition. If the OCD started when the person was a child, this likelihood increases by 10 times. Dizygotic twins have a concordance rate of 0.22, compared to monozygotic twins' 0.57. The *SLC6A4* gene [which affects serotonin transport and can influence OCD transmission through both genetic and epigenetic effects including deoxyribonucleic acid (DNA) methylation] as well as other serotonin system genes, such as *HTR2A*, *HTR1B*, and *HTR2C*, are some of the genes for OCD that are currently being studied. Research is also being done on the serotonin transporter polymorphism 5-HTTLPR and the HTR2A polymorphism rs6311 (or rs6313).[1]

Establishing Diagnosis: DSM-5 Diagnostic Criteria[2]

- Obsessions, compulsions, or both present:
  (1) and (2) define an obsession:
  1. Persistent and recurrent thoughts, urges, or images that most people experience as intrusive and unwanted at some point during the disturbance cause pronounced anger or distress.
  2. The person makes an effort to block out or suppress these urges, thoughts, or images, or to neutralize them with another thought or behavior (e.g., by engaging in a compulsion).

  (1) and (2) define compulsions:
  1. Repetitive actions that an individual feels compelled to carry out as a result of an obsession or in accordance with rules that must be followed strictly, such as handwashing, ordering, checking, or silently repeating words.
  2. The behavior or mental acts are intended to prevent or lessen anxiety or distress, or to avoid some terrifying event or circumstance; however, these behavior or mental acts are either obviously excessive or not connected in a realistic way to what they are intended to neutralize or prevent.

Note: Young children might not be able to express the purposes behind these actions or behaviors.

- The obsessions or compulsions take up a lot of time (for example, more than an hour a day), or they significantly impair social, occupational, or other important areas of functioning or cause clinically significant distress.
- The physiological effects of a substance (such as a drug of abuse, a medication, etc.) or another medical condition cannot be blamed for the obsessive-compulsive symptoms.
- The symptoms of another mental disorder, such as excessive worrying as in generalized anxiety disorder, obsession with appearance like in body dysmorphic disorder, difficulty in getting rid of or parting with possessions like in hoarding disorder, hair pulling like in trichotillomania (hair-pulling disorder), skin picking like in excoriation disorder (skin-picking disorder), stereotypies like in stereotypic movement disorder, or ritualized behavior like in ritualistic eating disorder, do not better explain the disturbance. Impulses, like those seen in conduct, disruptive, and impulse-control disorders; guilt-inducing thoughts, like those seen in major depressive disorder; thought insertion or delusional preoccupations, like those seen in schizophrenia spectrum and other psychotic disorders; or repetitive patterns of behavior, like those seen in autism spectrum disorder.
- *Specify if:* With good or fair insight.
- *Specify if:* Tic related.

Establishing Diagnosis: International Classification of Diseases 11th Revision (ICD-11) Diagnostic Criteria[3]

- The existence of enduring obsessions or compulsions
- Obsessions are unwelcome, intrusive thoughts (such as those about contamination), images (such as those of violent scenes), or impulses/urges (such as the desire to stab someone). They are frequently linked to anxiety. The person typically makes an effort to ignore, suppress, or neutralize obsessions by engaging in compulsions.
- Compulsions are repetitive behaviors or rituals, including repetitive mental acts, that a person feels compelled to carry out as a result of an obsession, in accordance with strict guidelines, or in order to feel "complete". The repetitive washing, checking, and ordering of objects are a few examples of overt behaviors. Analogous mental acts include reviewing a memory to ensure that one has not done any harm, mentally counting objects, and mentally repeating certain phrases to prevent negative outcomes. Compulsions are either not realistically connected to the feared event (such as symmetrically arranging objects to prevent harm to a loved one) or are obviously excessive (such as spending hours in the shower every day to avoid illness).
- Compulsions and obsessions take up a lot of time (e.g., more than an hour a day), cause a lot of distress, or significantly impair functioning in key areas, such as personal, family, social, educational, or occupational functioning. Only after putting in a lot more work is functioning maintained.
- Neither the symptoms nor the behaviors are a sign of another illness (such as basal ganglia ischemic stroke) nor are they brought on by a substance's or medication's effects on the central nervous system (such as amphetamine) including withdrawal symptoms.

CLINICAL FEATURES: OBSESSIONS AND COMPULSIONS[4]

Obsessive-compulsive disorders clinical symptoms are strikingly universal across ethnic groups and geographical regions. Through factor-analytical studies, common obsessions, compulsions, and symptom dimensions have been identified as:

Obsessions

Contamination-related Obsessions

- Anxiety or disgust with bodily excretions including stools and urine
- Aversion to grime, germs, or infections; worry about sticky materials
- Fear of contracting an illness as a result of contaminants (like AIDS).

Sexual Obsessions

- Thoughts, urges, or images that are inappropriately sexual about friends, family members, or strangers.
- Sexual ideas such as abusing children and sexual identity questions such as "am I gay"?

Harm/Aggression-related Obsessions

- Fear may cause one to harm oneself or others (e.g., the fear of hurting babies, stabbing a friend, or accidentally running over pedestrians while driving).
- Violent or gruesome pictures (accidents, mutilated bodies, and murders)
- Fear of using vulgar language.

Religious/Blasphemy

- Sacrifice and blasphemy (blasphemous thoughts and the reluctance to speak negatively about God)
- Excessive concern for morality and right and wrong.

Pathological Doubts about Daily Activities

Doubts of having not locked doors, or turned off gas knobs.

Need for Symmetry and Exactness

- Anxiety about something not being perfectly straight, symmetrical, accurate, or aligned
- With magical thinking (if the kitchen is not organized properly, the child could have an accident).

Miscellaneous

- Must know or remember number plates, advertisements, etc.
- Alarming nonviolent ideas and images
- Fear of superstitions (such as passing a cat or cemetery)
- Unlucky or lucky numbers and colors.

Compulsions

Cleaning and Washing

In response to contamination obsessions (excessive or ritualized handwashing, showering, bathing, brushing/excessive cleaning of home furnishings, floors, kitchenware, etc.).

Checking
- In response to pathological doubts (appliances, locks, stove, and doors)
- To avoid hurting oneself or others (verify that you were not at fault for the accident, look for injuries, etc.).

Repeating
- Writing or reading something again because you did not understand it or write it well.
- Repeating routine activities (going in and out of the doorway, sitting and standing up repeatedly, repeating till you feel just right).

Counting, e.g., money, or floor tiles.
Ordering and arranging (often until you find the perfect arrangement).

Miscellaneous
- Mental practices (prayer, perception good thoughts instead of negative ones)
- Superstitious practices
- Need to confess, tell, or ask.

Symptom Dimensions
- Fears of contamination and cleaning/washing
- Prohibited thoughts (violence, sexual, religious, and somatic obsessions) as well as compulsive checking
- Fears of contamination and cleaning/washing
- Symmetry (obsessions with symmetry and compulsions to repeat, order, and count)
- Hoarding (obsessions and compulsions with hoarding).

ASSESSMENT

Instead of the child's chronological age, the presentation of obsessive-compulsive (OC) symptoms may depend on the child's cognitive development. Some children may show symptoms as early as 2 years old. However, it is more common for symptoms to start between the ages of 6 years and preadolescence, as this is when they start to develop the maturity to carry out compulsions. Compared to rituals and compulsions at this age, pure obsessions are uncommon. Obsessions and compulsions may start to show up together as children get older, between the ages of 6 years and adolescence.[5]

The idea of "getting it just right" frequently arises in rituals. About one-third of pediatric patients have symptoms that are brought on by environmental factors. Additionally, a phenomenon known as a "sensory phenomenon" that resembles tics and frequently occurs in cases of preadolescent onset is reported. This phenomenon involves unpleasant or distressing sensations, perceptions, feelings, or urges that precede or accompany repetitive behaviors. Children may feel compelled to repeat compulsions until they are satisfied or the sensation goes away. These sensations can be either mental or physical. This may result in more distress from compulsions brought on by the sensory phenomenon.[5]

According to studies conducted in India, compulsions are more common in children and adolescents than obsessions. According to data from India, the most prevalent obsessions and compulsions among individuals 16 years of age or younger are obsessions with contamination (62%), aggression (57%), symmetry (34%), sex (22%), religion (22%), somatic (12%), and hoarding (7%). The most prevalent compulsions in terms of frequency are cleaning and washing (69%) and are followed by repeating (52%), checking (47%), ordering (29%), counting (15%), and hoarding (7%). The prevalence of various obsessions and compulsions is 65 and 47%, respectively, in the patients. Additionally, data from India suggests that cases with childhood onset have more severe symptoms than cases with adult onset. In India, children are less likely to experience aggressive and sexual obsessions than in the West.[5] **Table 1** lists the key points that need to be clarified during the assessment.[6]

Screening

If a child or adolescent presents with symptoms of disorders that are commonly comorbid with OCD, it may be necessary to suspect OCD. If the initial interview indicates a broad range of pathology, screening tools like the child behavior checklist and Spence Children's Anxiety Scale can be utilized. Specific screening tools, such as the parent/self-version of the Spence Children's Anxiety Scale and/or the short OCD screener, can be used if there are signs of OCD. Positive screening outcomes should trigger a more thorough evaluation of the child.[5]

History Taking

From the antenatal period up until the time of the clinical visit, a thorough history from a developmental perspective should be obtained (**Box 1**).[5]

Developmental and Medical Assessment

It is important to consider developmental perspectives and assess every aspect of a child's development and

Obsessive-Compulsive Disorder

TABLE 1: Issues that need to be clarified during assessment and before treatment.

Age of onset	Age when symptoms were first noticed by the patient or family
Degree of suffering, impairment and time consumed performing rituals	Important to distinguish OCD from transient obsessive or compulsive behaviors seen in the course of normal development
Insight	Poor insight is common in pediatric patients
Presence of sensory phenomena	Mental or physical premonitory urges often occur instead of obsessions
Family attitude toward the illness	Excessive criticism or high levels of accommodation of symptoms are associated with poorer outcome
Are there comorbid disorders?	Evaluate for the presence of comorbid conditions (e.g., anxiety disorders, mood disorders, tic disorders, ADHD, alcohol, and other substance use disorders)
History of psychiatric disorder in the family	Are family members affected with OCD or other psychiatric disorders?

(ADHD: attention-deficit hyperactivity disorder; OCD: obsessive-compulsive disorder)

BOX 1: Components of assessment of children and adolescents presenting with obsessive-compulsive symptoms.

- Detailed history taking
- Routine screening of a child with brief questioning from parents/child
- Use of screening instruments if there are initial hints of presence of obsessive-compulsive (OC) symptoms
- Detailed assessment of those found positive on initial screening
- Early developmental assessment from antenatal, perinatal, and postnatal period followed by medical history, examination, and organic factors such as streptococcal infections should be assessed
- A detailed assessment of child's symptoms with their form, content, severity, resistance offered, insight, role of environmental triggers, family involvement in rituals and their understanding of illness along with time spent and distress should be assessed
- Help of various scales and play observation/behavioral experiments must be taken
- Establish the diagnosis as per the prevailing diagnostic criteria
- Assess for suicidal behavior, substance use, child abuse/neglect, and comorbidities
- Detailed assessment of family environment, resources, and family accommodation
- Dysfunction in terms of impact of the symptoms on the educational attainment/performance, regularity in school/school refusal/inability to go to school
- Expectations of the family members from the treatment
- Relevant physical, biochemical, neuropsychological, neuroimaging testing, and immunological should be done as per the need of the case

medical history starting from the antenatal, perinatal, and postnatal periods. The presence of maternal infections, poor health, challenging labor, and hypoxic-ischemic injury must be thoroughly investigated. Additionally, it is crucial to evaluate a child's social, speech, language, fine motor, and gross motor development chronologically. Soft neurological signs found during physical examination require a reassessment of developmental history. In rare cases, symptoms may suddenly appear, with a rapid change in behavior and mood, and the sudden onset of severe anxiety. In such cases, a subtype of pediatric OCD caused by an infection (e.g., streptococcal throat) may be the culprit, which confuses the child's immune system into attacking the brain instead of the infection. Although neuroimaging may be taken into consideration in children and adolescents who present with atypical development, head injury, or other comorbidities, no imaging study is currently advised for the diagnosis of OCD.[5]

Family Evaluation

The child's OCD can be affected by how family members react, which in turn can impact the course of the disorder as well as its treatment and outcome. In some cases, family members may need to participate in rituals or provide reassurance to the child, and they may not always be aware of the illness or the best way to respond to it. To better understand how family members can help, it is important to assess each person's role in accommodating the child's OCD and to recognize any triggers that may exacerbate the condition. It is also important to consider the family dynamics and relationships, and to work with parents to develop effective strategies for addressing the child's condition.[5]

Educational Assessment

It is important to investigate the academic and cocurricular performance of children, as a decline in performance could indicate a more severe illness. Preadolescent OCD sufferers frequently also have a history of neurodevelopmental issues such as attention-deficit hyperactivity disorder (ADHD) and/or specific learning disorder (SLD), which can make it more difficult for them to benefit from cognitive-behavioral therapy (CBT). These children may struggle with visual memory, visual organization, and processing speed, which can impact their academic performance. It is recommended that children with prior academic difficulties receive a comprehensive assessment including neuropsychological testing to evaluate their intelligence, working memory, and specific learning problems.[5]

COMORBIDITY

All of the aforementioned evaluations provide cues for a number of disorders that may coexist with childhood OCD **(Box 2)**.[5] The diagnostic exercises that follow help to distinguish the hints from OCD and/or establish them as true comorbidities.

Assessment Scales

Rating scales can aid in obtaining detailed information regarding OCD symptoms, tics, and other aspects relevant to the diagnosis. Scales are also used to assess severity at baseline and to evaluate improvement in a more objective way during follow-up treatment. These questionnaires, only take 15–20 minutes to complete, are informant/parent-rated, trustworthy, valid, and helpful in clinical settings. The scales used to evaluate OCD in children and adolescents are listed in **Table 2**.[6]

DIFFERENTIAL DIAGNOSIS[5]

Distinguishing the OCD diagnosis from other disorders that may be the actual cause of the patient's symptoms rather than OCD is a crucial component of the OCD patient assessment.
- Continuity with normal behavior
- Subclinical compulsive behaviors
- The emergence of obsessive thoughts alongside another Axis I anxiety or depressive disorder
- Obsessive-compulsive spectrum disorders
- Neurodevelopmental disorders

MANAGEMENT

Selective serotonin reuptake inhibitors (SSRIs) and CBT are frequently combined in clinical practice to treat OCD in children and adolescents because there is strong evidence to support their use in this regard **(Table 3)**.

Psychological Management

Cognitive-behavioral therapy is frequently regarded as the main treatment option for kids and teenagers with mild to moderate OCD. When it comes to treating OCD, CBT has produced results that are comparable to or even superior to medication management. The effectiveness of other psychotherapies in treating pediatric OCD is not well established. Psychoeducation, cognitive retraining, and exposure response prevention are all components of CBT for OCD in children, according to studies. The Children's Yale-Brown Obsessive-Compulsive Scale (CY-BOCS) score and functional improvement can both significantly improve after just 5 weeks of treatment. Weekly CBT sessions are just as effective as daily sessions, and the CBT model frequently depends heavily on parental involvement and the positive interaction within the family.

Pharmacotherapy of OCD (Table 4)

Clomipramine was the first medication that showed clinical efficacy in treating pediatric OCD followed shortly by fluoxetine, but subsequent trials have also demonstrated the efficacy of fluvoxamine, sertraline, and paroxetine. However, response rates varied between 40 and 60% along with substantial number of nonresponders. Study design

---

BOX 2: Comorbidities.
- Comorbidity is very common in childhood OCD
- It is present in 60–80% of cases
- In particular, age at onset and chronological age at presentation may predict different comorbidity patterns
- The age of onset being associated with risk of various neurodevelopmental disorders, such as tic disorder/Tourette's syndrome, ADHD, learning disorders, separation anxiety, enuresis, and simple phobias
- Nearly 5% of autism cases have comorbid OCD
- Chronological age at presentation and diagnosis is mostly later than onset, with the emergence of generalized anxiety, panic disorder, substance use, mood (mainly depression), and psychotic disorders as comorbid disorders
- Neurodevelopmental conditions such as ADHD and/or SLD are frequently present in preadolescent OCD patients, which can make it more challenging for them to benefit from CBT
- Data varies from study to study but the highest comorbidity is with tic disorder, ADHD, other anxiety, OC spectrum, and mood disorders in this order reflecting shared development, biological, and genetic factors
- Comorbidity increases the severity of illness
- It has got diagnostic, prognostic, and management implications

(ADHD: attention-deficit hyperactivity disorder; OC: obsessive-compulsive; OCD: obsessive-compulsive disorder; SLD: specific learning disorder)

TABLE 2: Scales used for evaluation of OCD patients.

	CY-BOCS	DY-BOCS	YGTSS	USP-SPS	FAS
Author (Year)	Scahill et al. (1997)	Rosario-Campos et al. (2006)	Leckman et al. (1989)	Rosario et al. (2008)	Calvocoressi et al. (1999)
Aims	Assess presence and severity of obsessions and compulsions	Assess presence and severity of OCD symptom dimensions	Assess presence and severity of tics	Assess presence and severity of sensory phenomena	Assess levels of family accommodation
Administration time	15 minutes (excluding time to go over symptom checklist)	10 minutes for each dimension or 15 minutes for overall severity (excluding time to go over symptom checklist)	20 minutes (excluding time to go over symptom checklist)	20 minutes (excluding time to go over symptom checklist)	20 minutes (excluding time to go over symptom checklist)
Self-report	No	No	No	No	No
Valid and reliable	Yes	Yes	Yes	Yes	Yes
Clinically useful	Yes	Yes	Yes	Yes	Yes
Useful for research	Yes	Yes	Yes	Yes	Yes
Available in languages other than English	Yes	Yes	Yes	Yes	Yes

(CY-BOCS: Children's Yale-Brown Obsessive-Compulsive Scale; DY-BOCS: Dimensional Yale-Brown Obsessive-Compulsive Scale; FAS: Family Accommodation Scale; OCD: obsessive-compulsive disorder; USP-SPS: University of São Paulo Sensory Phenomena Scale; YGTSS: Yale Global Tic Severity Scale)

TABLE 3: Summary of recommendations for treatment of OCD.[6]

Type	Recommended treatment
Mild (CY-BOCS score: 16–19*)	CBT alone (single or group, minimum 10 sessions)
Moderate (CY-BOCS score: 20–29*)	CBT alone or combined with an SSRI (minimum 10-week trail)
Severe (CY-BOCS score: 30–40*)	CBT + SSRI (minimum 10-week trail)
Remission (CY-BOCS total score <10)	• Maintenance CBT (booster sessions for a minimum of 12 months) • Maintenance of SSRI at an optimal dose for a minimum of 12 months
Partial response (35–50% decrease in CY-BOCS score after achieving the optimal tolerated dose of SSRI for a minimum of 10 weeks)	• Switch to another SSRI • Augment with CBT (if not administered already) • Augment with atypical antipsychotic (e.g., risperidone, quetiapine, aripiprazole, or haloperidol) • Augment with clomipramine (ECG monitoring)
Nonresponse (<35% symptom remission)	• Review diagnosis, comorbidities, compliance, and family accommodation • Switch to another SSRI • Augment with CBT (if not administered already) • Augment with atypical antipsychotic (e.g., risperidone, quetiapine, aripiprazole or haloperidol) • Augment with clomipramine (ECG monitoring) • Treatment comorbid disorders concurrently

*March & Mulle (1998) severity criteria.[7]
(CBT: cognitive behavior treatment provided by a competent clinician trained in this form of treatment in sessions lasting at least 60 minutes; CY-BOCS: Children's Yale-Brown Obsessive Compulsive Scale scores, ECG: electrocardiogram; SSRI: selective serotonin reuptake inhibitor)

TABLE 4: Summary of pharmacotherapeutic agents in OCD patients.[6]

Medication	FDA approved for OCD in children	Minimum age (FDA)	Starting dose (mg/day)	Maximum dose (mg/day)
Clomipramine	Yes	5	12.5–25	300
Fluoxetine	Yes	8	2.5–10	80
Sertraline	Yes	6	12.5–25	200
Fluvoxamine	Yes	8	12.5–50	300
Paroxetine	Yes	8	2.5–10	60
Citalopram	No	N/A	2.5–10	60
Escitalopram	No	N/A	2.5–10	30

(FDA: Food and Drug Administration; N/A: not applicable; OCD: obsessive-compulsive disorder)

often excludes children and adolescents with comorbid psychiatric conditions, such as tic disorders, other primary mood disorders, and autism spectrum disorders.[1]

Augmentation Strategies

Even with sufficient treatment attempts, 40% of individuals with OCD experience ongoing symptoms that negatively impact their daily lives. Additional treatment options should be considered if a patient has not improved after two or more trials of SSRIs or clomipramine at the recommended dose and duration along with CBT **(Box 3)**. Newer neuromodulatory approaches, such as repetitive transcranial magnetic stimulation (rTMS) and deep brain stimulation (DBS) are promising but there are currently no randomized controlled trials of these methods among children and adolescents. Novel medications have been tried in children like D-cycloserine (DCS), riluzole, and N-acetyl cysteine (NAC), but none have shown a statistically significant benefit.[1] Most of the children and adolescents can be managed at the outpatient level. However, a few patients may require inpatient care.

BOX 3: Indications for hospitalization in children and adolescents with obsessive-compulsive disorder.[5]

- Client preference
- Needs diagnostic clarification and close observation
- Risk of harm to self and others due to comorbid depression and/or content of obsessive-compulsive disorder (OCD)
- Medical comorbidity requiring diagnostic clarification and management
- Difficulty in delivering treatment on an outpatient basis due to logistic reasons
- Intensive therapy is needed, need for electroconvulsive therapy (ECT) for comorbid disorders

COURSE AND PROGNOSIS

According to a study conducted by Marcia et al. in October 2015, the rate of partial or complete remission in youth with OCD was 0.53, which was significantly higher than that of adults in the same study (0.34). This indicates that youth recover from OCD at a faster rate than adults. About two-thirds of youth experienced sustained remission for an average of 2 years. The study found that the time taken to receive treatment and the extent of functional impairment predicted the course of the disorder. Youth who were less impaired and received early treatment had higher rates of remission. Overall, the study suggests that the prognosis for youth with OCD is better than that of adults. This emphasizes the importance of early recognition and intervention in pediatric OCD.[8,9]

CONCLUSION

Assumptions, obsessions and compulsions are all commonly observed in people, however, they might or not suffer OCD, which is ranked among top 10 most incapacitating disorders. The presentation of obsessive-compulsive (OC) symptoms depend on child's cognitive development rather than chronological age. Rituals and compulsions are common in younger children as compared to pure obsessions. Compulsions and obsessions start to show up together as child gets older. It is a cause of concern when such compulsions and/obsessions cause harm or distress to one self or family/community members. However, answer to these lies in CBT, psychotherapy and pharmacotherapy, alone or in combination. The outcome is much better in young children rather than in adults, thus important point to keep in mind is early recognition of such disorders.

REFERENCES

1. Nazeer A, Latif F, Mondal A, Azeem MW, Greydanus DE. Obsessive-compulsive disorder in children and adolescents: epidemiology, diagnosis and management. Transl Pediatr. 2020;9(Suppl 1):S76-S93.
2. American Psychiatric Association. Diagnostic and Statistical Manual of Mental Disorders, 5th edition. Washington, DC: American Psychiatric Association; 2013.
3. World Health Organization (2019/2021). ICD-11 for Mortality and Morbidity Statistics (ICD-11 MMS). [online] Available from: https://icd.who.int/browse11 [Last accessed October, 2023].
4. Janardhan Reddy YC, Sundar AS, Narayanaswamy JC, Math SB. Clinical practice guidelines for Obsessive-Compulsive Disorder. Indian J Psychiatry. 2017;59(Suppl 1):S74-S90.
5. International OCD Foundation. Diagnosis and Clinical Assessment for Mental Health Professionals. [online] Available from: https://kids.iocdf.org/professionals/mh/clinical-assessment-diagnosis/ [Last accessed October, 2023].
6. Avasthi A, Sharma A, Grover S. Clinical Practice Guidelines for the Management of Obsessive-Compulsive Disorder in Children and Adolescents. Indian J Psychiatry. 2019; 61(Suppl 2):306-16.
7. Narch JS & Mulle K. OCD in Children & Adolescents: a cognitive Behavioural treatment manual. 1998; New York: Guilford Press.
8. Alvarenga PG, Mastrorosa RS, Rosário MC. Obsessive Compulsive Disorder in Children and Adolescents. In: Rey JM (Ed). IACAPAP e-Textbook of Child and Adolescent Mental Health. Geneva: International Association for Child and Adolescent Psychiatry and Allied Professions; 2012.
9. Mancebo MC, Boisseau CL, Garnaat SL, Eisen JL, Greenberg BD, Sibrava NJ, et al. Long-term course of pediatric obsessive-compulsive disorder: 3 years of prospective follow-up. Compr Psychiatry. 2014;55(7):1498-504.

Phobias and Hallucinations

BS Karnawat, Mahesh Hemnani

"It is fear that is the great cause of mystery in the world and it is fearlessness that brings heaven even in a moment. Be not afraid my children. Look not up in that attitude of fear towards that infinite starry wall vault as if it would crush you."

—Swami Vivekananda

PHOBIAS

INTRODUCTION[1,2]

The canvas of human life is colored with different shades of emotions. Fear is one of the deepest emotions to evolve early in life. At as early as 6 months of age, an infant demonstrates *stranger anxiety* while approaching a stranger. It is mostly normal to have fear of darkness, wild animals, etc. Fear has a protective role in that it helps one to take appropriate precautions and safety measures as necessary.

Fear is the perception of a threat resulting from an actual stimulus, whereas anxiety is the feeling of unease caused by apprehension of danger, which can be internal or external. Worries are largely mental ruminations concerning the probability of bad outcomes from seemingly benign everyday events. Anxiety is normal to some extent and is typically transient. It can, however, be powerful, persistent, pervasive, and disturbing at times, demanding medical attention.

EPIDEMIOLOGY[1,3]

The most common age of onset of anxiety disorder is between 8 and 15 years, average being 11 years. In general, anxiety disorders are more common in girls exception being social phobias (SPs) which is twice more prevalent in boys. The prevalence varies from 0.9 to 1.9 though some conditions like separation anxiety disorder have prevalence as high as 5%. Many of these disorders can progress into adult life.

ETIOPATHOGENESIS[2,3]

It is observed that anxious parents beget anxious offspring. It is always a complex interplay between genetic and environmental factor that is operative in such cases. Common environmental triggers or stresses are change of school or place of residence, academic failure, parental overprotection, broken family situations, peer conflict, loss of a family member or of a pet, highly neurotic temperament, chronic physical illness, sexual abuse, etc. It has also been suggested that a broad spectrum of infectious agents may have the ability to trigger exacerbations in children with some neurobehavioral disorder.

CLINICAL FEATURES[1,3]

Anxiety disorders are defined by pathological anxiety, which persists in one or more areas of childhood, interfering with social relationships, growth, and overall quality of life. It can result in low self-esteem, social disengagement, and academic underperformance.

Anxiety may have somatic manifestations such as tachycardia, tremors, muscle cramps, paresthesias, hyperhydrosis, flushing, pallor, hyperreflexia, stomach upset, nausea, anorexia, or weight loss.

Different types of anxiety disorders seen in children are enlisted here:
- Specific phobia
- Social anxiety disorder (social phobia)
- Separation anxiety disorders (SAD)
- Selective mutism
- Acute stress disorder
- Post-traumatic stress disorder (PTSD)
- Generalized anxiety disorders (GAD)
- Adjustment disorder with anxiety
- Obsessive compulsive disorder (OCD)
- Pediatric autoimmune neuropsychiatric disorders associated with *Streptococcus pyogenes* (PANDAS)

- Panic disorder
- Agoraphobia.

Specific Phobia

Specific phobia is distinguished by strong fear when exposed to a specific stimulus or circumstance, or on occasion when thinking about or imagining the stimulus. Clinging, weeping, throwing a tantrum, or "freezing" are common manifestations of fear in children. Animals, heights, enclosed spaces, and exposure to injection or blood are all common specific phobias. Diagnostic criteria as per Diagnostic and Statistical Manual of Mental Disorders, Fifth Edition (DSM-5) for specific phobia are as follows:
- A certain stimulation causes intense terror.
- Almost always, the thing or scenario elicits immediate fear or anxiety.
- Stimuli are avoided or endured with significant apprehension.
- The fear is out of proportion to the threat.
- The fear persists 6 months or longer.

Social Anxiety Disorders (Social Phobia)

It is a distinctive phobia in which trigger is either a social or performance task. Diagnostic criteria include the following:
- Severe nervousness about one or more social situations.
- The individual is concerned that his or her actions will be judged unfavorably.
- Social circumstances nearly always cause worry or terror.
- Fear is exaggerated in relation to the actual threat posed by the social stimuli.
- Fear or anxiety persist 6 months or longer.

Social phobia most commonly manifests itself throughout the adolescence and is twice as likely in boys as in girls. Children with social anxiety frequently shun group play, prefer to be near familiar people, and look too hesitant in strange situations. Children may express somatic symptoms that go away when they are allowed to stay at home.

Separation Anxiety Disorder

Separation from a specific attachment figure is the primary anxiety in SAD. Separation anxiety is natural in infants and children aged 6–36 months, but it should be considered abnormal if it increases or persists beyond this age range. Diagnosis requires that at least three of following symptoms should be present for >4 weeks:
- Distress with separation
- Worry about losing loved ones
- Worry about an event causing separation
- Reluctance to be alone
- Refusal to sleep alone
- Repeated nightmares of separation
- Refusal to go away from home
- Somatic complaints when separation occurs or in anticipation.

Separation anxiety disorder has onset typically in early childhood. Such children may be more demanding or showing behavioral outburst resulting in family conflict.

School refusal, which occurs in approximately 1–2% of children, is associated with anxiety in 40–50% of cases, depression in 50–60% of cases, and oppositional behavior in 50% of the cases. Younger anxious children who refuse to attend school are more likely to have SAD, whereas older ones do so because of the social phobia. Somatic symptoms, especially abdominal pain or headaches, are common.

Selective Mutism

Patients with selective mutism have a persistent failure to speak in specific, but not in all situations. Children are often shy in public but controlling at home. Diagnostic criteria include the following:
- Consistent failure to speak in specific social situations
- Failure to speak interferes with achievement or social communication
- Duration of at least one month
- Failure to speak is not due to lack of knowledge or spoken language
- Disorder is not better explained by a communication or other neuropsychiatric disorder.

Acute Stress Disorder and Post-traumatic Stress Disorder

Phobias arising from traumatic events include *acute stress disorder* and *PTSD*. Exposure to real or threatened death, significant injury, or sexual violence is referred to as a traumatic event. Hyperarousal, avoiding situations that are reminiscent of the terrible experience, or reliving the incident through nightmares or flashbacks are all reactions to traumatic events. Both acute stress disorder and post-traumatic stress disorder (PTSD) are characterized by intense and persistent trauma reactions that impede function. The four groups of symptoms are intrusion, avoidance, a dramatic change in arousal and activity, and a negative change in cognition and mood. Regardless of the symptom cluster classification, acute stress disorder is defined as the persistence of at least 9 of the 14 described symptoms for 3 days to 1 month following exposure to a traumatic event. In contrast to acute stress disorder, PTSD must include symptoms from each of the separate symptoms' clusters.

Intrusion Symptoms

- Distressing memories of the event
- Dreams are related to events (in children, dreams are not necessarily related to an event)
- Dissociative reactions in which the patient feels the recurring flashbacks of the event (in children maybe reenactment in play)
- Psychological distress at exposure to reminders of the event
- Marked physiologic reactions to reminder of the event.

Avoidance Symptoms

- Avoidance of distressing memories (children may avoid places or physical reminder)
- Avoidance of external reminders (children may avoid people, conversation, or interpersonal relationships).

Negative Alterations in Cognition and Mood

- Inability to remember an important aspect of the traumatic event*
- Persistent and exaggerated negative beliefs*
- Persistent distorted thoughts about cause or consequences of trauma*
- Persistent negative emotional state (fear, guilt, sadness, and shame)
- Decrease interest in activities/play
- Feelings of detachment (social withdrawal behavior in children)
- Persistent inability to experience or express positive emotions.

Alterations in Arousal

- Irritable behavior and angry outbursts
- Reckless or self-destructive behavior (not applicable in children below 6 years of age)

- Hypervigilance
- Exaggerated startle response
- Problems with concentration
- Sleep disturbances.

While as many as 50% of the children will have some symptoms of acute stress disorder following a trauma, only 10% will meet the diagnostic criteria.

Generalized Anxiety Disorder

Generalized anxiety disorder is characterized by excessive worry and concern over many issues. GAD may lead to symptoms of depression or physical complaints. Diagnostic criteria are as follows:

- Excessive anxiety and worry about various issues for >6 months
- Difficulty in controlling the worry
- Anxiety and worry are associated with three of the following:
  - Restlessness
  - Being easily fatigued
  - Difficulty in concentrating
  - Irritability
  - Muscle tension
  - Sleep disturbance
- Anxiety, worry, or physical symptoms cause significant distress or impairment.

Adjustment Disorder with Anxiety

It is characterized by excessive worry or maladaptive response to a stressor that is out of proportion to that stressor. Of note, stressor should not represent a perceived threat to life of oneself or a loved one. DSM-5 diagnostic criteria are as follows:

- Symptoms develop within 3 months of the disease
- Significant impairment results
- The symptoms do not meet criteria for an alternative anxiety disorder.
- The symptoms abate 6 months after termination of the stress.

Obsessive Compulsive Disorder

Obsessive anxieties that are temporarily allayed by compensatory compulsive action are a hallmark of OCD. Obsessions are persistent, recurrent urges or images that a person tries to ignore or repress. The temptation to

---

*Symptoms are not criteria in children <6 years of age.

harm oneself or others, dread of illness or contamination, guilt about sexual fantasies, and images of violent or horrifying events are just a few examples of the common obsessions. Compulsions are repetitive, excessive behaviors that a person engages in to cope with the anxiety that an obsession causes. Compulsions might be physical behaviors such as checking locks and repeatedly washing your hands and they can be cerebral behaviors such as counting internally and repeating particular words. The compulsive behaviors must last more than an hour each day or interfere with the patient's regular activities in order to qualify as OCD. In the DSM-5, OCD and related disorders (such as trichotillomania) are listed separately and are no longer included under anxiety disorder.

Children generally present with vague anxiety symptoms or poor concentrations before clear OCD is seen. In children OCD is highly comorbid with Tourette-tic disorder and attention-deficit/hyperactivity disorder (ADHD).

Pediatric Autoimmune Neuropsychiatric Disorders Associated with *Streptococcus Pyogenes*

PANDAS is a term proposed for a group of neuropsychiatric disorder (particularly OSD and Tourette-tic disorder) for which a possible causal relationship with group A streptococcal infection has been hypothesized, but still remains to be proven.

Panic Disorder

Panic disorders are characterized by recurrent and unexpected panic attacks, the hallmark of panic disorder is persistent concern over having additional attacks, worrying about the consequences of an attack, or a significant change in behavior related to the attacks. A panic attack occurs suddenly; peak within 10 minutes, often resolves without intervention and consists of at least four of the following symptoms:
- Palpitations or tachycardia
- Diaphoresis
- Trembling or shaking
- Shortness of breath or sensation of a smothering
- Feeling of chocking
- Chest pain
- Nausea or abdominal discomfort
- Dizziness or feeling faint
- Chills or heat sensation
- Paresthesias
- Derealization (feeling of unreality) or depersonalization
- Fear of losing control or "going crazy"
- Fear of dying.

Agoraphobia

Agoraphobia is defined by crippling fear of experiencing a panic attack or other disabling or embarrassing symptoms in a situation from which the patient cannot flee or where assistance might not be accessible. Diagnosis requires that the anxiety manifests in at least two of the following situations:
- Riding public transport
- Being in open spaces
- Being in enclosed spaces
- Standing in line or in a crowd
- Being outside of the home alone.

Agoraphobia is typically preceded by panic disorder, phobias and separation anxiety disorder.

DIAGNOSIS[1,3]

To diagnose a particular anxiety disorder in a child there should be significant impairment in the child's psychosocial and/or academic or occupational functioning, which can occur even with subthreshold symptoms that do not meet criteria in the DSM-5 as described earlier. For practicing pediatricians, a simplified approach to diagnose these disorders is outlined in **Flowchart 1**.

It is prudent to rule out certain organic conditions before making a diagnosis of an anxiety disorder. These conditions include hyperthyroidism, caffeinism (carbonated beverages), hypoglycemia, central nervous system (CNS) disorders (such as delirium, encephalopathy, and brain tumors), migraine, asthma, lead poisoning, and cardiac arrhythmia. Rarely hyperparathyroidism, pheochromocytoma, porphyria, systemic lupus erythematosus (SLE), anaphylaxis may also be considered in differential diagnosis. Some drugs with side effect that can mimic anxiety include antihistamines, cold medicines, antiasthmatic agents, steroids, sympathomimetics, anticholinergic agents, etc.

Basic physical workup is needed only in order to consider primary or comorbid medical conditions. Unnecessary investigations only reinforce somatic symptoms in anxious patients and should be avoided. Appropriate psychological tests such as [Children's Apperception Test (CAT)/Thematic Apperception Test (TAT)] might throw more light on child' psychopathology.

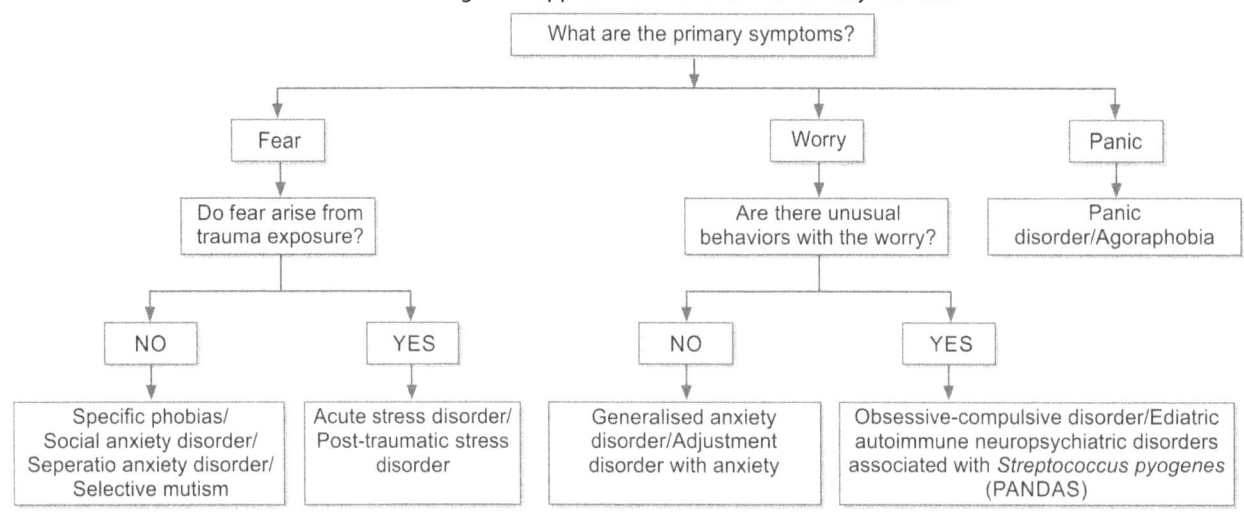

Flowchart 1: Diagnostic approach to the child with anxiety disorder.

TREATMENT

Management of anxiety disorders in children includes pharmacotherapy and psychotherapy, alone or in combination, along with counseling and relaxation training. A close collaboration between primary care pediatrician and mental health professional is warranted to obtain optimal beneficial result for the patient.

PHARMACOTHERAPY[2,4]

When a child reports recurring acute severe anxiety, antidepression, or anxiolytic medications is often necessary. In children <12 years of age small doses of tricyclic antidepressants such as imipramine or nortriptyline may be used. Selective serotonin reuptake inhibitors (SSRIs) such as fluoxetine, citalopram, sertraline, and escitalopram are useful in older children. The use of atypical antidepressant such as bupropion, duloxetine, and venlafaxine, should be reserved for more resistant cases. The tricyclic antidepressant (like clomipramine) is particularly useful in management of OCD. There is evidence that use of glutamine inhibitor (riluzole) may be beneficial in children with OCD.

Anxiolytic agents (including lorazepam, clonazepam, and hydroxyzine) have all been effectively used for acute situational anxiety, their efficacy as chronic medication is poorer.

Beta-adrenergic blocking agents like propranolol are used to treat social phobia particularly the subtype with performance anxiety and stage phobias. Clonidine or guanfacine may be helpful for sleep disturbances, persistent arousal, and exaggerated startle response in case of PTSD. Tics associated with OCD may be treated with dopamine receptor antagonist (haloperidol, pimozide, etc.). Pediatric dosages of commonly used psychotherapeutic drugs are given in **Table 1**.

PSYCHOTHERAPY[5]

Psychotherapy is the first line treatment for most child and adolescent disorders, because this type of treatment generally produces outcomes similar to pharmacotherapy, with less risk of harm. A variety of psychotherapeutic programs have been developed with varying levels of effectiveness in management of anxiety disorders. Commonly used are behavioral therapy (BT), cognitive behavior therapy (CBT), trauma-focused cognitive behavioral therapy (TF-CBT), family therapy, psychodynamic psychotherapy, supportive psychotherapy, and social effectiveness therapy for children (SET-C), alone or in combination.

Cognitive behavior therapy is a focused therapy that works on modifying the initial thought process, replacing negative thoughts with positive ones. Combination of CBT (plus parent components in some condition) and SSRI often result in a superior response in pediatric patients with anxiety disorder including GAD, panic disorder, social phobia, and SAD.

Systemic desensitization is form of behavior therapy that gradually exposes the patient to the fear inducing situations or object while simultaneously teaching relaxation techniques for anxiety management.

TABLE 1: Dosage of drugs used in childhood phobias and anxiety disorders.

Drug name	Pediatrics daily dosage range	Remarks
Imipramine	1–1.5 mg/kg	Maximum 5 mg/day
Nortriptyline	1–3 mg/kg	Maximum 150 mg/day
Fluoxetine	*Depression:* 10–20 mg Anxiety, OCD: 10–60 mg	Start with 10 mg OD increase dose if needed
Citalopram	10–40 mg	Start with 10 mg OD increase dose every 2 weekly if needed
Sertraline	12.5–200 mg	Start with 12.5 mg OD titrates by 25 mg/day at intervals of 1 week as needed
Escitalopram	5–20 mg	Start with 5 mg OD, increase by 5 mg/day at weekly intervals
Bupropion	150–300 mg	Start with 150 mg OD
Duloxetine	30–60 mg	Start with 30 mg/day for 2 weeks and increase up to 60 mg/day if needed
Venlafaxine	37.5–225 mg	Start with 37.5 mg OD for 1 week then titrate if needed
Clomipramine	25–200 mg	Start with 25 mg/day for 2 weeks and titrate weekly up to 200 mg/day if needed
Lorazepam	0.5–2 mg	Start with 0.5 mg HS
Clonazepam	0.5–1 mg	Start with 0.25mg BD (maximum 1 mg/day)
Hydroxyzine	Age <6 years: 50 mg Age >6 years: 50–100 mg	Start with 0.5 mg/kg/dose 6 hourly
Haloperidol	0.05–0.15 mg/kg	Start with 0.05 mg/kg/day in 2–3 divided doses for 1 week then titrate if needed up to max dose of 4 mg/day
Pimozide	0.05–0.2 mg/kg	Used in Tourette syndrome (>12 years of age) 0.05 mg/kg HS increased every third day if needed up to maximum of 0.2 mg/kg (10 mg/day)

Management of school refusal typically requires parental counseling and family therapy.

COMPLICATIONS[1,3]

The anxiety disorder if not treated well, results into complications such as school dropout, academic under-achievement, poor interpersonal relations, family crises, depression, suicidal behavior, and predisposition to alcohol abuse and drug abuse. Such patients generally have low esteem impairing work performance and overall quality of life.

Adverse childhood experiences, which include PTSD in addition to other substantial stressors, have been found to predispose kids to long-term physical and mental health issues. Ischemic heart disease, cancer, chronic lung disease, bone fractures, and liver disease are some of these illnesses.

FOLLOW-UP AND PROGNOSIS

Anxiety disorders generally run a chronic cause and many of these disorders progress to adult life, causing psychosocial impairment. Apart from appropriate management, prognosis also depends on the type of anxiety disorders and presence of comorbid disorders. Rational use of combination of pharmacotherapy and psychotherapy achieve recovery rate of 70–80% in most of childhood anxiety disorders.

PREVENTION[3]

Primary prevention of anxiety disorders in children would entail that every child and adolescent is reared up in a safe, secure, and supportive environment which is devoid of anxiety inducing stressors at home, school, and community. Due to obvious reasons it is a herculean task to accomplish; hence, focus should be on secondary prevention. For instance, when a child sustains some trauma, initial intervention should focus on reunification with a parent and attending to child's physical needs in a safe place. Along with these measures, aggressive treatment of pain and trauma might decrease likelihood of PTSD occurring.

CONCLUSION

Phobias are not uncommon in pediatric population. Equipping parents, educators and health care professionals with knowledge about phobias in cildren is essential. Pediatricians have to identify any other neurodevelopmental problem to manage patient accordingly. Understanding and managing phobias in children require a holistic and empathetic approach. Hence, early recognition, proper evaluation and appropriate management of fear/phobia, worry, anxiety, and panic would go a long way in reducing the burden of mental health problem in children and adolescents.

HALLUCINATIONS

INTRODUCTION

Hallucinations in children are usually either overlooked or missed as it is perceived to occur only in adults suffering with mental conditions/illness. Hallucinations are false perceptions (typically auditory, visual, tactile, or olfactory) that occurs in absence of any identifiable external stimuli. The occurence of hallucinations in children raises several questions and concerns regarding origin and its types to understand their potential impact on child's mental status and quality of life, which ultimately is important for management of such cases.[1,6]

EPIDEMIOLOGY[1,6]

Hallucinations occur in about 5% of the normal children. Sleep related hallucinations occur in as much as one-third of the children.

ETIOPATHOGENESIS[1,6]

Hallucinations in children may be an indication of a medical condition, poor visual or auditory function, the ingestion of a substance, or a psychotic illness. Among adults, hallucinations are viewed as synonymous with psychosis, but in children can be a part of normal development or can be associated with nonpsychotic psychopathology. Nonpsychotic hallucinations commonly occur in the context of severe traumatic stress, development difficulties, social and emotional deprivation, parents whose own psychopathology promote a breakdown in the child's sense of reality, cultural beliefs in mysticism, and unresolved mourning.

Medical conditions that can manifest with hallucination include drug intoxications [cannabis, 3,4-Methylenedioxymethamphetamine (MDMA), lysergic acid diethylamide (LSD), cocaine, amphetamine, and barbiturate], medication side effects (e.g., steroid, anticholinergic drugs, and stimulant drugs), and physical illness such as thyroid, parathyroid and adrenal disorder, fever, infection, Wilson disease, electrolyte imbalance, migraine, seizures, neoplasm, and mushroom (*Psilocybe* species) poisoning.

CLINICAL FEATURES[1,6]

- *Fantasy-based hallucinations:* Children progressively come to understand that reality and imagination are two distinct things. Children under the age of three sometimes mix these two, but by the time they are 8 years old, the majority of kids can usually accurately tell inner thoughts from voices. Some kids could use imagination for solace or enjoyment, but the majority of these kids go on to make healthy psychological adjustments.
- *Febrile hallucinations:* When they have a high temperature, young children may experience hallucinations. These hallucinations are transient and do not portend psychological issues in the future. The occurrence can be a minor case of delirium.
- *Phobic hallucinations:* Acute phobic hallucinations are periods of hallucination accompanied by dread and terror that affect preschoolers. These 10–60 minutes long hallucinations can happen at any time of day, but they tend to happen mostly at night. When an episode occurs, the youngster may cry out in terror or hide because they feel as though bugs are crawling all over them. Typically, symptoms appear for 1–3 days before going away over the course of a week.
- *Grief-induced hallucinations:* The grieving process following the death of a loved one may include visual or auditory hallucinations of the deceased. Some families may perceive these events as a supernatural or a religious experience.
- *Sleep-related hallucinations:* Hallucinations resembling dreams can happen at different phases of sleep. When sleep first begins, hypnagogic hallucinations happen, and when you first wake up, hypnopompic hallucinations happen. With a prevalence of 37% and 12.5%, respectively, hypnagogic and hypnopompic hallucinations are both extremely common. Hallucinations related to sleep may be more common in patients with insomnia or excessive daytime sleepiness. Additionally, patients with narcolepsy and PTSD may experience these hallucinations. Although they sometimes resemble hallucinations, night terrors

are a separate type of nonrapid eye movement that usually happen in the first hour of sleep. Over 30% of 18-month-old toddlers will have a night terror; by maturity, the rate drops to 2.2%.
- *Psychotic hallucinations:* Hallucinations along with delusions, disorganized thinking, grossly disorganized behavior, and negative symptoms are the key features which define psychotic disorders.

DIAGNOSIS[1,6]

The first step of evaluating hallucinations is to assess patient's mental status. Most children with hallucinations have otherwise normal mental status and they may hallucinate in the context of fantasy, grief, sleep, acute phobia, and fever **(Flowchart 2)**.

Medical delirium is taken into consideration if confusion is the main shift in mental status. Delusions or beliefs that are held on to while being objectively false according to reality, should cause one to think about schizophrenia or a mood condition. The majority of hallucinations connected to delirium are visual, while aural hallucinations are seen in mental disorders. Differential diagnosis of hallucinations comprises a broad range of mental ailments including diagnosis in which hallucinations may be viewed as associated symptoms (PTSD, nonpsychotic disorder, mood disorder, disruptive impulse-control, and conduct disorder); diagnosis that are defined by psychotic features (brief psychotic disorder, schizophrenia, major depression, or bipolar disorder with psychotic feature) and at risk clinical states (poor reality testing).

TREATMENT[6]

The line of treatment would depend on the underlying cause. Combination of disorder-specific psychotherapy (e.g., TF-CBT for PTSD) and adjunctive pharmacotherapy (e.g., antidepressant for depression or anxiety and brief trial of antipsychotic for agitation) would be needed to treat nonpsychotic hallucinations. True psychotic hallucinations would require antipsychotic medication. High dose of pyridoxine is indicated to treat hallucinations due to mushroom poisoning.

CONCLUSION

Hallucinatios are not very common in pediatric population, and in adults, they mostly harbinger of psychotic states. On the contrary, these may occur among chidren in absence of any psychiatric disorder. It becomes challenging for pediatrician to differentiate between the two, identify any other associated neurodevelopmental problem in the patient and manage appropriately. Encouraging open dialogue discussion and education about mental health froman early stage is crucial. Moreover, emphasizing support network involving parents, teachers, pediatrician, psychiatrist as well as psycho- analyst and the community at large can improve child's mental well being significantly. Rightly said ....

> *"vita-raga-bhaya-krodha man-maya mam upashritah bahavo jnana-tapasa puta mad-bhavam agatah"*
> —**Bhagavad Gita: Chapter 4, Verse 10**

(Being free from attachment, fear and anger becoming fully absorbed in Me, and taking refuse in Me, many persons in the past became purified by knowledge of Me, and thus attained My divine love)

REFERENCES

1. Burne R, Kirschner K. Unusual behaviors. In: Kliegman RM, Lye PS, Bordine BJ, Toth H (Eds). Nelson Pediatric Symptom-Based Diagnosis. Mumbai: Elsevier Publishers and RELX India Pvt. Ltd. Distributors; 2018. pp. 421-38.
2. Bhatawdekar M. Anxiety. In: Dalwani SH, Unni JC, Ahmed S, Singh K, Leena M, Leena D, et al. (Eds). IAP Handbook of Developmental and Behavioral Pediatrics, 1st edition.

Flowchart 2: Approach to evaluation of childhood hallucinations.

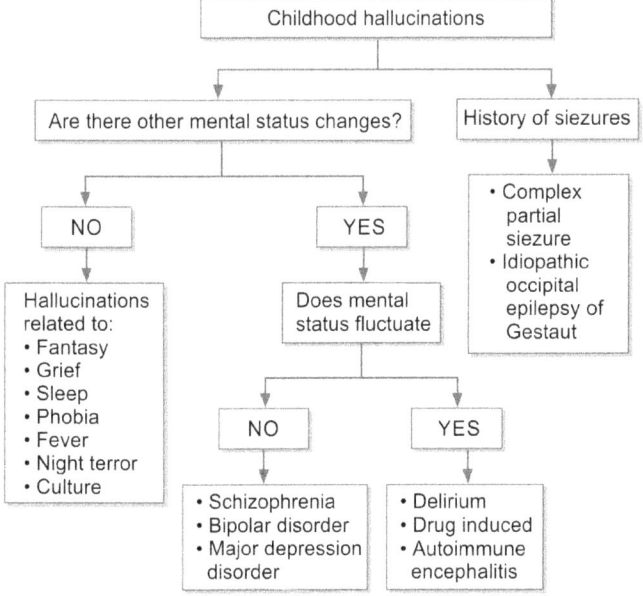

New Delhi: Jaypee Brothers Medical Publishers (P) Ltd; 2022. pp. 180-5.
3. Rosenberg DR, Chiriboga JA. Anxiety Disorder. In: Kliegman RM, St. Geme III JW, Blum NJ, Wilson K, Shah SS, Tasker RC (Eds). Nelson Textbook of Pediatrics, 21st edition. Philadelphia: Elsevier publisher; 2020. pp. 210-7.
4. DeMaso DR, Walter HJ. Psychopharmacology. In: Kliegman RM, St. Geme III JW, Blum NJ, Wilson K, Shah SS, Tasker RC (Eds). Nelson Textbook of Pediatrics, 21st edition. Philadelphia, Elsevier; 2020. pp. 189-96.
5. Walter HJ, DeMaso DR. Psychotherapy and psychiatric hospitalization. In: Kliegman RM, St. Geme III JW, Blum NJ, Wilson K, Shah SS, Tasker RC (Eds). Nelson Textbook of Pediatrics, 21st edition. Philadelphia, Elsevier. 2020; pp. 199-201.
6. Gongalez-Heydrich J, Walter HJ, DeMaso DR. Acute Phobic Hallucinations of childhood. In: Kliegman RM, St. Geme III JW, Blum NJ, Wilson K, Shah SS, Tasker RC (Eds). Nelson Textbook of Pediatrics, 21st edition. Philadelphia, Elsevier; 2020. pp. 250-2.

Chapter 10: Oppositional Defiant Disorder

Adhiraj Singh, Anurag Singh

INTRODUCTION

Oppositional defiant disorder (ODD) is a type of disruptive behavior disorder that is a commonly encountered but poorly dealt with condition in childhood. Parents usually find themselves unprepared, and clinicians are often ill-equipped to properly diagnose and counsel them. Many times this leads to a response that is further detrimental to the child. Children pass through phases of emotional development that takes them across various states of emotions ranging from love and compassion to spite and vengeance. Occasionally even the best-behaved children can experience an emotional outburst where they manifest anger or rage. Such occasional defiant behavior is not completely abnormal and does not denote a behavior disorder. Therefore, an occasional act of argument, aggression, acting angry or using defiant behavior toward adults cannot be considered as a disruptive behavioral disorder. A diagnosis of behavioral disorder must be entertained only when these disruptive behaviors are inappropriate for age and are severe or persistent.[1,2] The common disruptive behavioral disorders include ODD, conduct disorder (CD), attention deficit hyperactivity disorder (ADHD), intermittent explosive disorder (IED), and disruptive mood dysregulation disorder (DMDD). As there is an involvement of acting out by the child, these behavior disorders are also called *externalizing disorders*.[3,4]

Mental disorders in general are on the rise in India. If we look at the world's population, then it is evident that approximately one-third of it is in the younger age group of <15 years. Among this young population almost 5–15% are suffering with these disorders. The contribution of mental disorders to the total disability adjusted life years (DALYs) in India has almost doubled and has increased from 2.5% (2.0–3.1) in 1990 to 4.7% (3.7–5.6) in 2017.[5] The prevalence of ODD in India amongst the children studying in primary school is between 7 and 8%.[6]

In order to determine a diagnosis of behavioral disorder and eliminate other physical conditions or mental health disorders that may be causing symptoms, a detailed history, complete physical examination and laboratory tests are required to rule out any infirmity or substance abuse and categorically delineate the exact symptoms so that the criteria laid out in the Diagnostic and Statistical Manual of Mental Disorders, Fifth Edition (DSM-5) published by the American Psychiatric Association may be applied. In children suffering with behavioral disorders the aggressive episodes may be preceded or accompanied by:

- Rage
- Increased energy
- Irritability
- Racing thoughts
- Tremors
- Tingling
- Palpitations
- Chest tightness.

The violent verbal and behavioral outbursts are out of scale to the circumstance, with no consideration for the repercussions and can include:

- Temper tantrums
- Heated arguments
- Tirades
- Shouting
- Slapping, shoving, or pushing
- Physical fights
- Property damage
- Threatening or assaulting people or animals.

After the episode there may be a sense of tiredness and sometimes relief also. Later, he or she may feel remorse, regret, or embarrassment. Earlier it was considered that there is a hierarchical relationship between ODD and CD but Burke et al. showed that a substantive proportion of youths with onset of CD in adolescence did not have a diagnosis of ODD in their childhood. Based on these studies, there is a strong evidence against the previously considered hierarchical approach for considering the diagnosis of CD and ODD, and suggest that albeit lying in a continuum, the two are actually distinct disorders.[7] The exact cause of opposition defiant disorder is not known but some of the risk factors include:

- *Gender:* Boys are much more likely to suffer from opposition defiant disorder as compared to girls. It is not absolutely clear whether the cause is genetic or it is linked to experiences of socialization.
- *Gestation and birth:* The problematic behavior of the child in later life may have its roots in difficult pregnancy, prematurity, or being born with a low birth weight.
- *Temperament:* Oppositional defiant disorder is more likely to develop later in life in kids who are difficult to control, have challenging temperaments, or are violent from an early age.
- *Family life:* In dysfunctional homes, the likelihood of opposition defiant disorder is higher. A child is more at risk, for instance, in homes where domestic violence, poverty, inadequate parenting, or substance misuse are issues.
- *Learning difficulties:* Problems with reading and writing are often associated with behavior problems.
- *Intellectual disabilities:* Children with intellectual disabilities are twice as likely to have behavioral disorders.
- *Brain development:* Neuroimaging findings converge to implicate various parts of the prefrontal cortex, amygdala, and insula in children suffering with ODD.
- *Hormonal:* Alteration in cortisol levels has also been demonstrated consistently.
- *Genetics:* According to a study, ODD has got 61% heritability.[8] Oppositional defiant disorder shares 50% of its genes with CD; however, it does not have any unique component of genetic predisposition that is not shared by other psychopathologies.[9] One family-based linkage study of ADHD and comorbidities identified strong links among ADHD and ODD, ADHD and CD, ODD, and CD. Significant linkage results were obtained at 8q24. The linkage values were also suggestive at 6q23.3, 2p21–22.3, 14q21.1, 17p12, 17q25.1, and 19p13.2 in children having comorbidity with ODD.[10]

Oppositional defiant disorder usually manifests between 8 and 12 years of age. Children with ODD usually act defiant against people they know well such as teachers, family members, and usual care givers. Their oppositional behavior manifest more often than other children of their age and it causes serious problems at school, home, or with peers. Oppositional defiant disorder also includes a repetitive behavior pattern of being spiteful and seeking revenge, a behavior called *vindictiveness*. Examples of such defiant or oppositional behavior include:

- Loosing temper or often being angry.
- Refusing to comply with the rules set out by adults or arguing with them and not complying with their instructions.
- Often behaving in a spiteful or resentful manner.
- Getting ticked off easily or becoming annoyed or deliberately annoying others.
- Frequently blaming others for their own mistakes.

At times we may find it difficult to differentiate between an emotional or strong-willed child and the one with ODD, adding different facets to diagnostic criteria for ODD, as the recent evidence suggests that ODD could be multidimensional. The diagnostic criteria are divided into three groups as per the DSM-5—(1) angry/irritable mood, (2) vindictiveness, and (3) argumentative/defiant behavior. No emphasis has been kept on any of these particular dimensions for diagnosis; however, there is no significant change in the description and number of symptoms and the diagnostic threshold.

Unlike the DSM-IV, which was emphatic only about persistence of symptoms for >6 months, the DSM-5 has emphasized both persistence and frequency of behavior. For children below 5 years of age, the symptoms must be present on most days, and for those who are ≥5 years, symptoms must be present at least once per week (except for vindictiveness: Twice within the past 6 months). By doing this, the DSM-5 has made an attempt to differentiate disorder from normative behavior and is attentive to the developmental aspects.

Symptoms of ODD have an early onset, generally during preschool years. Sometimes ODD may develop a little later, but they almost always occur before the early teen years. There are resultant severe problems in social activities, relationships, school, and work. The child and the family both suffer. Emotional and behavioral symptoms of ODD generally last at least 6 months. They include angry and irritable mood, argumentative and defiant behavior, and hurtful and revengeful behavior.

ANGRY AND IRRITABLE MOOD
- The child loses temper often and very easily
- The child is frequently touchy and easily annoyed by others
- The child appears to be often angry and resentful.

ARGUMENTATIVE AND DEFIANT BEHAVIOR
- Often argues with adults, caregivers or people in authority
- Often actively defies or refuses to follow the rules set out by adults or requests made by them
- Frequently annoys or upsets people on purpose
- Often blames others for their own mistakes or misbehavior.

HURTFUL AND REVENGEFUL BEHAVIOR
- Resorts to saying mean and hateful things when upset.
- Tries to hurt the feelings of others and seeks revenge, or we may say is seen as being vindictive.
- There is evidence of vindictive behavior by the child at least two times in the past 6 months.

CLASSIFICATION OF ODD BASED UPON SEVERITY

Oppositional defiant disorder can be classified as mild, moderate, or severe based upon severity of the condition.
- *Mild:* Symptoms occur only in one setting, such as only at home, school, work, and with peers
- *Moderate:* Some symptoms occur in at least two settings
- *Severe:* Some symptoms occur in three or more settings.

For some children, symptoms may first be seen only at home. But with time, problem behavior also may happen in other settings, such as school, social activities, and with friends.

COMPLICATIONS

Children with behavior disorder have an increased risk of impaired interpersonal relationships. Children with behavior disorders are often perceived by others as always being angry. They may have frequent verbal fights or there can be physical abuse. These actions can lead to relationship problems and family stress. Other complications of behavior disorders may include school suspension, car accidents, financial problems, or trouble with the law. Mood disorders such as anxiety and depression can be often seen to coexist. Problems with alcohol and other substance abuse have also been reported. Adolescents suffering with behavior disorder are more likely to have problems with drugs or alcohol abuse as compared to their peers. These children are more prone to develop some medical condition such as high blood pressure, diabetes, heart disease, stroke, ulcers, and chronic pain. Self-harm in the form of intentional injuries to one self are seen and even suicide attempts can sometimes occur.

MANAGEMENT OF OPPOSITIONAL DEFIANT DISORDER

Psychotherapy

Cognitive behavioral therapy (CBT) is a tool which can be put to use to help children and adolescents learn the way to cope with thoughts and feelings that contribute to their feeling depressed or anxious. CBT for anxiety often includes exposing the child to situations that make them anxious so that they can learn to respond to those risk factors in children's behavioral disorders. Cognitive behavioral therapy is a common type of talk therapy (psychotherapy) provided by a mental health counselor (psychotherapist or therapist) in a structured way. CBT can help create awareness about inaccurate or negative thinking so the patient can view the challenging situations more clearly and respond to them in a more effective way.

Once a behavior disorder has been identified the treatment should be started as early as possible. The chances of successful treatment are better if it conforms to the specific needs of the child and the family. The first step in the management is talking with a health care provider. The specific diagnosis can be reached at by a mental health professional. One must ensure that the child does not have learning disabilities as the presence of same may also lead to difficulty in following rules at school. When the child is of the younger age group then behavior therapy training is required for the parents. Parents need to learn effective ways to strengthen the parent-child relationship and show correct response to the child's behavior. For slightly older age group such as school going children and teenagers, a combination of therapy and training may be required involving the child, the family and school.

Pharmacotherapy

Psychosocial approaches take precedence over drugs in management of ODD. It is only when aggression in an oppositional child is difficult to manage by psychosocial intervention that we must combine it with pharmacotherapy. We must focus on the treatment of comorbid conditions first. Secondly, we may add an atypical antipsychotic. If it still does not give the desired results, then it is better to change the medication rather than add another one. In case of partial response, a mood stabilizer might be required. Weight gain and sedation are the common side effects of these drugs and must be watched out for.[11]

When concomitant ADHD is present, methylphenidate, when compared to other drugs, provides the highest results against aggression. In cases with comorbid ADHD, nonstimulants such as guanfacine, atomoxetine, and clonidine show positive effects, with atomoxetine having the greatest outcomes. However, studies on these drugs have not explicitly focused on aggression as a side effect, therefore these therapies might be thought of as the second line of defense in the arsenal of antiaggression drugs.[12]

Risperidone, an atypical antipsychotic, has the best track record for treating aggression and irritability in young people, followed by aripiprazole, which some studies claim is risperidone's chemical equivalent.[13] Quetiapine has an enormous amount of result, but there are greater side-effect risks and the current trials are of poor quality, making it unpopular. According to numerous studies, common antipsychotics such as haloperidol have varying effects on aggression, making them less suitable for usage in children who are already aggressive. Lithium and valproate are the two mood stabilizers, with considerable effects but there are concerns regarding adverse effects and poor study quality. A conditional recommendation has been made for both, with valproate being favored over lithium. Carbamazepine has not shown to be very successful at reducing aggression in pediatric population.[14]

Different types of medications that may help in the treatment of intermittent explosive disorder include certain antidepressants—specifically serotonin reuptake inhibitors, anticonvulsants, and mood stabilizers. For ADHD the treatment may be done using methylphenidate or other drugs as detailed earlier. The clinician has to judiciously use them in conjunction with cognitive behavior therapy as per the need of the individual patient.

PREVENTION

Oppositional defiant disorder in children may arise for unknown reasons. Numerous factors, including biological and societal ones, may be causal. It is well recognized that children are more vulnerable to risk factors such as exposure to other forms of violence and criminal behavior, mistreatment, harsh or inconsistent parenting, and parental attention deficit hyperactivity disorder (ADHD). A child's propensity to develop behavioral issues can also be influenced by the quality of their early childhood care. There are techniques to reduce the likelihood that children will develop disruptive behavior disorders, but certain factors seem to enhance the risk.

In case a child has been diagnosed with behavior disorder, complete prevention of anger outbursts is beyond his or her control without getting treatment from a professional. Combined with treatment or even as a part of it, the following suggestions can help prevent some incidents from getting out of control:

- *Stick with treatment:* Regularly attending therapy sessions and practicing coping skills, and if medications are prescribed, then taking them regularly.
- *Taking maintenance medications:* In order to prevent the recurrence of explosive episodes, parents should be encouraged to maintain the drugs for as long as necessary before terminating them totally and should be advised to refrain from stopping the treatment abruptly.
- *Practicing relaxation techniques:* The youngster may benefit from regular practice of deep breathing, calming visualization, or yoga to maintain tranquility.
- *Developing new ways of thinking (cognitive restructuring):* Using logic, reasonable expectations, and rational thought to reframe one's perspective on a distressing situation might help one better understand it and respond to it. This is the foundation of cognitive restructuring technique.
- *Using problem solving:* This entails developing a strategy to figure out how to handle an annoying issue. Even if a solution is not possible immediately now, having a plan might help one concentrate their energies.
- *Learning ways to improve communication:* The youngster is encouraged to pay attention to the message the other person is attempting to convey before considering the best way to respond, rather than speaking on the spur of the moment.
- *Changing the environment:* When possible, the children are encouraged to leave or avoid situations that upset them. Also, scheduling personal time may enable a child to better handle an upcoming stressful or frustrating situation.
- *Avoiding mood-altering substances:* The children suffering with intermittent explosive disorder are

encouraged not to use alcohol or recreational or illegal drugs.

Public health approaches to prevent risks for ODD are:
- Positive parenting strategies for young children
- Positive parenting tips
- Child maltreatment prevention
- Youth violence prevention
- Mental health in adults
- Finding high quality child care.

MANAGING SYMPTOMS: STAYING HEALTHY

The importance of being healthy cannot be overemphasized in all the children and it can be especially important for children with behavior or conduct problems. In addition to taking help of behavioral therapy and medication, practicing certain healthy lifestyle behaviors may reduce challenging and disruptive behaviors in these children.

Some healthy behaviors that may help are:
- Physical activity, including aerobic and vigorous exercise
- Healthy diet including fruits, vegetables, whole grains, legumes (for example, beans, peas, and lentils), lean protein sources, and nuts and seeds.
- Getting adequate amount of sleep each night based on age
- Strengthening relationships with family members.

CONCLUSION

Oppositional defiant disorder in children is on the rise in India. They need proper recognition and an early diagnosis to avoid major harm to the child and the family. Treatment strategies include medications, CBT and parent, and teacher or healthcare professional driven counseling. Exercise and physical activity are having proven benefits. Alternate therapies such as yoga and meditation might be rewarding and may be used in conjunction with the established treatments.

REFERENCES

1. Centers for Disease Control and Prevention. (2023). Behavior or Conduct problems in Children. [online] Available from: https://www.cdc.gov/childrensmentalhealth/behavior.html [Last accessed October, 2023].
2. Better Health Channel. (2012). Behavioural Disorders in Children. [online] Available from: https://www.betterhealth.vic.gov.au/health/healthyliving/behavioural-disorders-in-children [Last accessed October, 2023].
3. Betterhelp. (2023). What are Behavioral Disorders? [online] Available from: https://www.betterhelp.com/advice/behavior/a-list-of-behavioral-disorders/ [Last accessed October, 2023].
4. India State-Level Disease Burden Initiative Mental Disorders Collaborators. The burden of mental disorders across the states of India: the Global Burden of Disease Study 1990-2017. Lancet Psychiatry. 2020;7(2):148-61.
5. Cleveland Clinic. (2022). Intermittent Explosive Disorder. [online] Available from: https://my.clevelandclinic.org/health/diseases/17786-intermittent-explosive-disorder [Last accessed October, 2023].
6. Mishra A, Garg SP, Desai SN. Prevalence of oppositional defiant disorder and conduct disorder in primary school children. Journal of Indian Academy of Forensic Medicine. 2014;36(3):246-50.
7. Burke JD, Waldman I, Lahey BB. Predictive validity of childhood oppositional defiant disorder and conduct disorder: implications for the DSM-V. J Abnorm Psychol. 2010;119(4):739-51.
8. Polderman TJ, Benyamin B, De Leeuw CA, Sullivan PF, Van Bochoven A, Visscher PM, et al. Meta-analysis of the heritability of human traits based on fifty years of twin studies. Nature Genet. 2015;47(7):702-9.
9. Krueger RF, Hicks BM, Patrick CJ, Carlson SR, Iacono WG, McGue M. Etiologic connections among substance dependence, antisocial behavior, and personality: modeling the externalizing spectrum. J Abnorm Psychol. 2002;111(3):411-24.
10. Coolidge FL, Thede LL, Young SE. Heritability and the comorbidity of attention deficit hyperactivity disorder with behavioral disorders and executive function deficits: A preliminary investigation. Dev Neuropsychol. 2000;17(3):273-87.
11. Rosato S, Correll N, Pappadopulos E, Chait A, Crystal S, Jensen PS, et al. Treatment of maladaptive aggression in youth: CERT guidelines II. Treatments and ongoing management. Pediatrics. 2012;129(6):1577-86.
12. Tourian L, LeBoeuf A, Breton JJ, Cohen D, Gignac M, Labelle R, et al. Treatment options for the cardinal symptoms of disruptive mood dysregulation disorder. J Can Aca Child Adolesc Psychiatry. 2015;24(1):41-54.
13. Safavi P, Hasanpour-Dehkordi A, AmirAhmadi M. Comparison of risperidone and aripiprazole in the treatment of preschool children with disruptive behavior disorder and attention deficit-hyperactivity disorder: a randomized clinical trial. J Adv Pharm Technol Res. 2016;7(2):43-7.
14. Gorman DA, Gardner DM, Murphy AL, Feldman M, Bélanger SA, Steele MM, et al. Canadian guidelines on pharmacotherapy for disruptive and aggressive behaviour in children and adolescents with attention-deficit hyperactivity disorder, oppositional defiant disorder, or conduct disorder. Can J Psychiatry. 2015;60(2):62-76.

Chapter 11

Conduct Disorders in Children

Pragya Chitlangia Somani

INTRODUCTION

Childhood is a phase characterized by the presence of mischievous behavior. In Indian mythology, the character of Krishna is portrayed as an exemplary child who demonstrates both intelligence and a mischievous nature simultaneously. During childhood and adolescence, it is not uncommon for individuals to engage in occasional rule-breaking and rebellious behavior. However, in the case of youth diagnosed with conduct disorder (CD), there is a notable distinction as their behaviors consistently and extensively infringe upon the rights of others.

DEFINITION

Conduct disorder is a descriptive term utilized in academic literature to denote a consistent and enduring pattern of dissocial conduct, wherein the individual recurrently violates societal norms and engages in aggressive behavior that causes distress to others.

EPIDEMIOLOGY

The prevalence of CD is observed to be higher in boys compared to girls, with a varying ratio that can range from 4:1 to as high as 12:1. The lifetime prevalence rate of CD in the general population can range anywhere between 2% and 10%, and this prevalence remains consistent across different racial and ethnic groups. Children diagnosed with CD often experience a continuity of antisocial behaviors into adulthood, where they may be diagnosed with antisocial personality disorder (ASPD).[1] Early onset of CD during childhood is associated with a poorer prognosis for the condition. Several socioeconomic factors contribute to an increased incidence of CD in children and adolescents, including parental substance-abuse disorders and involvement in criminal activities. In a study conducted in schools of rural India, the prevalence of CDs was 5.48%.[2]

ETIOPATHOGENESIS

The etiology of CD is a multifaceted process influenced by the interaction of various factors.

- *Biological factors:* Reduced activity of the noradrenergic system and lower levels of 5-hydroxyindoleacetic acid (5-HIAA) in cerebrospinal fluid are associated with aggression and violence during adolescence. Elevated testosterone levels have also been linked to increased aggression.
- *Parental and family factors:* An unstructured and poorly supervised home environment, frequent marital conflicts, and inconsistent discipline contribute to maladaptive behavior, and so does harsh parenting involving verbal and physical aggression toward children. Exposure to frequent domestic violence, family history of criminality and disruptive behaviors, parental substance abuse (particularly alcohol dependence) and living in low socioeconomic conditions (characterized by overcrowding, unemployment and socio-economic stress) lead to inadequate parenting, which in turn predispose to disruptive behavior.
- *Neurological factors:* There is a correlation between resting frontal brain electrical activity (EEG) and aggression in children. Neuropsychological insults in early life can result in deficits in language, memory, and executive functioning; impairing judgment; problem-solving; and crisis management skills. Developmental delays, including poor social skills, learning disabilities, and below-average intellectual capacity, contribute to academic difficulties, low self-esteem, and a propensity for disruptive behaviors. Aggression can be influenced by any history of traumatic brain injury, seizures, or other neurological damage.

- *School factors:* School environments characterized by large classroom sizes and a high ratio of children to teachers coupled with a lack of positive feedback from teachers, insufficient availability of supportive staff and counseling services to address socioeconomic challenges faced by children, and exposure to increased gang violence within the community are the factors at school that may lead to the development of CD.

Comorbid Conditions

Children with difficult temperaments, poor adaptability, specific anxiety disorders, depressive or bipolar disorders, substance-related disorders, learning disorders, and frequent negative emotions are prone to having CDs. Nearly one-third of children with attention-deficit/hyperactivity disorder (ADHD) exhibit symptoms of CD or other forms of central nervous system dysfunction or damage.

Trauma-related disorders, particularly repeated physical and sexual abuse and maltreatment, may lead to a diagnosis of post-traumatic stress disorder (PTSD) or other anxiety disorders.[1]

CLINICAL PRESENTATION

Conduct disorder's clinical characteristics emerge progressively over time. This progresses to a point where a persistent, regular pattern evolves that involves violating the fundamental rights of others. Less severe oppositional defiant disorders (ODDs) have a continuum of behavior development. Since some children exhibit these behaviors while they are still developing, it is crucial for the clinician to distinguish between normal and unhealthy behavior. Remote antisocial or illegal behavior is insufficient to support a CD diagnosis. CD needs to be distinguished from terms such as delinquency. Delinquency is a term used in the law, whereas CD is a mental and behavioral illness.[3]

DIAGNOSTIC CRITERIA (DSM-5 CRITERIA)

A. An ongoing and repetitive pattern of conduct where individuals consistently breach the fundamental rights of others or significant societal norms and age-appropriate regulations is evident when a minimum of 3 out of the 15 specified criteria have been observed within the previous 12 months, with at least 1 of these criteria being observed within the most recent 6-month period.

Aggression to people and animals:
1. Frequently engages in bullying, threats, or intimidation toward others
2. Regularly instigates physical altercations
3. Has employed a potentially lethal weapon to cause significant physical harm to others (such as a bat, brick, shattered bottle, knife, or firearm)
4. Has displayed physical cruelty toward individuals
5. Has demonstrated physical cruelty toward animals
6. Has committed theft while directly confronting a victim (such as mugging, snatching purses, extortion, or armed robbery)
7. Has coerced someone into engaging in sexual activity.

Destruction of property:
8. Has willfully participated in arson with the intent of inflicting substantial harm
9. Has intentionally damaged the property of others (excluding fire setting).

Deceitfulness or theft:
10. Has unlawfully entered another person's residence, structure, or vehicle
11. Frequently tells untruths to acquire goods or favors or to evade responsibilities, essentially deceiving others
12. Has taken items of significant value without direct confrontation with a victim (e.g., shoplifting without breaking and entering, or engaging in forgery).

Serious violations of rules:
13. Frequently disregards parental restrictions by staying out at night, starting prior to the age of 13 years
14. Has left home overnight without permission at least twice while residing with parents or parental guardians, or once without returning for an extended period
15. Regularly skips school, starting prior to the age of 13 years.

B. The disturbance in behavior causes clinically significant impairment in social, academic, or occupational functioning.

C. If the individual is of age 18 years or older, the criteria are not met for ASPD.

Subtypes (onset):
- *Childhood-onset type:* Before turning 10 years old, children exhibit at least one CD symptom.

- *Adolescent-onset type:* Before the age of 10 years, individuals do not exhibit any of the CD symptoms.
- *Unspecified onset:* The criteria for a diagnosis of CD have been satisfied, but there is insufficient information to establish whether the initial symptom onset occurred before or after the age of 10 years.

Individuals with childhood-onset CD are typically male, have troubled peer connections, may have experienced early childhood ODD, and typically exhibit all of the CD symptoms before puberty. Aggression toward others may be more common in people with the childhood-onset type than in people with the adolescent-onset type.

Specifiers:
- *With limited prosocial emotions:* To qualify for this specifier, an individual must have displayed at least two of the characteristics persistently over at least 12 months and in multiple relationships and settings.
- *Lack of remorse or guilt:* Does not feel bad or guilty when he or she does something wrong (exclude remorse when expressed only when caught and/or facing punishment).
- *Callous—lack of empathy:* Disregards and is unconcerned about the feelings of others.
- *Unconcerned about performance:* Does not show concern about poor/problematic performance at school, at work, or in other important activities. Even when expectations are clear, the person fails to put in the necessary effort to perform successfully and frequently places the blame for their poor performance on others.
- *Shallow or deficient affect:* Does not convey emotions or express feelings to others except in ways that come out as shallow, fake, or superficial.

Severity:
- *Mild:* Few, if any, conduct issues beyond those necessary for diagnosis are present, and those that are present tend to hurt others in very small ways (e.g., truancy, lying, staying out at night without permission, other rule breaking).
- *Moderate:* The amount of conduct issues and their impact on others fall in the middle of the "mild" and "severe" categories (e.g., vandalism, theft without confronting a victim).
- *Severe:* Many conduct issues are present that go beyond what is necessary to make the diagnosis, or these issues seriously affect other people (e.g., forced sex, use of a weapon, physical abuse, breaking and entering, stealing while confronting a victim).[4]

DIFFERENTIAL DIAGNOSIS (TABLE 1)
- Oppositional Defiant Disorder
- Attention-deficit/hyperactivity disorder
- Depressive and bipolar disorders
- Intermittent explosive disorders
- Adjustment disorders.[4]

ASSESSMENT

Although CD is a commonly encountered presentation in child and adolescent mental health settings, its manifestation is highly diverse, posing challenges in the assessment process. Assessing CD requires a comprehensive and multidimensional approach that involves interviews with the child, parents, and possibly other informants, along with collateral information from various sources. The inclusion of a physical examination and assessment of mental status, mood disturbances, impulsivity, and comorbidities further contribute to a thorough evaluation of the individual's condition.[5]

The following organized diagnostic schedule might be used during the assessment procedure:
- Diagnostic interview schedule for children (DISC-IV)

TABLE 1: Differential diagnosis of conduct disorders.		
Differential diagnosis	**Similarity**	**Difference**
ADHD	Hyperactivity/impulsive behavior	Does not violate societal norms or the rights of others
ODD	Symptoms that bring conflict with adults and other authority figures	Less severe, no aggression toward others, no destruction
Depressive and bipolar disorders	Aggressive/irritability	Mood disturbance
Intermittent explosive disorders	Aggression	Limited to impulsive aggression and not premediated
Adjustment disorders	Conduct disturbances	Not repetitive or persistent
(ADHD: attention-deficit hyperactivity disorder; ODD: oppositional defiant disorder)		

- Diagnostic interview for children and adolescents (DICA)
- Schedule for affective disorders and schizophrenia for school-age children (K-SADS)
- Child and adolescent psychiatric assessment (CAPA).

DISC-IV and DICA are structured interviews and do not require trained professionals to be administered, while K-SADS and CAPA should be administered by trained professionals.[3]

The Achenbach's child behavior checklist had an Indian-adapted version and is known as childhood psychopathology measurement schedule (CPMS). It is a semi-structured interview schedule having 75 symptoms and has a designated section on CD symptoms, and it gives a dimensional score. It is standardized on Indian children with good reliability (0.88–0.98) and validity. With a cutoff score of >10, CPMS has 82% sensitivity and 87% specificity.[3]

MANAGEMENT

Early Intervention

Early intervention is crucial for addressing anger, aggression, and antisocial behavior in youth. Providing an opportunity for open dialogue and assessment within the primary care setting allows a pediatrician to take the following steps:
- Establishing therapeutic rapport
- Assessing symptoms and associated factors
- Guided self-help intervention
- Special school-based education evaluation
- Media-based parenting intervention.[5]

Guided self-help interventions involve providing educational material such as pamphlets, books, videos, and online resources. When problematic behavior predominantly occurs at school, a special education evaluation's role can be explained to parents. The plan, which has the potential to be formalized under an individualized education program (IEP) or a 504 plan, aims to avoid disciplinary proceedings. Similarly, an example of media-based parenting intervention is Positive Parenting Program (Triple P).[5]

Primary care settings with integrated mental health clinicians can offer brief parent training programs to all parents of young children (universal prevention) and such programs, which are designed for children ranging from toddlers to 12 years old, have demonstrated their effectiveness in enhancing parenting abilities, bolstering parental mental well-being, and addressing emotional and behavioral issues. As an example, the Incredible Years program offers a universal prevention variant consisting of six to eight sessions. This program is specifically tailored to empower parents in fostering emotional regulation, nurturing social competence, facilitating effective problem-solving, and promoting early reading readiness among children aged 2–6 years old. A longer 12–20-session version focuses on strengthening parent–child interactions, reducing harsh discipline, and fostering emotional, social, and language development in toddler to school-age children.

For young individuals who persist in displaying mild to moderate behavior issues following guided self-help or brief parent training, or for those who initially manifest moderate to severe behavior problems, comorbid conditions, or have a history of child maltreatment, severe family dysfunction, or psychopathology, it becomes imperative to conduct a thorough assessment and administer treatment in specialized mental health settings. In this context, the involvement of qualified mental health clinicians with expertise in child and adolescent mental health is crucial for delivering comprehensive care to these individuals.

Cognitive-behavioral Therapy

Cognitive-behavioral therapy (CBT) appears to be effective in addressing disruptive behavior in youth. Typical CBT techniques encompass various strategies, such as identifying the triggers and outcomes of disruptive or aggressive behavior, acquiring skills for recognizing and managing anger expression, problem-solving, employing cognitive restructuring techniques, and practicing modeling and rehearsal of socially acceptable behaviors to replace aggressive reactions. CBT programs usually consist of a series of 16–20 weekly sessions for effective implementation.

Multicomponent Treatments

Multicomponent treatments aim to address the broader social context of CD. For instance, one approach, known as multidimensional treatment foster care, involves a range of interventions. This includes training and providing support for foster parents, offering family therapy for biological parents, teaching youth anger management, social skills, and problem-solving techniques, implementing school-based interventions, providing academic support, and offering psychiatric consultation with

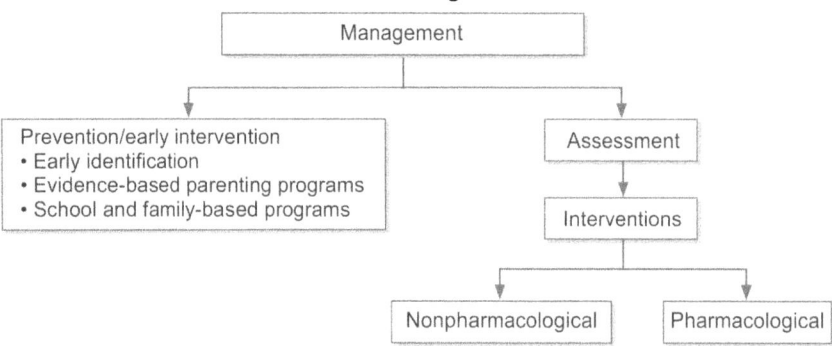

Flowchart 1: Assessment and management of conduct disorders.

medication management when necessary. Another approach is multisystem therapy, which typically spans 3–5 months and incorporates various components such as social competence training, parent and family skills training, medication management, academic engagement strategies, school interventions, peer mediation, mentoring, and collaboration with child-serving agencies.

It is worth noting that while these multicomponent programs have been classified as "probably efficacious," the supporting evidence is limited in terms of rigor. Certain factors that may predict nonresponse to multicomponent treatments include a higher frequency of rule-breaking behavior and predatory aggression, elevated psychopathy scores, and the presence of comorbid mood disorders.

Pharmacotherapy

Stimulants and atypical antipsychotics are two kinds of drugs that have a great track record of controlling impulsive, enraged aggression, although they are not approved by the Food and Drug Administration (FDA) for this specific indication. In resource-limited settings, primary care providers may provide pharmacotherapy with regular consultation from a child and adolescent psychiatrist to ensure safety and efficacy. In children with ADHD, stimulants have had positive effects on aggressive and oppositional behavior. The dosages prescribed for aggression are comparable to those prescribed for ADHD (the typical methylphenidate dosage is 1 mg/kg/day). Children aged 5–18 years have shown that risperidone is effective in lowering aggression and behavioral issues. For children and teenagers, the recommended typical daily dose of risperidone is 1.5–2 and 2–4 mg, respectively, for extreme aggressiveness. Children and adolescents are given the initial starting dosages of 0.25 and 0.5 mg, respectively, and are thereafter titrated up to the recommended daily amount as needed and tolerated.[5]

In order to ensure reliability and effectiveness, trials of medications should be conducted in a methodical manner and for an appropriate amount of time. For atypical antipsychotics, a general trial period of 6–8 weeks is recommended to accurately determine the effectiveness of the medication. The main goal of the short-term treatment phase is to reduce aggressive symptoms by at least 50%, as measured using a standardized rating scale. Remission of symptoms is the main objective of treatment, which means that the symptoms fall below the clinical cut point on the rating scale.

If there is insufficient evidence of response to the maximum tolerated dose within 8 weeks, it may be appropriate to consider trying a second medication from the same class. However, it is important to exercise caution to avoid unnecessary polypharmacy. This can be achieved, in part, by discontinuing medications that have not shown significant benefits.

It is important to note that discontinuation of the medication should be considered after a symptom-free period has been achieved, indicating that the medication is no longer necessary **(Flowchart 1)**.

FOLLOW-UP

These children and their families should be on regular follow-up by a multidisciplinary team. It should be ensured that they return to their routine activities including schools and social interactions.

PROGNOSIS

The presence of positive role models in a child's life, affectionate parenting, and emotional regulation skills, including self-soothing early intervention and effective parenting strategies, protects against the development of CD. People with the childhood-onset type are more likely than those with the adolescent-onset type to develop chronic CD into adulthood. Adolescent-onset CD sufferers frequently exhibit conduct issues around other people, but they tend to have more normative peer connections.[4]

PREVENTION

The prevention of CD is a crucial aspect of intervention, and the integration of multiple intervention strategies can yield additional benefits. Addressing multiple risk factors in interventions has shown increased effectiveness.

The FAST Track (Families and Schools Together) Program is a preventive intervention program for managing CD that was created by the Conduct Problems Prevention Research Group. The goal of this program is to improve the child's psychosocial competence in a variety of contexts, including the home and classroom. This preventive strategy can lower the incidence of behavior issues, strained social ties, and school dropout rates. The 10-year program featured instruction for parents on behavior management as well as instruction for kids on enhancing their social and cognitive abilities. The initiative included a universal school program, home visits, mentorship, and tutoring. The biggest impacts were shown after grade 9, with the results showing a substantial interaction between the intervention and the original risk level at each age. The intervention group showed notable improvements, particularly in fewer diagnoses of CD and other externalizing illnesses, as well as in fewer instances of antisocial behavior. The people who were initially at the greatest risk felt these consequences the most strongly.

CONCLUSION

Early adolescent substance use, high-intensity argumentative/defiant behavior, aggression toward people/animals (both low and high intensity), deceitfulness/stealing (high intensity), peer problems (high intensity), destruction of property (high intensity), and inappropriate sexual behavior are just a few examples of risk factors connected to the future development of CD. It is crucial to identify these risk factors. These elements need to be recognized and targeted for quick action. Evidence-based parenting programs have proved cost-efficiency and effectiveness in lowering the persistence of CD throughout adulthood, particularly ASPD. Additionally, numerous school-based initiatives have demonstrated efficacy in avoiding CD.[3]

REFERENCES

1. Mohan L, Yilanli M, Ray S. Conduct disorder. In: StatPearls [Internet]. Treasure Island (FL): StatPearls Publishing; 2023.
2. Mishra N, Mishra A and Dwivedi R. Prevalence of conduct disorder in primary school children of rural area. J Evol Med Dent Sci. 2015;4(12):1977-22.
3. Sagar R, Patra BN, and Patil V. Clinical Practice Guidelines for the Management of Conduct Disorder. Indian J Psychiatry. 2019;61(Suppl 2):270-6.
4. Burke JD, Burt SA, Coccaro EF, Grant JE. Disruptive, impulse-control and conduct disorders. American Psychiatric Association. Diagnostic and Statistical Manual of Mental Disorders DSM-5-TR, 5th edition. Washington, DC: American Psychiatric Publishing; 2013. pp. 738-47.
5. Heather J. Walter and David R. DeMaso. Disruptive, impulse-control, and conduct disorders. In: Kliegman RM, St Geme III JW, Blum NJ, Shah SS, Tasker RC, Wilson K (Eds). Nelson Textbook of Pediatrics, 21st edition. Philadelphia: Elsevier; 2020. pp. 236-40.

Chapter 12: Substance Abuse in Children: A Growing Concern

PC Khatri, Nimish Khatri, Shaina Raheja

INTRODUCTION

Substance use among children and adolescents is a public health concern all across the globe.[1] The onset of substance abuse during the formative years interferes with academic, social, and life skills development and warrants both primary and secondary prevention.[2] The incidence of drug abuse among children and adolescents is higher than the general population as adolescence age is a period for experimentation and identity forming.

From time immemorial in our country, many substances have been in practice to get happiness and have been labeled as "joy giver" and "liberator". The Vedas, the sacred texts of our country, describe *somras* and cannabis (*bhang*) for this purpose. Still, many Sadhus or ascetics consume these to experience hallucinations and a sense of timelessness. Bhang drinking has social acceptance in many parts of India.[3]

The current scenario concerning drug abuse and dependency among adolescents has evolved into a global concern and has reached a worrying level in India as well. This escalation can, in part, be attributed to the aging baby boomer generation, which had great exposure to drugs, alcohol, and tobacco from a younger age.[4,5] Such early exposure is reported to be a risk factor for the subsequent use and abuse of these substances. It is imperative to address substance abuse promptly due to the changing trends in the prevalence of substance use and the increasing magnitude of this issue.

Every year, on June 26, the International Day Against Drug Abuse and Illicit Trafficking is observed to raise awareness, particularly among young people, about the dangers of drug abuse. This observance draws inspiration from Lin Zexu's efforts to combat the scourge of drug abuse.

PREVALENCE IN INDIA

One of the major issues affecting children's and adolescents' health and behavior is substance misuse. As high as 22.8% of Indian population is of adolescents; hence, the issue should have raised alarms but on the contrary the issue is poorly recognized and grossly underestimated.[6,7] It is crucial to note that substance abuse commences during adolescence in as high as 70% cases. A study conducted by Reddy and Chandrashekhar in 1998 unveiled an overall substance-use prevalence of 6.9 per 1,000 individuals in India, with urban and rural rates standing at 5.8 and 7.3 per 1,000 population, respectively. The problem is more common in males (11.9%) than in females (1.7%). Additionally, the prevalence of inhalant abuse among individuals aged 10–17 years is 1.17%, which surpasses the prevalence in the age group above 18 years (0.58%). Opioid abuse is prevalent in 1.8% of individuals aged 10–17 years, similar to the prevalence in the age group above (2.1%). Furthermore, alcohol abuse affects 1.3% of children aged 10–17 years, while cannabis abuse is seen in 0.9% of this same age group.[8]

In India, both street kids and enrolled students take a variety of drugs. The prevalence rate for street kids has been shown to be as high as 82.98%, whereas the corresponding figure for school kids is 18%.[9,10] The ratio of in-school children to out-of-school or street children in a major, nationwide study (2013) of substance-abusing youngsters was 0.37.[11]

WHAT IS SUBSTANCE ABUSE?

Substance abuse refers to the nonmedical use of chemical substances with the goal of altering one's psychological functioning.

It is characterized by a pattern of drug use that leads to significant impairment or distress, as outlined in the DSM-5 (Diagnostic and Statistical Manual of Mental Disorders, Fifth Edition).[12] To diagnose a substance-use disorder (SUD), an individual must exhibit at least two of the following symptoms within a given year:[12]

1. Increased use of a substance than initially planned or for a longer duration than intended
2. Inability to reduce substance use despite a desire to do so
3. Spending a considerable amount of time acquiring, using, or recovering from substance use
4. Experiencing cravings or intense urges to use
5. Continued substance use causing difficulties in meeting important social, professional, or personal obligations
6. Persistent use despite the awareness that it is causing problems at work, school, or home
7. Giving up or reducing involvement in important social, professional, or leisure activities due to substance use
8. Using substances in physically hazardous situations or causing physical or mental harm
9. Continued use despite awareness of substance-related physical or mental problems
10. Developing tolerance, requiring increasing amounts of a substance to achieve desired effects
11. Experiencing withdrawal symptoms as substance levels decrease in the body.

SYMPTOMS AND SIGNS OF SUBSTANCE ABUSE

- Increased tolerance or the need for higher doses to achieve the desired effect
- Appearance of withdrawal symptoms once the dose of substance is reduced
- Unsuccessful attempts to decrease substance use
- Spending excessive time acquiring substances
- Withdrawal from social and recreational activities, even with awareness of related physical or psychological problems
- Regular intoxication or drug-induced highs
- Deceptive behavior, particularly concerning the extent of substance use
- Avoidance of friends and family members
- Avoidance of eye contact and physical contact with parents
- Changes in eating or sleeping patterns
- Changes in peer groups
- Shifted preferences for music and movies toward those featuring drug use
- Abandoning previously enjoyed activities, such as sports or spending time with friends
- Alterations in daily routines, such as late nights and sleepovers
- Attempts to mask substance-related smells (e.g., using perfume, chewing peppermint, mouth rinsing)
- Belief that substance use is necessary for fun
- Trouble at school or with the law
- Risky behaviors, including unsafe sex or driving under the influence
- School suspension due to substance-related incidents
- Decline in academic performance
- Neglect of grooming, poor hygiene, and changes in eating and sleeping habits
- Increased isolation in the bedroom or bathroom
- Detection of injection marks, known as "track marks" (dark linear marks) commonly on the nondominant hand
- Stealing to support substance use
- Experiencing feelings of depression, hopelessness, or suicidality
- Physical symptoms such as headaches, sore throat, worsening asthma, chronic cough, chest pain, gastritis, hepatitis, needle puncture marks, and pancreatitis may indicate drug abuse.

RISK FACTORS

The substance use/abuse has no bars affecting all age groups, both sexes, and persons from all socioeconomic groups. However, certain factors as depicted below may increase the risk:

- Family history of addiction
- Mental health disorders, such as depression, attention-deficit/hyperactivity disorder (ADHD), or post-traumatic stress disorder (PTSD)
- Peer pressure is important in both drug use and abstinence.[13]
- *Familial causes:* Child–parent disharmony, poor parental supervision, child neglect, or maltreated or punished child all increase the incidence.[14,15]

TYPES OF SUBSTANCE ABUSE

- *Alcohol* intoxication leads to several behavior issues and mental changes. Coma, permanent brain damage, or even death may occur due to high alcohol levels in blood.

Early onset and heavy alcohol use in adolescents can have numerous adverse effects on their physical and psychological wellbeing. Some of these effects include the following:
- *Impaired memory function:* Excessive alcohol consumption during adolescence can lead to impaired memory function, affecting a young person's ability to learn and retain information effectively.[16,17]
- Hippocampus (a critical part of the brain responsible for memory and learning) can be damaged leading to long-lasting consequences on cognitive abilities.[18]
- Heavy alcoholic teenagers often experience a decline in school performance compared to their peers who abstain from alcohol.[17] This can result in lower grades and academic setbacks.
- Drinking is always associated with an increased risk of road accidents, physical fights, and unintentional injuries due to impaired judgment and coordination while under the influence of alcohol.[7]
- Drunk teenagers have a high incidence of engaging in risky sexual behaviors leading to early pregnancies (teen pregnancies) and exposure to sexually transmitted infections due to impaired decision-making and reduced inhibitions when intoxicated.[19]
- *Alcohol withdrawal* symptoms can occur within several hours to 4–5 days later. Signs/symptoms include sweating, rapid heartbeat, hand tremors, sleeping problems, nausea, vomiting, hallucinations, restlessness, agitation, anxiety, and occasionally seizures.

- *Marijuana, hashish, and other cannabis-containing substances:* Cannabis is consumed through smoking, ingestion, or inhaling a vaporized form. It is frequently used alongside other substances such as alcohol or illicit drugs and is often the initial drug experimented with. Persons may shift to marijuana or hashish.
- *Barbiturates, benzodiazepines, and hypnotics:* They are central nervous system (CNS) depressants:
  - *Barbiturates*—phenobarbital
  - *Benzodiazepines*—include sedatives, such as diazepam, alprazolam, lorazepam, clonazepam, and chlordiazepoxide
  - *Hypnotics*—this group encompasses drugs that induce sleep such as zolpidem and zaleplon.
- *Methamphetamines, cocaine, and other stimulants:* Stimulants encompass substances such as amphetamines, meth (methamphetamine), cocaine, methylphenidate, and amphetamine–dextroamphetamine. They are frequently used/misused to seek a "high", enhance energy, improve performance, or control appetite and weight.
- *Hallucinogens:* Lysergic acid diethylamide (LSD) and phencyclidine (PCP) are the most prevalent hallucinogens.
- *Inhalants:* Inhalant usage symptoms vary based on the substance, which may include glue, paint thinners, correction fluid, marker fluid, gasoline, cleaning products, and household aerosols. Due to their toxicity, users may experience brain damage or sudden fatality.
- *Opioid painkillers:* Opioids (narcotics and painkillers) are derived from opium or synthetically produced and encompass drugs such as heroin, morphine, codeine, methadone, fentanyl, and oxycodone. Nearly 70% of drug abuse deaths are due to opioids and about 30% of these deaths are due to their overdose.[20]
- *Tobacco* is an agricultural crop. Nicotine, a highly addictive substance comparable to heroin and cocaine, is found in tobacco. It is typically smoked, but can also be chewed or absorbed through the gums.[21] The mean age of initiation is 18 years (8.4% students are in 13–15 years age) in India and the mean age of initiation of tobacco abuse in Rajasthan is 18.4 years (4.1% of students are in 13–15 years age).[22] *Bidis* are thin, hand-rolled, filter-less cigarettes consisting of flavored or unflavored tobacco wrapped in a tendu or temburni leaf, commonly used by the lower socio-economic class as a source of tobacco.
- *E-cigarettes/vaping/hookahs* are devices that produce an aerosol by heating a liquid containing nicotine and other chemicals. They represent an alternative form of nicotine consumption.

LEGAL SYSTEM IN INDIA

The Narcotic Drugs and Psychotropic Substances (NDPS) Act of 1985, applicable to all states and union territories, prohibits the production, possession, cultivation, sale/purchase, transport, store, and consumption of narcotic drugs and psychotropic drugs.[23] Additionally, six drugs (morphine, fentanyl, methadone, oxycodone, codeine, and hydrocodone) used in medical science were included under this Act.[24] National programs such as

Rashtriya Kishor Swasthya Karyakram (National Adolescent Health Policy) and Scheme of Prevention of Alcoholism and Substance (Drugs) Abuse (SPASA) have been designed to prevent the menace of drug use/abuse.[25]

SCREENING OF SUBSTANCE ABUSE IN ADOLESCENTS[26,27]

The National Institute of Drug Abuse (NIDA) has introduced two online screening tools for providers to assess SUD risk among adolescents aged 12–17 years. These tools, S2BI (Screening to brief Intervention) and BSTAD (Brief Screener for Tobacco, Alcohol, and other Drugs), categorize patients based on risk levels. Depending upon the frequency of usage in the past year, they are classified into no reported use, low-risk, and high-risk groups.

How does One Decide on which Tool to Select?

It is crucial to choose an empirically validated tool based on provider preference. These tools can be self-administered and serve to normalize discussions about substance use, promote healthy behaviors, identify at-risk individuals, and guide interventions. The advantages inherent in the utilization of these tools encompass the following:

- Facilitating open dialogues with adolescents regarding substance use in a manner that fosters normalization
- The endorsement and encouragement of salubrious behaviors and decision-making
- The discernment of adolescents who may exhibit susceptibility to SUD
- Providing guidance for the implementation of concise interventions and the facilitation of referrals for appropriate treatment when warranted.

PREVENTION AND INTERVENTION IN INDIA

Nonschool and street children are significant contributors to the issue of SUDs. Community-based prevention has been the primary focus in India, with a higher prevalence noted among these children.[9,11] Strategies targeting both educational institutions and the broader community seem imperative. Pertinently, the 2015 revision of the SPASA, under "preventive education and awareness generation", mentions targeting children both "in and outside educational institutions".[28] Instating "inside", i.e., school-based prevention (SBP) programs, in addition to the already in-place "outside", i.e., community-based prevention, for substance use seems to be definitely necessary.

Universal and selected SBP models in India are guided by three key approaches: Social resistance skills training (SRST), normative education (NE), and competence enhancement skills training (CEST).[29] These models detailed in **Table 1** aim to address substance-use issues.

Among the various programs evaluated for their effectiveness in universal SBPs, a Cochrane systematic review identified the "good behavior game (GBG)", "life skills training (LST)", and the "unplugged" programs

TABLE 1: Principal approaches guiding universal and selected prevention of substance use disorders in schools.

	Assumption	Training methods
SRST	Adolescents begin to use drugs largely because they lack the confidence or skills to resist social influences to smoke, drink, or use illicit drugs	• Teaching students to recognize high-risk situations • Increasing the awareness of media influences • Refusal skills training
NE	Adolescents generally overestimate the prevalence of smoking, drinking, and illicit drug use among other adolescents and adults	• Information about the prevalence of drug use from national or local surveys • Conduct own surveys
CEST	Drug-use behavior is learned through a process of modeling, imitation, and reinforcement and is influenced by an adolescent's prodrug cognitions, attitudes, and beliefs	• Self-management and social skills • Decision-making and problem-solving skills • Assertiveness skills • Increasing personal control • Enhancing self-esteem • Adaptive coping strategies for managing stress and anxiety

(CEST: competence enhancement skills training; NE: normative education; SRST: social resistance skills training)
Source: Adapted from Pattojoshi A, Tikka SK. School-based substance use disorder prevention in India: A brief appraisal. Indian J Psychiatry. 2020;62(4):427-30.

as the most successful.[30] The GBG, implemented in first- and second-grade classrooms in elementary schools, focuses on promoting positive classroom behaviors such as "working quietly" and "being polite to others". It is a straightforward behavior management method provided by teachers. LST primarily targets middle-school children but also extends its reach to elementary and high-school students. It involves a curriculum spanning 30 class sessions over 3 years. School teachers primarily deliver this program, although peer leaders and health professionals can also be involved.

The United Nations Office on Drugs and Crime (UNODC) and the Ministry of Social Justice and Empowerment, Government of India, have launched a life skills-based, teacher-conducted school drug awareness program called "I Decide - I Will Not Take Drugs". Additionally, there is the "Project-Mobilizing Youth for Tobacco-Related Initiatives (MYTRI)" in India.

MANAGEMENT OF SUBSTANCE ABUSE

In cases of intoxication, a systematic approach known as ABCDE should be employed for patient assessment. Early resuscitation plays a critical role in saving the lives of intoxicated patients. The primary management of substance overdose involves providing supportive care.[31]

Airway and antidotes: Intoxication often leads to CNS depression, altered consciousness, and increased secretions compromising the airway. Airway patency management may require intubation. In cases of secured airway, consider administering antidotes as needed.

Breathing: Support breathing with supplemental oxygen and monitor oxygen saturation during treatment. Ventilator support may be necessary in severe intoxication.

Circulation: Initiate cardiac monitoring and conduct ECG. Secure intravenous access for fluid administration. Adequate hydration is crucial in cases of intoxication.

Disability: Create a calm environment for managing the patient. Initial management of agitation should involve verbal de-escalation. If there is a poor response or aggressive behavior, consider pharmacological management, including the use of benzodiazepines. Rule out hypoglycemia, a rapidly reversible cause of agitation. Actively manage seizures with benzodiazepines and address cardiac dysrhythmias and metabolic abnormalities.

Exposure: Manage hyperthermia by employing effective cooling measures and treat any associated injuries. Various signs and symptoms of substance use in adolescents are summarised below **(Table 2)**.

TABLE 2: Acute signs and symptoms of substance use in adolescents.

	RS	CVS/autonomic	CNS	GIT
Cannabis	Frequent respiratory infections, cough	Tachycardia, sweating, tremors, high fever, chills	*Psychological disturbances:* Depersonalization, decreased inhibition, disorientation, altered mood, lack of attention, memory impairment	Pain in the abdomen, vomiting
Opioids (heroin, morphine, codeine, oxycodone, fentanyl)	Respiratory depression, pulmonary edema	Miosis, sweating, hypothermia, bradycardia, hypotension	*CNS depression:* Drowsiness to coma	Dry mouth, nausea, vomiting, constipation
Stimulants (cocaine, amphetamine, and MDMA)	Pulmonary edema, respiratory distress due to pulmonary barotrauma	*Autonomic effects:* Mydriasis, hyperthermia, flushing, diaphoresis, hypertension, tachycardia, arrhythmias, and myocardial depression	*CNS excitation:* Agitation, euphoria, delirium, hallucination, psychosis, seizures, hyperreflexia, tremors	Nausea, stomach pain
Benzodiazepines (lorazepam, alprazolam, diazepam, clonazepam)	Respiratory depression	Hypotension, bradycardia	CNS depression, slurred speech, ataxia, drowsiness, confusion, impaired judgment	

(CNS: central nervous system; CVS: cardiovascular system; GIT: gastrointestinal tract; RS: respiratory system)
Source: Adapted from Sathanantham S, Dayasiri K, Thadchanamoorthy V. Approach to the adolescent with substance use in the acute setting. Cureus. 2021;13(7):e16309.

MANAGEMENT OF SPECIFIC SUBSTANCES

- *Cannabis:* In cases of cannabis intoxication, benzodiazepines can be helpful in controlling agitation.
- *Opioids:* Naloxone, an opioid antagonist, is used to treat opioid intoxication and should be administered according to respiratory effort and rate.
- *Stimulants (amphetamines, cocaine, MDMA):* For substances such as amphetamines, cocaine, and MDMA, benzodiazepines are the first-line medication to manage agitation or aggressive behavior. Neuroleptics can be considered if delusions or hallucinations are present. Hyperthermia, a potentially fatal complication, should be actively treated.
  - *Benzodiazepines:* In cases of severe intoxication associated with respiratory and neurological depression due to benzodiazepines, flumazenil, a benzodiazepine antagonist, can be used.

MANAGEMENT OF CHRONIC ABUSERS[32]

Treatment for SUD often requires ongoing care because SUD is a chronic condition with the potential for both recovery and relapse. It is generally more effective to treat co-occurring mental health conditions alongside SUD rather than separately. The three primary forms of treatment are as follows:

1. *Detoxification:* This involves discontinuing the use of the substance(s), allowing them to leave the body. Depending on the severity of SUD, a substance may be tapered off to mitigate withdrawal effects. Detoxification marks the initial significant step in SUD treatment.
2. *Cognitive and behavioral therapies:* Psychotherapy, or talk therapy, can effectively address SUD and co-existing mental health conditions. Therapy also teaches healthy coping strategies. One may recommend cognitive and behavioral therapies alone or in combination with drugs. Some examples of effective therapies are as follows:
   - *Cognitive-behavioral therapy (CBT):* It is a disciplined, outcome-driven kind of psychotherapy. An expert can assist in closely examining the thoughts as well as feelings. Negative attitudes and habits can be unlearned and the patient may learn to develop better through processes and routines.
   - *Dialectical behavior therapy (DBT):* It is useful for persons who find difficulty in controlling and regulating their emotions.
   - *Assertive community treatment (ACT):* It provides mental health services in a community setting rather than a residential or hospital setting.
   - *Therapeutic communities (TCs):* It is a long-term residential treatment program that focuses on supporting individuals with SUD in changing their attitudes and actions toward substance used and other co-occurring mental health problems.
   - *Contingency management (CM):* It promotes positive behavior by providing rewards for positive actions.
   - *Adolescent community reinforcement approach (A-CRA):* Achieve and maintain abstinence from drugs by replacing influences in their lives that had reinforced substance use.
3. *Medication-assisted therapies:* Medicine may be recommended as part of opioid addiction treatment. While medicines do not cure opioid addiction, they can aid in recovery by reducing cravings and preventing relapse. Medications for opioid addiction may include buprenorphine, methadone, naltrexone, and combinations like buprenorphine and naloxone.

Substance-use disorder patients should be managed by a team of multiple disciplines (primary care physicians, psychiatrists, etc.). Management must focus on treating person as a whole and not simply his/her substance use. The majority of these teenagers have underlying psychological issues that must be addressed. Depending upon the severity for treatment and follow-up, specialized mental health counseling or specialized treatment plans or inpatient drug rehabilitation facilities may be required.

The burden of adolescent substance use on the healthcare system is growing. A precise risk assessment, knowledge of a substance's pharmacological characteristics, and adequate supportive care are necessary for the effective management of acute substance intoxication. All concerned (patient, their caretakers, friends, and community) must be educated about both short-term and long-term effects of this menace.

KEY GAPS IN CURRENT INFRASTRUCTURE, FACILITIES, TECHNOLOGIES, POLICIES, AND PROGRAMS[33]

Several challenges and gaps exist in the current infrastructure and policies for addressing SUDs. These include a lack of adequate treatment facilities, insufficient knowledge and skills among medical personnel, fragmentation among different agencies dealing with SUDs, nonuniform policies on alcohol, limited awareness of available treatment options, insufficient community support for treatment and aftercare, lack of regulation for some treatment centers, and inadequate focus on SUDs at the state level amidst competing priorities.

LIFE-CHANGING COMPLICATIONS

Getting an infectious disease: Substance users (especially teenagers) are more likely to go for unsafe sex or sharing needles with others which ultimately may lead to infectious diseases such as human immunodeficiency virus (HIV).

Accidents: Drug-dependent children are more prone to undertaking dangerous activities under the influence.

Suicide: Drug addicts are more likely to commit suicide than nonaddicts.

Family problems: Substance usage promotes disharmony both within the house and at place of work leading to multiple family issues.

Work issues: Drug use usually declines performance at work, increases absenteeism, and ultimately may lead to loss of employment.

Problems at school: Drug usage spoils scholastic performance.

Legal issues: Possession of illegal drugs, their purchase and stealing done to fund the purchase, and driving under the influence of drugs/alcohol all may have legal consequences.

Financial problems: Allocating financial resources to sustain drug consumption diverts funds from other essential requirements potentially culminating in indebtedness and prompting engagement in illicit or morally questionable conduct.

CONCLUSION

To prevent substance abuse in adolescents, it is important to communicate with them about the risks of drug use, be supportive in their efforts to resist peer pressure, set a positive example by not misusing alcohol or drugs, strengthen the parent–child bond, and provide parental monitoring and supervision. Encourage appropriate behavior, be aware of your child's activities and friends, establish rules and consequences, monitor media exposure, and enhance their self-esteem and self-confidence through skill development, assertiveness training, critical thinking, and communication skills.

REFERENCES

1. CASA. (2011). Adolescent substance use: America's #1 public health concern. The National Centre on Addiction and Substance Abuse. Columbia University, New York. [online] Available from: https://drugfree.org/wp-content/uploads/drupal/Adolescent-substance-use-americas-no-1-public-health-problem.pdf [Last accessed October, 2023].
2. Squeglia LM, Jacobus J, Tapert SF. The influence of substance use on adolescent brain development. Clin EEG Neurosci. 2009;40:31-8.
3. Nehra KD, Sharma V, Mushtaq H, Sharma N, Sharma M, Nehra S. Emotional intelligence and self-esteem in Cannabis abusers. J Indian Acad Appl Psychol. 2012;38:385-93.
4. Gfroerer J, Penne M, Pemberton M, Folsom R. Substance abuse treatment need among older adults in 2020: The impact of the aging baby-boom cohort. Drug Alcohol Depend. 2003;69:127-35.
5. Colliver JD, Compton WM, Gfroerer JC, Condon T. Projecting drug use among aging baby boomers in 2020. Ann Epidemiol. 2006;16:257-65.
6. Ahmad Nadeem, Bano Rubeena, Agarwal VK, Kalakoti Piyush. Substance Abuse in India. Available from WHO Techn. Res Series No. 886:1999. p. 48.
7. Hingson R, Heeren T, Zakocs R. Age of drinking onset and involvement in physical fights after drinking. Paediatrics. 2001;108:872-7.
8. Ministry of Social Justice and Empowerment. (2019). [online] Available from: https://socialjustice.gov.in/whats-new/1494 [Last accessed October, 2023].
9. Sharma N, Joshi S. Preventing substance abuse among street children in India: A literature review. Health Sci J. 2013;7:137-8.
10. Pal R, Tsering D. Tobacco use in Indian high-school students. Int J Green Pharm. 2009;3:319-23.
11. Dhawan A, Pattanayak RD, Chopra A, Tikoo VK, Kumar R. Pattern and profile of children using substances in India: Insights and recommendations. Natl Med J India. 2017;30:224-9.
12. American Psychiatric Association. Diagnostic and Statistical Manual of Mental Disorders, 5th edition. Arlington, VA: American Psychiatric Association; 2013.
13. Belcher HM, Shinitzky HE. Substance abuse in children: prediction, protection and prevention. Arch Pediatr Adolesc Med. 1998;152(10):952-60.
14. Bennett EM, Kemper KJ. Is abuse during childhood a risk factor for developing substance abuse problems as an adult? J Dev Behav Pediatr. 1994;15:426-9.

15. Wilsnack SC, Vogeltanz ND, Klassen AD, Harris TR. Childhood sexual abuse and women's substance abuse: national survey findings. J Stud Alcohol. 1997;58:264-71.
16. Harris S K, Csemy L, Sherrit L, Starostova O, Van Hook S, Johnson J, et al. Computer-facilitated substance use screening and brief advice for teens in primary care: an international trial. Pediatrics. 2012;129(6):1072-82.
17. Brown SA, Tapert SF. Health consequences of adolescent alcohol involvement. In: Bonnie RJ, O'Connell ME (Eds). National Research Council (US) and Institute of Medicine (US) Committee on Developing a Strategy to Reduce and Prevent Underage Drinking. [online] Available from: https://www.ncbi.nlm.nih.gov/books/NBK37610/. [Last accessed October, 2023].
18. De Bellis MD. Hippocampal volume in adolescent onset alcohol use disorders. Am J Psychiatry. 2000;157: 737-44.
19. Tapert SF, Aaron GA, Sedlar GR, Brown SA. Adolescent substance use and sexual risk-taking behaviour. J Adolesc Health. 2001;28:181-9.
20. UNODC. (2020). World Drug Report. [online] Available from: https://wdr.unodc.org/wdr2020/index2020.html. [Last accessed October, 2023].
21. National Center for Chronic Disease Prevention and Health Promotion (US) Office on Smoking and Health. Preventing Tobacco Use among Youth and Young Adults: A Report of the Surgeon General. Atlanta (GA): Centers for Disease Control and Prevention (US); 2012. [online] Available from: https://www.ncbi.nlm.nih.gov/books/NBK99237/. [Last accessed October, 2023].
22. Global Youth Tobacco Survey (GYTS). (2019). Fact Sheet India 2019. [online] Available from: https://ntcp.mohfw.gov.in/assets/document/National_Fact_Sheet_of_fourth_round_of_Global_Youth_Tobacco_Survey_GYTS-4.pdf. [Last accessed October, 2023].
23. Central Bureau of Narcotics. Department of Revenue Gazette Notification: NDPS Rules 2015. [online] Available from: http://cbn.nic.in/en/notifications/acts_rules/ [Last accessed October, 2023].
24. Central Bureau of Narcotics. Department of Revenue Gazette Notification: Essential Narcotic Drugs [online] Available from: http://cbn.nic.in/en/notifications/circulars_notifications/ [Last accessed October, 2023].
25. Rashtriya Kishor Swasthya Karyakram (RKSK). Ministry of Health and Family Welfare, Government of India, draft 2015. [online] Available from: http://nhm.gov.in/rashtriya-kishor-swasthya-karyakram.html [Last accessed October, 2023].
26. Kelly SM, Gryczynski J, Mitchell SG, Kirk A, O'Grady KE, Schwartz RP. Validity of brief screening instrument for adolescent tobacco, alcohol, and drug use. Pediatrics. 2014;133(5):819-26.
27. Levy S, Weiss R, Sherritt L, Ziemnik R, Spalding A, Van Hook S, et al. An electronic screen for triaging adolescent substance use by risk levels. JAMA Pediatr. 2014;168(9):822-8.
28. Ministry of Social Justice and Empowerment. Central sector scheme of assistance for prevention of alcoholism and substance (drugs) Abuse and for Social Defence Services Ministry of Social Justice and Empowerment, Government of India; 2015.
29. Botvin GJ. Preventing drug abuse in schools: Social and competence enhancement approaches targeting individual-level etiologic factors. Addict Behav. 2000;25: 887-97.
30. Foxcroft DR, Tsertsvadze A. Universal school-based prevention programs for alcohol misuse in young people. Cochrane Database Syst Rev. 2011;5:CD009113.
31. Maldonado JR. An approach to the patient with substance use and abuse. Maldonado JR. Med Clin North Am. 2010; 94:1169205.
32. Cleveland Clinic. Substance use disorder. [online] Available from: https://my.clevelandclinic.org/health/diseases/16652-drug-addiction-substance-use-disorder-sud [Last accessed October, 2023].
33. National Academy of Medical Sciences (India), Directorate General of Health Services. (2023). Report of Task Force on Alcohol, Substance Use Disorders and Behavioural Addictions in India. [online] Available from: https://www.nams-india.in/downloads/Taskforce/04%20NAMS%20Task%20force%20repoAlcohol%20Substance%20Abuse.pdf [Last accessed October, 2023].

Chapter 13: Feeding and Eating Disorders

Kapil Jetha, Neeraj Gupta

INTRODUCTION

Eating disorders (EDs) are complex medical illnesses characterized by disturbance in body image, weight control, and/or dietary patterns. EDs affect the biopsychosocial aspect of health causing a negative impact on physical, mental, and emotional health and ability to function in important areas of life.

Diagnostic and Statistical Manual of Mental Disorders, Fifth Edition (DSM-5),[1] summarizes feeding disorders and ED that include the following:
- Anorexia nervosa (AN)
- Bulimia nervosa (BN)
- Binge eating disorders (BED)
- Avoidant/restrictive food intake disorder (ARFID)
- Pica
- Rumination disorder
- Other specified feeding or eating disorder (OSFED)
- Unspecified feeding or eating disorder (USFED).

DSM-5 emphasizes more on behavioral criteria than on physical and cognitive criteria, indicating that body or weight distortion should not be the main/only criterion. Early identification is important as early intervention improves outcome.

EPIDEMIOLOGY

Eating disorders in children are a growing concern with an increasing number of cases being reported worldwide. However, the research is limited in children, and available data provide some insights into the prevalence and patterns of ED in children. Prevalence estimates range from 0.3% to 2.6% in children aged 8–14 years;[2] however, these estimates may vary depending on the diagnostic criteria and methodology used. A population-based study from Germany[3] reported that 4.98% of participants displayed a recurrent pica behavior and 1.49% displayed a rumination behavior in children aged 7–14 years.

Anorexia nervosa typically starts in late childhood or early adolescence, while ARFID can appear in early childhood.[4] Gender distribution is almost equal in younger children with ED, particularly for ARFID.[2,5] The exact cause of ED is unknown. Risk factors include genetics, family factors, social pressures, and psychological factors such as perfectionism and body dissatisfaction.[6,7] ED often co-occur (>70%) with psychiatric comorbidities, which include anxiety disorders, substance abuse, obsessive–compulsive disorder (OCD), and attention deficit hyperactivity disorder (ADHD) in children.[7-9] Any psychiatric disorder increases the risk of ED. People with diabetes have an increased prevalence of ED and an increased risk of diabetic complications and premature death, especially if insulin omission is used to compensate for eating.[10-14] Rarely ED may be seen along with celiac and other autoimmune disorders such as Crohn's (bidirectional associations).[15]

There is a paucity of research from India; Srinivasan et al.[16] found that 14.8% of study population had the syndrome of eating distress in a research conducted on 210 medical students in Chennai utilizing the eating attitudes test (EAT) and BITE self-report questionnaires. Iyer et al.[17] recently conducted a research on 332 students at a medical college in South India; 13% of students had a high risk of developing eating problems. Males and females were nearly equally affected. A significant level of stress and serious body image problems were linked to an increased risk of EDs. History of therapy, peer pressure, excessive exercise, and any behavioral signs, such as the use of laxatives and diet medications, were additional indicators.

A BRIEF DISCUSSION ON VARIOUS EATING DISORDERS

Anorexia Nervosa

Anorexia nervosa is characterized by a significantly low weight for age (the weight that is less than minimally normal), fear of gaining weight (despite being underweight), and a disturbance in the perception of body shape or weight (e.g., a denial of the medical seriousness of being underweight or feeling fat despite emaciation).[1]

Anorexia nervosa can be further divided into two types: restrictive type and binge eating/purging type. The restrictive type will have nonpurging behaviors to control weight such as fasting, skipping meals, and excessive physical activity, while binge eating/purging type will have behaviors such as diuretic abuse, laxative and/or enema abuse, and self-induced vomiting (use of ipecac abuse) to purge calories to reduce weight.[1]

The minimum level of severity of AN has been defined based on body mass index (BMI) for adults and corresponding BMI percentiles (for children and adolescents)[1] **(Table 1)**.

Bulimia Nervosa

Bulimia nervosa is characterized by recurrent binge eating along with inappropriate compensatory behaviors to control weight or to purge calories consumed during the binge. To meet the diagnostic criteria, these behaviors must occur at least once/week for 3 months. BN is also accompanied by excessive influence of weight and/or shape on body image.[1] Binge eating is defined as consumption of excessive amounts of food during a discrete period and accompanied by the feeling that eating cannot be controlled.

Severity of BN is based on the frequency of inappropriate compensatory behaviors[1] **(Table 2)**.

Binge Eating Disorder

Binge eating disorder is one in which binge eating is not followed by inappropriate compensatory behaviors. BED can be differentiated from nonpathologic overeating by associated symptoms, including rapid eating, eating irrespective of hunger or satiety, eating alone because of shame, and negative feelings after a binge.

Avoidant/Restrictive Food Intake Disorder

Avoidant/restrictive food intake disorder has been recently introduced as a type of feeding disorder and ED

TABLE 1: Severity of anorexia nervosa (AN) has been defined based on body mass index (BMI).

Severity of AN	BMI (kg/m^2)
Mild	17–18.5
Moderate	16–16.99
Severe	15–15.99
Extreme	<15

Courtesy: Dr Jinali Sheth.

TABLE 2: Severity of bulimia nervosa (BN) is based on the frequency of inappropriate compensatory behaviors.

Severity of BN	Inappropriate compensatory behaviors
Mild	1–3 episodes/week
Moderate	4–7 episodes/week
Severe	8–13 episodes/week
Extreme	14 or more episodes/week

Courtesy: Dr Jinali Sheth.

in DSM-5. ARFID should be considered in those who have food restrictions or avoidance without shape or weight concerns or without intentional efforts to lose weight.[1] Absence of body image concerns differentiate ARFID from other EDs. ARFID may result in significant weight loss, nutritional deficiencies, and impaired functioning.[18]

The exact causes of ARFID are not known but may involve sensory sensitivity, negative food experiences, anxiety and genetic factors, and are usually associated with disturbances in psychological development and functioning.[19]

Patients may have highly selective eating, limited food acceptance, neophobia (fear of new things) related to food types, and high sensitivity for food tastes, textures and appearances. It also applies to individuals who have a lack of interest in eating or have a low appetite. As this is a new entity, the exact prevalence is not known, but most are cases that were diagnosed as unspecified or nonspecific feeding disorder in DSM-IV. ARFID affects individuals of all ages but is more common in children and adolescents. Estimates suggest a prevalence of 5–14% in ED clinics. Certain reports have found very high prevalence, ranging between 20% and 30%.

Treatment typically includes psychobehavioral therapy with a multidisciplinary approach for nutrition, exposure therapy, and cognitive behavioral therapy (CBT). Medications also help in managing ARFID. Drugs such as olanzapine, cyproheptadine, fluoxetine, risperidone, and aripiprazole have been tried successfully in case reports.[20]

Pica

Pica is a condition characterized by persistent ingestion of nonfood/non-nutritive items (dirt, chalk, paint chips, hair, paper, etc.) over a period of at least 1 month and is commonly seen in young children.

Etiology is most likely to be multifactorial but may include exploratory behavior, self-stimulation or seeking sensory feedback, self-soothing, or nutritional deficiencies. Occasional mouthing of nonfood objects is considered normal in children <2 years of age; pica becomes a concern when it occurs regularly and persists beyond toddlerhood. It is often associated with nutritional deficiencies, developmental disorders, psychiatric disorders such as OCD, schizophrenia, or sensory issues (autism).

Pica can lead to serious health risks, including poisoning, intestinal blockages, anemia, dental injury, or infections. It might be associated with other feeding disorders. In terms of treatment, the current focus is predominantly on behavioral interventions and appropriate management of environment.[21,22] Evidence is limited for the use of medical management in the treatment of pica.[23]

Rumination Disorder

Rumination disorder is a type of ED in which there is repetitive regurgitation and rechewing of food that has already been swallowed. It typically affects infants, children, and individuals with intellectual disabilities and children with abuse or neglect. The regurgitated food may be spat out or reswallowed. It usually looks like a habit disorder and is often perceived as pleasurable by the child, with increase in intensity during stress and anxiety. Unlike vomiting, which is involuntary and usually organic, rumination is a deliberate behavior.

The exact cause of rumination disorder is unclear, but it is believed to be influenced by a combination of physiological, psychological, and environmental factors. It can lead to weight loss, malnutrition, persistent smell of gastric acid from mouth, dental decay due to enamel erosion, and social difficulties. Diagnosis is usually straightforward with good history, but sometimes high-resolution esophageal manometry is required.[24] Gastroesophageal reflux is an important differential.

Treatment involves mainly behavioral approaches with habit-reversal training and cognitive behavioral therapy in older children. There is a limited role of pharmacological treatment and is not recommended as first-line intervention. **Table 3** summarises important clinical features of various feeding and eating disorders which can be of help in exact diagnosis of the condition.

SCREENING TOOLS FOR EATING DISORDERS

Several tools are available to assist in the early detection of EDs. They cannot be used as a diagnostic tool and should be used to identify when a comprehensive evaluation is required.

The eating disorder screen for primary care (ESP),[25] SCOFF,[26] and eating disorders examination questionnaire (EDE-Q)[27] are commonly used validated tools **(Table 4)**.

DETAILED EVALUATION

A detailed evaluation includes a thorough medical, nutritional, and psychiatric history followed by a detailed

TABLE 3: Distinguishing features of feeding and eating disorders.

Type of ED	Importance of weight	Restrictive-pattern eating	Binge eating behavior	Purging behavior	Body image concern
AN	Significantly underweight	Typically	May be present	May occur in half of the cases	Yes
BN	Usually normal weight or overweight	May occur as a behavior to control weight	Must occur at an average of once per week for at least 3 months	Must occur on an average of once per week to meet diagnostic criteria	Yes
BED	Usually overweight or obese	No	Must occur at an average of once per week for at least 3 months	No	Yes
ARFID	Significantly underweight	Typically	No	No	No
Pica	Variable	No	No	No	No
Rumination disorder	Variable	No	No	No (voluntary regurgitation occurs)	No

(AN: anorexia nervosa; ARFID: avoidant restrictive food intake disorder; BED: binge eating disorder; BN: bulimia nervosa; ED: eating disorder)

TABLE 4: Tools to assist in the early detection of EDs.

ESP	SCOFF	EDE-Q

• Are you satisfied with your eating patterns?
• Do you ever eat in secret?
• Does your weight affect the way you feel about yourself?
• Have any members of your family suffered with an eating disorder?
• Do you currently suffer with, or have you ever suffered in the past, with an eating disorder?
  – A "no" to question 1 is classified as an abnormal response
  – A "yes" to questions 2–5 is classified as an abnormal response
  – Any abnormal response indicates that the client needs further assessment
	• S: Do you make yourself Sick because you feel uncomfortably full?
	• C: Do you worry you have lost Control over how much you eat?
	• O: Have you recently lost more than One stone (6.35 kg) in a 3-month period?
	• F: Do you believe yourself to be Fat when others say you are too thin?
	• F: Would you say Food dominates your life?
	• An answer of "yes" to two or more questions indicates the need for a more comprehensive assessment.[28] A further two questions with SCOFF have been shown to have a high sensitivity and specificity to bulimia nervosa. These questions are not diagnostic but would indicate further questioning and discussion is required: 1. Are you satisfied with your eating patterns? 2. Do you ever eat in secret?
		Can be accessed by this link https://insideoutinstitute.org.au/assessment?started=true Or by scanning this QR code 

(ESP: eating disorder screen for primary care; EDE-Q: eating disorders examination questionnaire)

clinical examination. In adolescents, a full psychosocial assessment including home, education, activity, drugs/diet, sexuality, suicidality/depression (HEADSS) assessment is important.

A thorough clinical examination with close attention to anthropometry (weight and BMI) and vitals is extremely important and tells about signs of medical compromise in EDs **(Table 5)**. Low resting heart rate, resting BP, and low body temperature for age suggest energy restriction. Orthostatic hypotension and tachycardia [heart rate (HR) and blood pressure (BP) taken after 5 minutes of supine rest and then repeated after 3 minutes of standing revealing tachycardia or a drop of systolic BP >20 mm Hg or drop of diastolic BP >10 mm Hg] indicate either volume depletion due to restricted fluid intake or purging, or a compromised cardiovascular status.[29]

TABLE 5: Relevant signs of eating disorder.

Features related to reduced energy intake	*Features related to purging*	*Features related to overeating and excess energy intake*
• Poor growth trajectories • Abnormal vitals (hypotension, resting bradycardia, orthostatic tachycardia or hypotension, hypothermia) • Flat/anxious appearance • Pallor, dull, yellow or pale brown skin, carotenemia—palm and soles • Cachectic, wasting, loss of subcutaneous fat, facial wasting • Dull, dry, thin, lusterless scalp hairs, lanugo • Cardiac murmur (one-third with mitral valve prolapse), cool extremities, acrocyanosis, poor perfusion • Stool mass left lower quadrant • Delayed or interrupted pubertal development • Small breasts; vaginal dryness • Small testes	• *Abnormal vital signs:* Orthostatic increase in HR (>40 beats per min) or decrease in BP (>10 mm Hg in diastolic) • Angular stomatitis • Palatal scratches; dental enamel erosions • Russell's sign (abrasion or callous on knuckles from self-induced emesis) • Salivary gland enlargement (parotid and submandibular) • Epigastric tenderness • Bruising or abrasions over the spine (related to excessive exercise or sit-ups)	• Deviation from previous growth trajectory when plotted on growth charts • Obesity • Elevated BP or hypertension • Acanthosis nigricans, acne, hirsutism • Hepatomegaly • Premature puberty • Musculoskeletal pain

Relevant history points
1. How long is the illness?
2. History of weight trend/weight loss—highest recorded weight, its date, any history with symptom of bingeing or purging, ask methods used to lose weight—laxatives, diuretics, diet pills, increased exercise
3. Diet history—emphasis on carbs restriction, fasting, reducing food portion, increasing intake of fluids
4. Exercise—if yes, then ask for intensity, type, duration, and frequency
5. Menstrual history—oligo/amenorrhea
6. Any history of anxiety, depression, obsessive–compulsive disorder, sexual/physical abuse, substance abuse, psychiatric illness
7. Family history of obesity, psychiatric illness

Laboratory evaluation is not required for diagnosis but to rule out complications or alternative diagnoses. Typical initial tests include complete blood count, serum electrolytes, liver function tests (LFTs), calcium, phosphorous, blood glucose, thyroid function test, and urinalysis.[30] Normal tests do not exclude the presence of complications or need for hospitalization for medical stabilization. Additional tests can be planned according to signs and symptoms (e.g., urine pregnancy test, serum gonadotropin levels and serum prolactin for amenorrhea, ECG for cardiovascular compromise or electrolyte imbalance, serum estradiol levels—baseline levels, and reassessment during recovery may serve as a marker for improvement,[31] testosterone levels for boys with delayed puberty, DEXA for amenorrhea >6–12 months,[32,33] and tests for specific vitamin and mineral deficiencies). If the diagnosis is uncertain, then other studies such as testing for inflammatory markers, test for celiac disease, and serum cortisol concentration can be planned.

Indications for hospitalization:[34]

- Dehydration
- Electrolyte disturbance (hypokalemia, hyponatremia, hypophosphatemia)
- ECG abnormalities (e.g., prolonged QTc or severe bradycardia)
- Physiologic instability
  - Severe bradycardia (HR <50 beats/min daytime, <45 beats/min at night)
  - Hypotension (BP <90/45 mm Hg)
  - Hypothermia (body temperature <96°F/ 35.6°C)
  - Orthostatic increase in pulse (>40 beats/min) or decrease in BP (>20 mm Hg systolic or >10 mm Hg diastolic)
- Arrested growth and development
- Failure of outpatient treatment
- Acute food refusal
- Uncontrollable binge eating and purging
- Acute medical complications of malnutrition (e.g., syncope, seizures, cardiac failure, pancreatitis)

> **BOX 1:** Differential diagnosis of EDs and complications of EDs.
>
> *Anorexia nervosa:*
> - ARFID
> - Rumination disorder
> - Any medical illness leading to weight loss, loss of appetite—celiac disease, Addison disease, inflammatory bowel disease, thyroid disease, connective tissue disorder, cystic fibrosis, diabetes, occult malignancy
>
> *Bulimia nervosa and binge eating disorder:*
> - Anorexia nervosa—binge purge type
> - Subthreshold BED or BN
> - Purging behavior
> - CNS tumors
> - Klüver–Bucy syndrome
> - Kleine–Levin syndrome
>
> *ARFID:*
> - Anorexia nervosa
> - Autistic spectrum disorder
> - Neurodevelopmental disorders
> - Anxiety disorders
>
> *Complications of eating disorders and malnutrition:*
> - Acute complications:
>   – Cool peripheries with poor perfusion
>   – Bradycardia
>   – Amenorrhea
>   – Constipation and abdominal bloating
>   – Alopecia
>   – Electrolyte disturbances (hypokalemia from purging or hyponatremia from polydipsia)
>   – Micronutrient deficiencies (commonly vitamin D)
>   – Dry skin, lanugo hair
>   – Dependent edema
>   – Mood changes (increased irritability, being withdrawn and low mood)
>   – Low metabolic rate
> - Long-term complications:
>   – Osteopenia
>   – Constipation
>   – Delayed growth and puberty
>   – Infertility
>   – Chronic eating disorder and psychiatric disorder

- Comorbid psychiatric or medical condition that prohibits or limits appropriate outpatient treatment (e.g., severe depression, suicidal ideation, obsessive–compulsive disorder, type 1 diabetes mellitus). Differential diagnosis for various Eating Disodrers and commonly associated complications have been listed in **Box 1**.

MANAGEMENT PRINCIPLES

The treatment goal is to nourish them back to their full healthy weight and growth trajectory, to normalize their eating pattern and behavior, and to establish a healthy relationship with food and body image as well as healthy sense of self. Irrespective of the DSM-5 diagnosis, treatment focuses on nutritional rehabilitation and psychological therapy. Medications may be required in selected cases. Management often requires a multidisciplinary team comprising a pediatrician, a psychologist/psychiatrist, and a dietician or ED specialist. The first task is to determine a treatment goal weight (in range). This is usually based on age, height, premorbid growth trajectory, pubertal stage, and menstrual history.[35,36]

Once a goal weight range is determined, re-establish a regular eating pattern. Stepwise introduce meals and snacks, with three meals and frequent snacks daily. The key message should be "food is the medicine that is required for recovery."

Vitamins and mineral supplements may be added as per associated signs of deficiencies. For constipation, dietary modification is the treatment of choice; however, if it still persists, then use of osmotic (polyethylene glycol) or bulk forming laxatives is preferred over stimulant laxatives to prevent cathartic colon syndrome and electrolyte imbalance. For bloating discomfort caused by slow gastric emptying, counseling should be done that it is temporary and will improve with regular eating. For dental care, patients who vomit should use a topical fluoride gel or 5,000 ppm fluoride toothpaste. Brushing should not be done immediately after vomiting as this will accelerate enamel erosion. Just rinse the mouth with clean water.

Psychotherapeutic options:

- *Family-based treatment (FBT)* proposes that parents are not to be blamed for their child's illness and they play an essential role in recovery. FBT consists of three phases: phase 1 is weight restoration, phase 2 is transferring responsibility of eating on own, and phase 3 is to address other issues of adolescent psychosocial development.
- *Parent-focused therapy* is similar to FBT. Here, the therapist supports the parents to renourish the patient and limit weight-control behaviors but meets only with the parents after initial appointment.
- *Cognitive behavioral therapy*—mainly for BN and BED
- *Interpersonal therapy*

Pharmacological options: There is a minimal role for drugs in the management of EDs. No drugs have been approved for the management of AN, pica, rumination disorders, OSFED, and USFED. ARFID is a relatively new entity and demands more evidence. For BN and BED, the Food and Drug Administration (FDA) has approved fluoxetine and lisdexamfetamine in adults to reduce binge and purging episodes. As fluoxetine is approved for depression in children and adolescents, and for OCDs, giving a trial of fluoxetine may be considered after failure of other therapies. Patients may be advised for day treatment programs, residential treatment, or hospital-based stabilization in certain cases.

CONCLUSION

Pediatricians play a significant role as they are usually the first point of contact. A high index of suspicion is required in all cases as early diagnosis and intervention are critical for a better outcome.[37,38] Patients with medical complications may require early referral. Delay in diagnosis can be hazardous as EDs are serious illnesses and have the highest mortality rate among all psychiatric disorders. Mortality can be because of either physical or psychiatric complication.

For early identification of these disorders, a pediatrician should follow the following:
- Incorporate screening tools for ED in history sheet in all children and adolescents for early identification.
- Always monitor BMI and not only height and weight. During pubertal growth spurt, there is a rapid increase in height so absolute weight loss may get missed.
- Any child with symptoms of weight loss, disordered eating (positive screening tools), or medical complications of malnutrition require a detailed assessment. Details should be asked in a nonjudgmental, empathetic manner.
- Body image concerns and related dietary habits should not be dismissed as a normal phase of adolescent development.

REFERENCES

1. Arlington VA, American Psychiatric Association. Diagnostic and statistical manual of mental disorders. American Psychiatric Association. 2013;5:612-3.
2. Vaidyanathan S, Kuppili PP, Menon V. Eating disorders: An overview of Indian research. Indian Journal of Psychological Medicine. 2019;41(4):311-7.
3. Hartmann AS, Poulain T, Vogel M, Hiemisch A, Kiess W, Hilbert A. Prevalence of pica and rumination behaviors in German children aged 7-14 and their associations with feeding, eating, and general psychopathology: a population-based study. Eur Child Adolesc Psychiatry. 2018;27(11):1499-508.
4. Katzman DK, Norris ML. Feeding and eating disorders. In: Feldman M, Friedman LS, Brandt LJ (Eds). Sleisenger and Fordtran's Gastrointestinal and Liver Disease, 11th edition. Philadelphia: Elsevier; 2020 pp. 117-32.e6
5. Swanson SA, Crow SJ, Le Grange D, Swendsen J, Merikangas KR. Prevalence and correlates of eating disorders in adolescents. Results from the national comorbidity survey replication adolescent supplement. Arch Gen Psychiatry. 2011;68(7):714-23.
6. Treasure J, Claudino AM, Zucker N. Eating disorders. The Lancet. 2010;375(9714):583-93.
7. Hudson JI, Hiripi E, Pope HG Jr, Kessler RC. The prevalence and correlates of eating disorders in the National Comorbidity Survey Replication. Biol Psychiatry. 2007;61(3):348-58.
8. Keski-Rahkonen A, Mustelin L. Epidemiology of eating disorders in Europe: prevalence, incidence, comorbidity, course, consequences, and risk factors. Curr Opin Psychiatry. 2016;29(6):340-5.
9. Udo T, Grilo CM. Psychiatric and medical correlates of DSM-5 eating disorders in a nationally representative sample of adults in the United States. Int J Eat Disord. 2019;52(1):42-50.
10. Wisting L, Wonderlich J, Skrivarhaug T, Dahl-Jorgensen K, Ro O. Psychometric properties and factor structure of the diabetes eating problem survey - revised (DEPS-R) among adult males and females with type 1 diabetes. J Eat Disord. 2019;7:2.
11. de Jonge P, Alonso J, Stein DJ, Kiejna A, Aguilar-Gaxiola S, Viana MC, et al. Associations between DSM-IV mental disorders and diabetes mellitus: a role for impulse control disorders and depression. Diabetologia. 2014;57(4):699-709.
12. Treasure J, Kan C, Stephenson L, Warren E, Smith E, Heller S, et al. Developing a theoretical maintenance model for disordered eating in Type 1 diabetes. Diabet Med. 2015;32(12):1541-5.
13. De Paoli T, Rogers PJ. Disordered eating and insulin restriction in type 1 diabetes: A systematic review and testable model. Eating Disorders. 2018;26(4):343-60.
14. Staite E, Zaremba N, Macdonald P, Allan J, Treasure J, Ismail K, et al. 'Diabulima' through the lens of social media: a qualitative review and analysis of online blogs by people with Type 1 diabetes mellitus and eating disorders. Diabet Med. 2018;35(10):1329-36.
15. Hedman A, Breithaupt L, Hubel C, Thornton LM, Tillander A, Norring C, et al. Bidirectional relationship between eating disorders and autoimmune diseases. J Child Psychol Psychiatry. 2019;60(7):803-12.

16. Srinivasan TN, Suresh TR, Jayaram V, Fernandez MP. Eating disorders in India. Indian J Psychiatry. 1995;37(1):26-30.
17. Iyer S, Shriraam V. Prevalence of eating disorders and its associated risk factors in students of a medical college hospital in South India. Cureus. 2021;13(1):e12926.
18. Norris ML, Robinson A, Obeid N, Harrison M, Spettigue W, Henderson K. Exploring avoidant/restrictive food intake disorder in eating disordered patients: A descriptive study. Int J Eat Disord. 2014;47(5):495-9.
19. Thomas JJ, Lawson EA, Micali N, Misra M, Deckersbach T, Eddy KT. Avoidant/Restrictive Food Intake Disorder: a Three-Dimensional Model of Neurobiology with Implications for Etiology and Treatment. Curr Psychiatry Rep. 2017;19(8):54.
20. Bryant-Waugh R, Loomes R, Munuve A, Rhind C. Towards an evidence-based out-patient care pathway for children and young people with avoidant restrictive food intake disorder. J Behav Cogn Ther. 2021;31(1):15-26.
21. Saini V, Greer BD, Fisher WW, Lichtblau KR, DeSouza AA, Mitteer DR. Individual and combined effects of non-contingent reinforcement and response blocking on automatically reinforced problem behavior. J Appl Behav Anal. 2016;49(3):693-8.
22. Hauptman M, Woolf AD. Childhood ingestions of environmental toxins: what are the risks? Pediatr Ann. 2017;46:e466-71.
23. McNaughten B, Bourke T, Thompson A. Fifteen-minute consultation: the child with pica. Arch Dis Child Educ Pract Ed. 2017;102:226-9.
24. Righini Grunder F, Aspirot A, Faure C. High-resolution esophageal manometry patterns in children and adolescents with rumination syndrome. J Pediatr Gastroenterol Nutr. 2017;65:627-32.
25. Cotton M, Ball C, Robinson J. Four simple questions can help screen for eating disorders. J Gen Intern Med. 2003;18(1):53-6.
26. Luck AJ, Morgan JF, Reid F, O Brien A, Brunton J, Price C, et al. The SCOFF questionnaire and clinical interview for eating disorders in general practice: comparative study. BMJ. 2002;325(7367):755-6.
27. Fairburn CG. Eating Disorder Examination Questionnaire (EDE-Q 6.0). In: Fairburn CG (Ed). Cognitive Behaviour Therapy and Eating Disorders. New York: Guilford Press; 2008.
28. Hay P, Chinn D, Forbes D, Madden S, Newton R, Sugenor L, et al. Royal Australian and New Zealand College of Psychiatrists clinical practice guidelines for the treatment of eating disorders. Aust N Z J Psychiatry. 2014;48(11):977-1008.
29. Hornberger LL, Lane MA; Committee on Adolescence. Identification and Management of Eating Disorders in Children and Adolescents. Pediatrics. 2021;147(1):e2020040279.
30. Academy for Eating Disorders Medical Care Standards Committee. Eating Disorders: A Guide to Medical Care, 3rd edition. Reston, VA: Academy for Eating Disorders; 2016. [online] Available from: https://www.aedweb.org/learn/publications/medical-care-standards. [Last accessed October, 2023].
31. Committee on Adolescent Health Care. ACOG Committee opinion no. 740: gynecologic care for adolescents and young women with eating disorders. Obstet Gynecol. 2018;131(6):e205-13.
32. Misra M, Klibanski A. Anorexia nervosa and its associated endocrinopathy in young people. Horm Res Paediatr. 2016;85(3):147-57.
33. Misra M, Golden NH, Katzman DK. State of the art systematic review of bone disease in anorexia nervosa. Int J Eat Disord. 2016;49(3):276-92.
34. Golden NH, Katzman DK, Sawyer SM, Ornstein RM, Rome ES, Garber AK, et al. Society for Adolescent Health and Medicine. Position paper of the Society for Adolescent Health and Medicine: medical management of restrictive eating disorders in adolescents and young adults. J Adolesc Health. 2015;56(1):121-5.
35. Golden NH, Katzman DK, Sawyer SM, Ornstein RM, Rome ES, Garber AK, et al. Update on the medical management of eating disorders in adolescents. J Adolesc Health. 2015;56(4):370-5.
36. Norris ML, Hiebert JD, Katzman DK. Determining treatment goal weights for children and adolescents with anorexia nervosa. Paediatr Child Health. 2018;23(8):551-2.
37. Le Grange D, Accurso EC, Lock J, Agras S, Bryson SW. Early weight gain predicts outcome in two treatments for adolescent anorexia nervosa. Int J Eat Disord. 2014;47(2):124-9.
38. Madden S, Miskovic-Wheatley J, Wallis A, Kohn M, Hay P, Touyz S. Early weight gain in family-based treatment predicts greater weight gain and remission at the end of treatment and remission at 12-month follow-up in adolescent anorexia nervosa. Int J Eat Disord. 2015;48(7):919-22.

Hysterical Conversion Disorder in Children

Pradeep Kumar Gunasekaran, Lokesh Saini

INTRODUCTION

Conversion disorder (CD) or functional neurological disorder (FND) is defined by neurological symptoms inconsistent or incompatible with recognized patterns of neurologic disease and cannot be explained by organic pathology.[1-3] The term "conversion disorder" was first coined by an Austrian Neurologist and Psychoanalyst, Sigmund Freud. In the Diagnostic and Statistical Manual of Mental Disorders, Fifth Edition (DSM-5), CD is classified under the somatic symptom and related disorders (SSRDs), which also include factitious disorders, illness anxiety disorders, and other specified/unspecified somatic symptom disorders.[1] The DSM-5 criteria for CD are summarized in **Box 1**. In DSM-5, *"la belle indifférence"* has been removed as a diagnostic criterion. Hysterical CD represents "functional" or unexplained neurological symptoms, including sensory or motor symptoms that are not explained by organic lesions but arise in the context of "psychogenic" stress or emotional conflicts.[4-6] It has a wide spectrum of presentation including motor weakness; loss of sensory functions such as sight, touch, or hearing impairment; and nonepileptic seizures.[6,7] In the pediatric age group, the presentation of CD is complex and varied. In addition, anxiety and depression are common among children with CD that makes the presentation more confusing.

EPIDEMIOLOGY

The prevalence of CD varies greatly between studies based on the population and geographic settings. The prevalence of CD among children is estimated at 2-15% in outpatient pediatric neurology settings, 5-14% in inpatient settings, and 5-25% in outpatient psychiatry settings.[2,3] The prevalence of CD among adolescents is estimated at 0.3-10%.[3] The frequency and heterogeneity of complaints increase with age, with symptoms more frequently among girls. The variations in the prevalence estimation are influenced by the diversity of study populations, level of awareness of CD, sociocultural environment including the socioeconomic class and education status, rural or developing areas, and patriarchal family, study sampling technique, and the diagnostic criteria used.[3] CD is rare under 7 years of age and most commonly occurs during puberty and adolescence and is postulated due to externalization of impulses by children under the age of 7 years.[3] The rate of misdiagnosis of CD is estimated at 0.4-4%.[8]

ETIOPATHOGENESIS

In many children with CD, there is a history of abuse in childhood (sexual and emotional), trauma, acute/chronic stressor, or any other adverse life event. The CD is

> **BOX 1:** DSM-5 criteria for conversion disorder or functional neurologic symptom disorder.
>
> - One or more symptoms of altered voluntary motor or sensory function
> - Clinical findings provide evidence of incompatibility between the symptom and recognized neurologic or medical conditions
> - The symptom is not better explained by another medical or mental disorder
> - The symptom causes clinically significant distress or impairment in social, occupational, or other important areas of functioning or warrants medical evaluation
>   - *Specify symptom type:* Weakness or paralysis, abnormal movements, swallowing symptoms, speech symptom, attacks/seizures, anesthesia/sensory loss, special sensory symptom (e.g., visual, olfactory, hearing), or mixed symptoms

(DSM-5: Diagnostic and Statistical Manual of Mental Disorders, Fifth Edition)

precipitated and perpetuated by psychosocial, social, and biological factors (**Fig. 1**). The CD is also associated with anxiety, depression, and personality disorders and is likely to present with multiple somatic symptoms, including generalized fatigue, pain, or weakness. The main proposed hypotheses/models for CD include[4]:

- *Psychodynamic models:* This model postulates that CD symptoms are a product of emotional conflict, which is repressed into the unconscious mind and gets converted to presenting symptoms. These are defense mechanisms to the negative feelings induced by emotional conflict as a coping mechanism or behavior.
- *Cognitive behavioral models:* This model postulates that the specific CD symptoms are due to exposure to specific information, thereby creating representation in the memory and getting activated due to excessive worrying. After crossing of a specific threshold, this activation overrides the sensory inputs and presents as an actual symptom. This model hypothesizes that perceptual and behavioral processing occurs automatically and is beyond the awareness of the individual, and the symptoms may also occur due to psychological influences at a lower level of processing.
- *Neurobiological models:* The model suggests that CD results from high-order cortical processing changes. There is an enhanced functional connectivity of the regions of the brain involved in emotion processing, movement control, and sensory information processing, resulting in the generation of a multitude of sensory-motor symptoms during stress episodes.[9,10] The activation of brain's frontal and subcortical areas by emotional stress gives rise to input to the inhibitory basal ganglia—thalamocortical circuits—thereby reducing conscious motor or sensory processing.[4] There can be an abnormal correlation between the amygdala activation and the supplementary motor area.

For nonepileptic seizures, it is also postulated that it is secondary to hyperventilation or fear-triggered bradycardia during the perceived psychological or physical threat, thereby reducing blood flow or oxygen availability to the brain. The recent model is that CD is a disorder of cognitive control, and during the acute symptoms, they have reduced capacity to manipulate/retain the information, block/stop the interfering information, and inhibit responses that are required for memory, effective attention, and executive function.[6]

CLINICAL FEATURES

Conversion disorder represents a constellation of symptoms that together points toward the diagnosis. CD cannot be considered a diagnosis of exclusion. In CD, almost any neurological symptom can be the initial presentation along with multiple symptoms.[11] These neurological symptoms significantly impact these children out of proportion to its severity.[11] The reliable indicators for diagnosing CD can be symptoms inconsistent with the history, normal laboratory investigations, and normal neuroimaging, with/without a history of psychiatric disorders. If the symptoms are present for ≤6 months, it is defined as acute CD, while the presence of symptoms for >6 months indicates persistent CD. The symptoms of CD are summarized in **Table 1**. The most common subtype

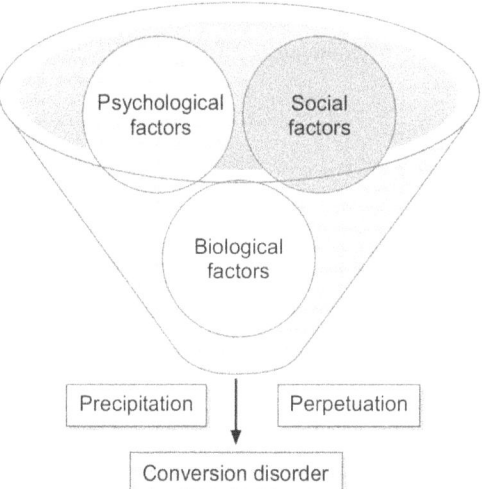

Fig. 1: Etiological factors in conversion disorder.

TABLE 1: Symptoms of conversion disorder (CD).

Positive symptoms	Negative symptoms
• Nonepileptic seizures	• Focal weakness
• Dystonias	• Imbalance
• Myoclonus	• Paresthesia/sensory loss
• Tremors	• Blindness
• Ataxia	• Deafness
• Gait disorder	• Anosmia
• Dizziness	• Mutism
• Breathlessness	• Memory deficits
• Tunnel vision	• Attention deficits
• Double vision	• Chronic fatigue
• Swallowing disturbances	
• Dysphonia	
• Dysarthria	
• Foreign accent syndrome	

of CD is psychogenic nonepileptic seizures (PNES), followed by paralysis or weakness. In younger children, negative symptoms including loss of function such as weakness, imbalance, or loss of vision are more common. Positive symptoms, including nonepileptic seizures and psychogenic movement disorders, are more common in older children or during puberty.[11] Pal et al. reported a high (84%) presence of a social or environmental stressor, illness, and preceding event, before the occurrence of CD.[2] The symptoms often develop suddenly and are linked to a stressful event. Children with CD may have a low desire to attend school and participation in activities, while adolescents may verbally state to desire to attend them.[11]

DIAGNOSIS

The most essential tools for diagnosing CD are appropriate history-taking with a specific focus on the time frame of symptoms along with context and physical examination. The clinician should explore for any history of abuse in childhood (both emotional and sexual), trauma, acute/chronic stressors, or any psychiatric disorder(s). The family history should be explored for any psychiatric disorder/chronic medical illness of parents, and any frequent unexplained symptoms. The common presentation patterns include: (1) chronic symptoms with a sudden onset at the maximum intensity that persists since the onset, and (2) paroxysmal symptoms that exclusively occur in the presence of family or friends.[11] CD is no more considered a diagnosis of exclusion but it is a positive diagnosis relying on excluding neurological illnesses, identifying inconsistencies on examination, and clinical signs and symptoms not suggestive of organic disorders.[4] The DSM-5 diagnostic criteria are summarized in **Box 1**. The various examination findings and tests that are done to differentiate organic disorders and CD are summarized in **Table 2**. The investigations are varied based on the

TABLE 2: Examination findings and tests for diagnosing conversion disorder (CD).

Positive symptoms	
Psychogenic nonepileptic seizures	Generalized nonrhythmic limb thrashing, prominent involvement of truncal muscles (hip thrusting, lateral rolling of head and body), no postictal confusion, moaning vocalizations, response to noxious stimuli, no paroxysmal activity on electroencephalogram (EEG), forced eye closure
Dystonias	Severe pain in affected limb, clenched fist, fixed posture during sleep, inverted foot, and resolution of symptoms on general anesthesia, placebo
Myoclonus	Inconsistent frequency/amplitude, exaggerated startle response, stimuli sensitive, long and variable latency from stimulus, anticipatory jerk by stopping reflex hammer just short of contact
Tremors	Abrupt and unilateral onset, maximum severity, varying direction, amplitude, and frequency, subsides with distraction, amplification with attention, entrainment
Ataxia/gait disorders	Atypical pattern, sudden knee buckling, "walking-on-ice" pattern, excessively slow gait initiation, pseudoataxia
Swallowing symptoms	Globus sensation/globus pharyngeus occurrence between meals, absence of odynophagia/dysphagia
Speech symptoms	Hoarseness/whispering, dysarthria
Negative symptoms	
Paralysis/focal weakness Tests	• Nonspecific anatomical pattern, inconsistent and give-way weakness, no atrophy, normal deep tendon reflexes, normal Babinski reflex • Hoover sign, co-contraction sign, arm drop test, sternocleidomastoid test, collapsing weakness
Paresthesia/Sensory loss	Atypical dermatological patterns, nonanatomic distribution, hemisensory syndrome with ipsilateral hearing/vision problems, affected area changes over time
Olfactory/hearing disturbances	Normal sense of taste on anosmia testing, blink or startle response on loud sounds
Visual disturbances	• Complete blindness with normal pupillary reflex, preserved optokinetic nystagmus, and flinching to bright light, no difficulty in maneuvering with no superficial bruises/wounds, diplopia persisting with one eye closed
Tests	• Mirror test, fingertip test, signature test, optokinetic test, menace reflex, tearing reflex

clinical presentation and may include electroencephalogram (EEG), electromyogram (EMG), and magnetic resonance imaging (MRI). The common bedside clinical tests include:

- *Hoover's test:* This is based on the fact that patients extend their hip when the contralateral hip flexes against resistance. This test is helpful in patients presenting with functional weakness of lower limbs. Patient is made to lie supine, the examiner's hand is placed under the affected heel, and the patient is asked to lift their unaffected leg against resistance. Patients with functional weakness will have downward pressure on the affected heel.
- *Arm-drop test:* The patient's outstretched arm is held in front by the examiner and then released. In functional weakness, jerky motion or slow descent of the arm onto the patient's lap is seen.

The barriers to establishing CD diagnosis include anticipation of confusion, potential misperception, and anger from the family, time taken to communicate the diagnosis, lack of knowledge or expertise for diagnosis, and medicolegal concerns.[11] The diagnosis should be clearly stated to them, which further helps the clinician to evaluate other comorbidities, including anxiety and mood disorders. Early diagnosis and timely intervention are crucial in reducing the morbidity encountered in children with CD.[12] The common differential diagnoses for CD are psychiatric disorders that include factitious disorder, somatic symptom disorder, illness anxiety disorder, and malingering, and also neurological disorders, including multiple sclerosis, epilepsy, myasthenia gravis, stroke, spinal disorders (cervical myelopathy, spinal stenosis), and movement disorders. The differentiating features for common differentials include generalized limb shaking, hip thrusting, no loss of bowel or bladder control, forced eye closure, lack of postictal confusion, and no response to antiseizure medications in case of PNES. In functional paralysis or weakness, there will be inconsistency in weakness with no anatomical pattern. There will be no specific dermatomal patterns in functional anesthesia or sensory loss.

TREATMENT

The first step in managing children with CD is providing support to the family/children for understanding the diagnosis, accepting the diagnosis, and providing a detailed effective explanation availability of effective treatment, failure of which results in the prolongation of maladaptive coping. This helps establish trust and a solid therapeutic alliance with the family and the children. The clinical approach suggested for managing CD is VEER (validate, educate, empathize, rehabilitate).[11] Psychotherapy is the first-line treatment for CD, of which cognitive behavioral therapy (CBT) is the most effective. Predisposing factors should be analyzed. Tailored CBT is beneficial in patients with PNES attacks.[13] The other therapies that can be used include psychodynamic psychotherapy, group therapy, and family therapy. Physiotherapy is used with CBT in children with motor symptoms, including weakness, gait, and movement disorders.[14] Pharmacotherapy is used for comorbid psychiatric illnesses, including anxiety and depression. The commonly used classes of drugs are antidepressants, including serotonin and norepinephrine reuptake inhibitors, mood stabilizers, anxiolytics, and neuroleptics. Regular monitoring for the side effects of these drugs is advised and compliance should be assessed on every follow-up visit. Hypnotherapy is considered effective in sensory loss, speech symptoms, and associated comorbidities, including chronic pain conditions. The list of therapies used in CD is summarized in **Table 3**.

FOLLOW-UP

These children, along with family, should be on regular follow-ups of a multidisciplinary team, as rehabilitation plays a crucial role in the management. It should be ensured that these children return to their routine, including eating, sleep habits, schooling, and other activities.

COMPLICATIONS

The common complications in children with CD are permanent disability and poor quality of life. These children have comparable or higher rates of physical disability and psychological disorders compared to children with neurological disorders.[4]

PROGNOSIS

The poor prognostic factors in CD include PNES, polysymptomatic presentation, severe internal conflict, comorbid medical/psychiatric illnesses, and severe family dysfunction. Favorable outcomes in CD are associated with early diagnosis, younger age at diagnosis, reasonable premorbid adjustment, easily identifiable stressors, and good cooperation of the child and family.[15]

TABLE 3: Treatment of conversion disorder (CD).

Treatment/Management of CD

Psychotherapy:
- Cognitive behavioral therapy
- Psychodynamic psychotherapy

Hypnotherapy

Physical therapy

Occupational therapy

Speech and language therapy

Pharmacological therapy*

Antidepressants

• Amitriptyline	1–1.5 mg/kg/day Q12H
• Nortriptyline	1–3 mg/kg/day Q6-8H
• Escitalopram	10 mg once daily/max 20 mg/day
• Fluoxetine	10–20 mg once daily

Anxiolytics

• Clonazepam	*Initial:* 0.01–0.05 mg/kg/day Q8-12H
• Diazepam	*Maintenance:* 0.1–0.2 mg/kg/day
	0.1–0.8 mg/kg/day Q6-8H

Mood stabilizers

• Lithium	15–60 mg/kg/day Q6-8H
• Carbamazepine	10–30 mg/kg/day Q8H
• Gabapentin	10–40 mg/kg/day Q8H

Neuroleptics

• Haloperidol	0.05–0.15 mg/kg/day Q8-12H
• Aripiprazole	*Initial:* 2 mg/day/max 30 mg/day
• Risperidone	*Initial:* <20 kg–0.25 mg/day;
	>20 kg–0.5 mg/day
	Maximum: <20 kg–1 mg/day;
	>20 kg–2.5 mg/day

Transmagnetic stimulation (TMS)

*Drug dosage references: The Harriet Lane Handbook, 21st Edition.

CONCLUSION

The parents of these children should be educated on active distraction techniques to help these children to focus on developmentally appropriate leisure activities to prevent symptoms.

REFERENCES

1. American Psychiatric Association. Diagnosis and Statistical Manual of Mental Disorders, 5th edition. American Psychiatric Publishing: Washington DC; 2013. pp. 309-27.
2. Pal R, Romero E, He Z, Stevenson T, Campen CJ. Pediatric functional neurological disorder: demographic and clinical factors impacting care. J Child Neurol. 2022; 37(8-9):669-76.
3. Boz S, Mungo A, Delhaye M. Conversion disorder in children and adolescents: definition, diagnosis, treatment, and clinical illustration. Ment Health Fam Med. 2020;16: 1012-7.
4. Peeling JL, Muzio MR. Conversion Disorder. [Updated 2022 May]. In: StatPearls [Internet]. Treasure Island (FL): StatPearls Publishing; 2023 Jan. [online] Available from: https://www.ncbi.nlm.nih.gov/books/NBK551567/. [Last accessed October, 2023].
5. Vuilleumier P. Hysterical conversion and brain function. Prog Brain Res. 2005;150:309-29.
6. Kozlowska K, Palmer DM, Brown KJ, Scher S, Chudleigh C, Davies F, et al. Conversion disorder in children and adolescents: a disorder of cognitive control. J Neuropsychol. 2015;9(1):87-108.
7. Krasnik C, Grant C. Conversion disorder: not a malingering matter. Paediatr Child Health. 2012;17(5):246.
8. Stone J, Smyth R, Carson A, Lewis S, Prescott R, Warlow C, et al. Systematic review of misdiagnosis of conversion symptoms and "hysteria". BMJ. 2005;331(7523):989.
9. Voon V, Brezing C, Gallea C, Ameli R, Roelofs K, LaFrance WC Jr, et al. Emotional stimuli and motor conversion disorder. Brain. 2010;133(Pt 5):1526-36.
10. Van der Kruijs SJ, Bodde NM, Vaessen MJ, Lazeron RHC, Vonck K, Boon P, et al. Functional connectivity of dissociation in patients with psychogenic non-epileptic seizures. J Neurol Neurosurg Psychiatry. 2012;83(3):239-47.
11. Krasnik CE, Meaney B, Grant C. (2013). A clinical approach to paediatric conversion disorder: VEER in the right direction. [online] Available from: https://cpsp.cps.ca/uploads/publications/RA-conversion-disorder.pdf. [Last accessed October, 2023].
12. Ndukuba AC, Ibekwe RC, Odinka PC, Muomah RC, Nwoha SO, Eze C. Knowledge of conversion disorder in children by pediatricians in a developing country. Niger J Clin Pract. 2015;18:534-7.
13. Goldstein LH, Robinson EJ, Chalder T, Reuber M, Medford N, Stone J, et al. Six-month outcomes of the CODES randomised controlled trial of cognitive behavioural therapy for dissociative seizures: A secondary analysis. Seizure. 2022;96:128-36.
14. Lehn A, Gelauff J, Hoeritzauer I, Ludwig L, McWhirter L, Williams S, et al. Functional neurological disorders: mechanisms and treatment. J Neurol. 2016;263(3):611-20.
15. Pehlivantürk B, Unal F. Conversion disorder in children and adolescents: a 4-year follow-up study. J Psychosom Res. 2002;52(4):187-91.

Chapter 15: Somatic Symptom and Related Disorders in Children

Adarsh Purohit

"Medicine is not only a science; it is also an art. It does not consist of compounding pills and plasters; it deals with the very processes of life, which must be understood before they may be guided."
—**Paracelsus**

INTRODUCTION

There are a number of children who present in emergency room (ER) with a variety of discomforts which prove to be a challenge for the pediatrician as even after a thorough history and clinical examination and after an exhausting list of investigations, the origin of discomfort still remains a mystery, not fitting into any specific disease or illness. The child reacts excessively to the physical symptoms, may it be pain at any of the body sites, breathing difficulty or sometimes weakness of any body part. The problem may be of short history or many times, there have been multiple visits to the ER with the same problem or sometimes a variety of problems which could never be explained by any specific medical condition. Some children may even have a diagnosed medical condition, but the reaction of the child to that problem is often out of proportion. Most of these children, after exclusion of any serious medical condition, are placed under Somatoform Disorders.

DEFINITION

Somatoform disorders are those group of mental and behavioral problems in which the child's reaction to the physical symptom is excessively heightened to that what can be perceived after examination and investigations. Child as well as the parents keep worrying about the symptoms, while the symptoms cannot be explained by any specific medical disease and any organic cause cannot be detected. The only thing that is persistent is distress and worry associated with the symptoms.

It is a group of disorders which under ICD-10 (International Classification of Diseases, 10th Revision) was labeled as Somatic Symptom and Related Disorders, which were further classified into:
- Somatization disorder
- Undifferentiated somatoform disorder
- Hypochondriacal disorder
- Somatoform autonomous dysfunction
- Persistent somatoform pain disorder
- Other somatoform disorder
- Somatoform disorder, unspecified.

Similarly, under DSM-IV (Diagnostic and Statistical Manual of Mental Disorders, Fourth edition), there were seven classes of *somatoform disorders* as following:
1. Somatization disorder (disorder with symptoms involving multiple body systems)
2. Conversion disorder (voluntary motor and/or sensory symptoms)
3. Pain disorder (consists of pain with a strong psychological component)
4. Hypochondriasis (unrealistic fear of having some serious illness)
5. Body dysmorphic disorder (overly occupied with an imaginary or real body defect)
6. Undifferentiated somatoform disorder (similar to somatization disorder with fewer symptoms)
7. Somatoform disorder not otherwise specified (does not fulfill criteria for any of the above-mentioned disorders).

Under DSM-IV, these were labeled as *"Somatoform Disorders,"* which was changed to *"Somatic Symptom and Related Disorder"* in DSM-5 (Diagnostic and Statistical Manual of Mental Disorders, Fifth Edition), while in ICD-11 (International Classification of Diseases, 11th Revision), they have been renamed as *Bodily Distress Disorder (BDD)*, which is further divided into mild, moderate, and severe bodily distress disorder. The major change in ICD-11 from the previous one is that Hypochondriasis has been removed from this list of disorders. DSM-5 also removed body dysmorphic disorder from the list of somatic symptom and related disorder to obsessive compulsive disorder (OCD). Under DSM-IV for diagnosis of Somatoform Disorder, it required a patient to have at least four pain symptoms (at different sites), two gastrointestinal symptoms other than pain, one sexual symptom (in adults) and at least one pseudo neurological symptom, but these all have been removed in DSM-5 and now it requires only a somatic symptom which is distressing to the child and the family resulting in disruption of the routine activity of the child.[1-6] The following disorders have also been excluded from bodily distress disorder in ICD-11:

- Tourette syndrome
- Hair-pulling disorder
- Dissociative disorders
- Hair-plucking
- Hypochondriasis
- Body dysmorphic disorder
- Excoriation disorder
- Gender incongruence
- Sexual dysfunctions
- Tic disorders
- Sexual pain-penetration disorder
- Postviral fatigue syndrome
- Chronic fatigue syndrome
- Myalgic encephalomyelitis.

EPIDEMIOLOGY OF SOMATOFORM DISORDERS

There are very few studies from India depicting exact prevalence of somatoform disorders in children. Besides, exact diagnosis and prevalence have been difficult to extract because of varied presentations (symptoms confused many times as organic disease) and changing criteria over the time (most of the time, the criteria have been developed as per the need of the adult population, which were later applied over pediatric age group). The prevalence of somatoform symptoms has been reported ranging from 5 to 83% in various studies worldwide, while the prevalence of somatoform disorders has been reported ranging from 0.5 to 13%. Overall, both the symptoms and disorder have been reported to be more common in females than males (ratio of girls to boys reported to be as high as 5:1). Among girls, the onset is usually around 9–10 years of age, which keeps on increasing consistently till adulthood while in boys, it starts at an almost similar age, but it begins to fall post-puberty, i.e., around 13–14 years of age. Amongst different age groups, pain disorders have a higher incidence in older age groups and are the most common among teenagers and adolescents. Recurrent abdominal pain and headache are the two most commonly presented symptoms, followed by dizziness, fatigue, and pain in limbs. Polysymptomatic presentation has mostly been found to be higher than the persistent monosymptomatic disorder. These data show it to be a highly prevalent problem among children in all societies. These children form a large chunk amongst the patients who repeatedly present in medical outdoors and emergencies increasing the overall load on healthcare sector.[7-10]

ETIOLOGY OF SOMATOFORM DISORDERS

Somatoform symptoms are physical manifestations of ongoing subconscious stress in a person and many times associated with some secondary gains. Multiple factors are responsible for somatoform disorders, which include individual factors and surrounding or environmental factors. *Individual factors* may be genetic makeup of the child, which predisposes him/her to psychiatric or behavioral disorders or any chronic illness (physical or mental) which acts as a stressor predisposing the child for somatoform issues. Somatoform disorders have been reported to be more common in children with borderline or low intelligence. Substance abuse in a child also predisposes him to such issues.

Environmental factors mainly comprise family harmony, environment in school, and relationship with peers. If there is disturbed family harmony such as multiple fights among parents, divorced parents or single parent, there are greater chances of the child being affected. Besides, either the child is overlooked and is not getting appropriate care or time and attention by any of the parents, or is too pampered and parents are too anxious regarding the smallest of issues, then also the child may develop such somatoform symptoms, mostly triggered by secondary gains. If there is a history of mental health issues in the family, there are chances of the child acquiring similar somatoform symptoms. It is a known fact that there is a significant relationship between anxiety in mothers and colicky pain in infants. If either parent is having mental health issues, their child also has a greater chance of suffering from poor mental health and it may further predispose her/him to develop somatoform symptoms and disorder in addition to the primary mental health issue. Children suffering from psychiatric disorders such as anxiety, depression, OCD, and post-traumatic stress disorder (PTSD) have a higher incidence of somatoform disorders. In addition to all these factors, any stressors like separation or loss of a close family member, friend, or pet can aggravate such symptoms.[3,5,8,11]

Children exposed to bullying in school, those who are pressurized excessively regarding studies or other performances, those who come across some incidents in school or neighborhood which have a long-lasting fearful impact on the psyche, those who have been victims of physical or sexual abuse, or some similar adverse incidents develop somatoform disorders in the long run. Studies have reported a higher incidence of somatoform symptoms in children with poor peer relationships and those exposed to community violence. Children suffering from social anxiety have been reported to have somatic complaints more often than other children of the same age. Boys and girls may be affected differently by peer pressure and relationship with their peers. Absence of social support may be the cause behind somatization and adequate social support may be the only treatment required for these children.[12-14]

CLINICAL PRESENTATION

The child may present with a single symptom repeatedly or with a vague variety of symptoms each time, and for most of the symptoms, no organic disease could be diagnosed. It has been reported that younger children present with single symptoms repeatedly rather than multiple bodily symptoms. Multiple bodily symptoms are more common in adolescents. The commonly reported symptoms are headache, pain abdomen, nausea, dizziness, fatigue, difficulty in breathing, pain in any of the limbs, or rarely symptoms related to the nervous system such as fainting, loss of speech, hearing loss, and paresthesia. Adolescents may present with sexual symptoms at times such as erectile dysfunction, ejaculatory dysfunction, irregular menses, or menorrhagia. Most of the time, there is an exaggerated and out-of-proportion response to milder problems and distress is much more prominent than the symptom itself. One of the main features is a significant amount of distress to the child and/or the parents hampering the routine activity of the child and the family. Most of the times, child and parents are adamant that the child has some severe physical illness and the idea of consulting a psychologist for an assessment is rejected by them. They would go for a battery of tests again and again in spite of no significant findings in the investigations performed. Failure to get any specific cause for the symptoms further increases the family's anxiety and at times, they would believe that the physician is not competent enough to detect the disease of the child.[1,2,15,16]

DIAGNOSIS OF SOMATOFORM DISORDER/ BODILY DISTRESS DISORDER

The International Classification of Diseases has provided essential diagnostic criteria which must be met before a final diagnosis of *somatoform disorder* is established, which are as following:

- The patient is in distress because of the physical symptoms and which may vary from time to time. Sometimes, the patient may have a single symptom only as fatigue or pain.
- Excessive attention is being paid to the symptoms and it affects the routine activity of the child, like missing school or play days. Even if there is a preexisting medical condition, the attention given to the specific symptom and negative thoughts are out of proportion to that what is there and this may lead to frequent visits to the healthcare provider.
- Excessive attention toward the symptom persists even after a thorough clinical examination and necessary investigations.
- Bodily symptoms (single or multiple) are present consistently over a period of the last 3 months.
- Excessive attention toward the symptoms significantly affects the family and educational, social, and emotional functioning of the patient.
- The symptoms cannot be explained by any physical or mental disorder (i.e., schizophrenia or mood disorder).

The International Classification of Diseases has further classified bodily distress disorder into *mild*, *moderate*, and *severe* depending upon the distress felt by the patient, hampering of routine activity and number of visits to the healthcare facilities, but as such, there are no clear-cut boundaries between the three. Those with mild BDD would spend less time focusing on their symptoms while those with severe BDD would be totally preoccupied with their symptoms and would repeatedly visit healthcare providers, ask for investigations frequently, or try different alternative forms of therapy. Similar to ICD, DSM-5 has described somatic symptom and related disorder as overfocusing on the somatic symptoms leading to functional impairment in various domains of life with an absence of any identifiable physical illness for the same.[1,2,15,17]

Clinicians must be very vigilant while diagnosing somatoform disorder and should not hurry in disclosing their diagnosis to the patient and/or the parents. Most of the times, disclosing the diagnosis on 1st meeting itself is met with disbelief and denial. Most parents cannot believe that their child may have any psychological disorder, as still in many parts of the world, psychological disorder is considered insanity, making it a taboo for the child in society. Pediatrician must listen to all the issues with empathy, do a thorough physical examination as in any other disorder and go for necessary investigations before reaching the diagnosis and as over next 2-3 meetings, he/she earns the trust of the family, then only a diagnosis of somatoform disorder should be the discussed first with the family. We propose a sample questionnaire for children suspected of having somatization disorder to help clinicians in diagnosing the disorder (**Annexure 1**).

DIFFERENTIAL DIAGNOSIS

- Mood disorders
- Generalized anxiety disorder
- Panic disorder
- Hypochondriasis
- Factitious disorder imposed on self.

All of these psychological disorders can have somatic symptoms at a given point of time and the physician has to differentiate amongst them very subtly as the difference is very fine at times. There will be persistence of somatic symptoms in a child with bodily distress disorder while these will subside in patients with mood disorders when the episode is over. Patients with generalized anxiety disorder are not that preoccupied with their bodily symptoms, although they are having some or other physical symptoms and besides, they do not reject that somatic symptoms are because of psychological causes. Somatic symptoms are transient in cases with panic disorder, although the presentation of a patient with panic disorder may be similar at the time of the attack, but once the attack is over, they do not have bodily symptoms, but only the fear of the recurrence of symptoms. Patient with hypochondriasis are not preoccupied with the symptoms itself, but with the false idea that they are having some serious disease, so they are more concerned about the disease than the symptoms and mostly, they want repeated reassurance that they do not have the disease.[3]

ANNEXURE 1: Sample questionnaire for parents/patients.

Over the last 1 month have the child suffered the following symptoms often:

Physical symptoms   Yes   No

1. Stomach pain
2. Nausea
3. Chest pain
4. Sudden difficulty in breathing
5. Cough
6. Pain in limbs
7. Headache
8. Back pain
9. Menstrual pain
10. Pain in eyes
11. Poor vision
12. Fatigue
13. Dizziness
14. Fainting episodes

Behavioral symptoms

1. Restlessness
2. Significant change in appetite
3. Refusing to go to school
4. Feeling low or lethargic
5. Unexpected emotional outbursts
6. Episodes of crying
7. Loss of interest in activities
8. Disturbed sleep

If the child exhibit any of the physical symptoms frequently with or without any of the behavioral symptoms often, over the last 1 month, for which there is no medical explanation then diagnosis of somatoform disorder needs to be considered. Identification of a trigger or a stressor helps in confirming the diagnosis. Assessing behavioral symptoms is useful in quantifying the distress cause by the symptom and identifying any comorbid condition like anxiety or depression.

TREATMENT

Once the diagnosis has been established and accepted by the parents, it gets easier to treat the child, but still, it requires a multi-disciplinary approach for effective management. Till the time the diagnosis and presence of psychological factors are accepted by the parents, it is prudent to treat the child symptomatically rather than dismissing the physical symptoms, as it will stifle the building of trust between the physician and the parents and/or the child. Frequent follow-ups during the early days of management are necessary, which will help in identifying the stressors, evaluating the response to the symptomatic treatment and helping the parents understand the nature of the disorder. Physician must treat the patient with empathy and must take the complaints of the patient seriously even after knowing that it is primarily a psychosomatic case. Management of these cases include psychological and pharmacological treatment, of which the former is the mainstay of therapy.[3] Kallivayalil and Punnoose have described three types of approach for managing these patients:

1. *Reattribution approach:* The patient/parents are taught to identify the link between the bodily symptoms and stressors in life, which help them later to develop the proper coping strategies.
2. *Psychodynamic approach:* It helps in developing a faithful bonding between the patient and the physician which is especially helpful in the management of chronic cases.
3. *Directive approach:* In cases where the parents reject the involvement of psychological factors in the development of bodily symptoms, it is better to treat the symptoms as real, providing symptomatic treatment until there is acceptance.[18]

Psychological Treatment

Behavior management is the mainstay of treatment for somatoform disorders. *Cognitive behavior therapy* (*CBT*) helps in changing the behavioral pattern and developing adequate coping strategies. Goals must be divided into short-term, mid-term, and long-term goals and then child psychologists work on the approach to meet those goals. It is crucial to detect the stressor which may be the basic cause of physical symptoms. CBT may also be useful in patients having comorbid problems such as generalized anxiety or depression. The challenge for psychologists providing CBT is to identify the thought and emotional process of children as it is difficult for young children to identify their own thoughts and emotions and may be misguided by the suggestions given to them by parents or even the psychologist. Cognitive function of children below the age of 7 years is not appropriately matured which is required for rational thinking, expressing themselves, and reflecting their emotions and this is why CBT has been found to be more effective in adolescents than in younger children. A psychoeducational program for parents may also be required at times, within the CBT framework to involve them in child's therapy. By the use of active CBT techniques, the child's dysfunctional beliefs are gradually replaced by more adaptive ones and illness behavior is remodeled into a healthy behavior pattern. Group CBT involving children, parents and at times, school teachers has also been tried by some with success.[18-21]

Family therapy is a structured form of psychotherapy that has been found to be of particular use where family disharmony is the basic stressor leading to psychosomatic problems. Mullins and Olson proposed that dysfunctional family harmony is an important factor in the development of somatoform disorder in children. Families with too much strictness or too much attention to a child predispose them for developing somatoform disorders. Family therapy helps improve communication amongst the family members and improves functionality reducing stress and conflicts in the family. Family therapy focuses on improving interpersonal problems and rather than being concerned only about the one person in the family, it works on the whole family. Removing the reinforcement for the child's somatic behavior and rather supporting the healthy positive behavior is also emphasized to the family members.[3,22,23]

Child-centered play therapy is a novel form of child psychotherapy where parents are also involved in structured play therapy techniques combining them with ordinary plays. Studies have shown that it can be particularly useful for children between age of 4 and 10 years who have difficulty identifying and expressing their emotional disturbance. Child-centered play therapy when combined with functional parental counseling can give impressive results in young children with somatoform disorders.[24,25]

Relaxing techniques such as box breathing, guided imagery, progressive muscle relaxation (PMR), and yoga and mindfulness practice have been reported as useful adjuncts in the management of adolescents, especially those experiencing pain symptoms or those having associated anxiety.[3,25] A meta-analysis by Hamdani et al.

TABLE 1: Pharmacological agents for somatic pain and related disorders.[28-30]

Name of drug	Class	Dose	
Fluoxetine Brand name: Fludac • Suspension containing 20 mg/5 mL • Capsule 10, 20 and 60 mg Dawnex • Tablet 10 mg	SSRI	*6–12 years:* 10 mg once daily in morning *12–18 years:* 20 mg once daily in morning	Has been approved for use in children >6 years age
Fluvoxamine Brand name: Fluvoxin • Tablet 50 and 100 mg	SSRI	*6–18 years:* 25–50 mg after meals twice daily *12–18 years:* 100 mg once daily after meals; can be increased up to 300 mg/day	Approved by the FDA for use in children above 6 years age
Citalopram Brand name: Citara • Tablet 20 and 40 mg Citadep • Tablet 10, 20, and 40 mg	SSRI	*12–18 years age:* 10 mg once daily in morning; can be increased to maximum of 40 mg/day	Approved for use in young adolescents
Escitalopram Brand name: Nexito • Tablet 5, 10, and 20 mg Esdep • Tablet 5, 10, and 20 mg	SSRI	*12–18 years age:* 5 mg once daily in morning; can be increased up to 20 mg daily	Approved for use in young adolescents above 12 years

(FDA: Food and Drug Administration; SSRI: selective serotonin reuptake inhibitor)

reported relaxing techniques to be effective in adolescents in tackling anxiety and reducing stress.[26]

Pharmacological Treatment

Pharmacological treatment has been used as an adjunct to psychological treatment in cases not responding to psychological treatment alone, in severe cases or those having associated mental health problems such as anxiety or depression. It has been proven that there is dysregulation of serotoninergic and noradrenergic transmission in patients presenting with somatic symptoms. Neuroimaging and genetic studies have demonstrated the role of reduced serotonin (5-HT) and norepinephrine (NE) signal transmission and diminished receptor binding in these cases. It has been proposed that 5-HT and NE can play a role in diminishing painful symptoms by affecting the spinal cord inhibitory descending pain pathway. Antidepressants may also be helpful in alleviating symptoms such as fatigue and disturbed sleep through immunoregulatory effects. However, most data regarding the use of antidepressant medicines in somatoform disorders have been from studies on adult population and there have been few studies on usefulness of these medicines in children. Selective serotonin reuptake inhibitor (SSRI) and serotonin and norepinephrine reuptake inhibitor (SNRI) have been shown to be some benefit in these cases with benefits but have been advised to be used only when psychotherapy fails, however, SNRIs are not yet approved for use in children.[3,27] A list of SSRIs that have been approved in children for use as antidepressants and in other mental health disorders has been described in **Table 1**.

PROGNOSIS

Cognitive behavior therapy is the mainstay of therapy in patients with somatic pain and as per literature, there is immediate relief as the CBT is started, but for the long-term management, it may require 6–16 sessions of therapy with a trained mental health professional. Proper engagement of the patient and the family is absolutely necessary because it is not just the problem of the child and the cause as well as treatment may lie in the family dynamics and functionality. With long-term behavioral management therapy, patient is able to identify the stressors and becomes efficient in relating the physical symptoms to the stressor. Once the patient is able to identify the problem, he/she may use relaxation techniques and healthy coping strategies learnt during the therapy to tackle the symptoms.[3,8,15]

CONCLUSION

Somatoform disorders or bodily distress disorder, as the name suggests, is a distressing situation for the child and the family and puts a great deal of burden on the psyche of everyone closely related to the child. Besides, there is a loss of time and money because of frequent visits to healthcare providers and multiple investigations to find an organic symptom to answer the cause of the symptoms. Clinician after diagnosing the disorder as psychological, should first develop a rapport and trusting relationship with the child and the family and over the next few visits, describe the psychological component using the serotoninergic and noradrenergic models to provide an explanation for the disease and reassure that there is no serious health problem and the symptoms are manageable with behavioral therapy. It would be prudent for the family physician to be involved with the family even when the child is in therapy with a mental health professional, as it would strengthen the belief of the family and improve the compliance to the therapy.

REFERENCES

1. Disorders of bodily distress or bodily experience. ICD-11 for Mortality and Morbidity Statistics (Version:01/2023). [online] Available from: https://icd.who.int/browse11/l-m/en#/http%3a%2f%2fid.who.int%2ficd%2fentity%2f794195577 [Last accessed October, 2023].
2. Bodily distress disorder. ICD-11 for Mortality and Morbidity Statistics (Version:01/2023). [online] Available from: https://icd.who.int/dev11/f/en#/http%3A%2F%2Fid.who.int%2Ficd%2Fentity%2F767044268 [Last accessed October, 2023].
3. Agarwal V, Srivastava C, Sitholey P. Clinical practice guidelines for the management of somatoform disorders in children and adolescents. Indian J Psychiatry. 2019;61: 241-6.
4. Elia J. Somatic Symptom and Related Disorders in Children. [online] Available from: https://www.msdmanuals.com/en-in/home/children-s-health-issues/mental-health-disorders-in-children-and-adolescents/somatic-symptom-and-related-disorders-in-children [Last accessed October, 2023].
5. Shanker G, Sharma I. Study of Determinants of Somatoform Disorders in Children. Cureus. 2023;15(3):e36447.
6. Impact of the DSM-IV to DSM-5 Changes on the National Survey on Drug Use and Health [Internet]. National Library of Medicine. [online] Available from: https://www.ncbi.nlm.nih.gov/books/NBK519704/table/ch3.t31/#_ncbi_dlg_citbx_NBK519704 [Last accessed October, 2023].
7. Vesterling C, Wilke J, Baker N, Bolz T. Epidemiology of somatoform symptoms and disorders in childhood and adolescence: A systematic review and meta-analysis. Health Soc Care Community. 2023;6242678:1-16.
8. Mohapatra S, Deo SJK, Satapathy A, Rath N. Somatoform disorders in children and adolescents. Ger J Psychiatry. 2014;17:7-10.
9. Mullick MS. Somatoform disorders in children and adolescents. Bangladesh Med Res Counc Bull. 2002;28(3): 112-22.
10. Konichezky A, Gothelf D. Somatoform disorders in children and adolescents. Harefuah. 2011;150(2):180-4, 203.
11. Yeung AS, He DJ. Somatoform disorder. Western J Med. 2002;176:253-6.
12. Hart SL, Hodgkinson SC, Belcher HME, Hyman C, Cooley-Strickland M. Somatic symptoms, peer and school stress, and family and community violence exposure among urban elementary school children. J Behav Med. 2013;36(5):454-65.
13. Jellesma F, Rieffe C, Terwogt M. My peers, my friend, and I: Peer interactions and somatic complaints in boys and girls. Soc Sci Med. 2008;66(11):2195-205.
14. Das S, Mandal US, Nath S. Relationship between perceived social support and severity of symptoms in persons with somatoform disorder. J Evolution Med Dent Sci. 2020;9(06):320-3.
15. Oyama O, Paltoo C, Greengold J. Somatoform disorders. Am Fam Physician. 2007;76(9):1333-8.
16. Spitzer RL, Williams JB, Kroenke K, Linzer M, deGruy FV 3rd, Hahn SR, et al. Utility of a new procedure for diagnosing mental disorders in primary care: The PRIME-MD 1000 Study. JAMA. 1994;272(22):1749-56.
17. Heimann P, Herpertz-Dahlmann B, Buning J, Wagner N, Stollbrink-Peschgens C, Dempfle A, et al. Somatic symptom and related disorders in children and adolescents: evaluation of a naturalistic inpatient multidisciplinary treatment. Child Adolesc Psychiatry Ment Health. 2018; 12:34.
18. Kallivayalil RA, Punnoose VP. Understanding and managing somatoform disorders: Making sense of non-sense. Indian J Psychiatry. 2010;52(1):S240-5.

19. Halder S, Mahato AK. Cognitive behavior therapy for children and adolescents: Challenges and gaps in practice. Indian J Psychol Med. 2019;41:279-83.
20. Spence SH. Cognitive therapy with children and adolescents: from theory to practice. J Child Psychol Psychiatry. 1994;35(7):1191-228.
21. Matthys W, Schutter DJG. Increasing effectiveness of cognitive behavioral therapy for conduct problems in children and adolescents: What can we learn from neuroimaging studies? Clin Child Fam Psychol Rev. 2021; 24:484-99.
22. Mullins LL, Olson RA, Chaney JM. A social learning/family systems approach to the treatment of somatoform disorders in children and adolescents. Fam Syst Med. 1992;10:201-12.
23. Varghese M, Kirpekar V, Loganathan S. Family interventions: Basic principles and techniques. Indian J Psychiatry. 2020;62:S192-200.
24. Dutta R, Mehta M. Child-centered play therapy in management of somatoform disorders. J Indian Assoc. Child Adolesc Ment Health. 2006;2(3):85-8.
25. Norelli SK, Long A, Krepps JM. Relaxation Techniques. In: StatPearls [Internet]. Treasure Island (FL): StatPearls Publishing; 2023.
26. Hamdani SU, Huma ZE, Zafar SW, Suleman N, Baneen UU, Waqas A, et al. Effectiveness of relaxation techniques as an active ingredient of psychological interventions' to reduce distress, anxiety and depression in adolescents: A systematic review and meta-analysis. Int J Ment Health Syst. 2022;16:31.
27. Liu Y, Zhao J, Fan X, Guo W. Dysfunction of serotonergic and noradrenergic systems and somatic symptoms in psychiatric disorders. Front Psychiatry. 2019;10:286.
28. DeMaso DR, Walter HJ. Psychopharmacology. Kliegman RM, St. Geme JW, Blum NJ, Shah SS, Tasker RC, Wilson KM (Eds). Nelson Textbook of Pediatrics, 21st edition. Philadelphia: Elsevier; 2020. pp. 189-96.
29. Drug Monograph. In: Unni JC, Nair MKC, Menon PSN, Bansal CP (Eds). IAP Pediatric Drug Formulary 2015 with IAP Recommendations on Drug Therapy for Pediatric Illnesses. 4th edition Cochin: A Project of IAP Computer and Medical Informatics Chapter; 2015. pp. 343-6.
30. Tripathi KD (Ed). Drugs used in mental illness: Antidepressant and antianxiety drugs. Essentials of Medical Pharmacology, 8th edition. New Delhi/London: Jaypee Brothers Medical Publishers (P) Ltd.; 2019. pp. 481-96.

Chapter 16: Sleep Disorders in Children

Manish Parakh, Ankit Kumar Meena, Bhanu Pratap Rathore

INTRODUCTION

Between the age of 1 and 5 years, 20–30% of children experience sleep issues such as settling problems and frequent night awakenings. However, cultural variations may also play a role. Even after 15 months, 40–80% of children still have chronic sleep difficulties that may continue into adulthood.[1] Toddlers often face settling and night-waking issues, with rates ranging from 20 to 25%. Adolescents experience their second peak of sleep issues during delayed sleep phase syndrome, struggling to fall asleep, and wake up in the morning for school. Children with epilepsy, learning disabilities, physical disabilities, or attention deficit hyperactivity disorder often experience more frequent sleep issues.[1]

This chapter explores healthy sleep in childhood, including age-appropriate sleep durations, changes in sleep architecture with age, the significance of sleep for learning, and various sleep disorders.

MECHANISM OF SLEEP

It is widely known that gamma-aminobutyric acid (GABA) is the main inhibitory neurotransmitter in the central nervous system, and activating GABA-a receptors promotes sleep.[2] Sleep-promoting neurons in the anterior hypothalamus release GABA, suppressing wake-promoting areas in the hypothalamus and brainstem.[3] Adenosine effectively supports sleep by inhibiting the neurons that encourage wakefulness in various brain regions, such as the basal forebrain, tuberomammillary nucleus, and lateral hypothalamus.[4] To maintain alertness, certain neurochemicals, including acetylcholine (ACh), dopamine (DA), norepinephrine (NE), serotonin (5-HT), histamine (HA), and the neuropeptide hypocretin are responsible.[3] The levels of cortical ACh release are highest during waking and lowest during rapid eye movement (REM) sleep.[5]

TABLE 1: Summary of various sleep and wakefulness-promoting agents and their location in the brain.

Sleep-promoting agents	Wakefulness-promoting agents
• *GABA:* Anterior hypothalamus • *Adenosine:* Basal forebrain	• *Acetylcholine:* Cortex • *Dopamine:* Median raphe nucleus • *Norepinephrine:* Locus ceruleus • *Serotonin:* Dorsal raphe nucleus • *Histamine:* Posterior thalamus (tuberomammillary nucleus) • *Hypocretin:* Dorsolateral hypothalamus

While the neurons in the locus ceruleus (LC) release NE, the neurons in the dorsal raphe nucleus release 5-HT. The LC's noradrenergic cells project to various brain areas that regulate arousal, including the basal forebrain, thalamus, hypothalamus, and cortex. They promote wakefulness and inhibit REM sleep. The production of HA is a result of histamine-containing neurons located in the posterior thalamic tuberomammillary nucleus. The dorsolateral hypothalamus contains the cells that produce hypocretin; these cells send projections to key brain regions that regulate arousal **(Table 1)**.[4]

Newborns and Infants (Birth—1 Year) (Table 2)

During the first few weeks of life, neonates have an irregular sleep pattern with no fixed schedule for sleeping or waking up. This means that they sleep intermittently both during the day and night. Babies typically sleep 16–18 hours daily, in short and irregular periods. Their longest stretch of sleep typically lasts around 2.5–4 hours. Newborns experience three different types of sleep: (1) Silent sleep, which is similar to nonrapid eye movement (NREM); (2) active sleep, which is similar to REM; and (3) indeterminate sleep. It is important to note that newborns

TABLE 2: Recommended sleep duration for various age groups (As per the American Academy of Sleep Medicine guidelines).

Age	Recommended sleep hours
4–12 months	12–16 hours (including naps)
1–2 years	11–14 hours (including naps)
3–5 years	10–13 hours (including naps)
6–12 years	9–12 hours
13–18 years	8–10 hours

BOX 1: International Classification of Sleep Disorder-3.
- Insomnia
- Sleep-related breathing disorders
- Central disorders of hypersomnolence
- Circadian rhythm sleep-wake disorders
- Parasomnias
- Sleep-related movement disorders
- Other sleep disorders

BOX 2: Classification of insomnia.
- Chronic insomnia disorder
- Short-term insomnia disorder
- Other insomnia disorder

enter sleep through REM rather than NREM, and their sleep episodes typically only consist of one or two cycles. This is a crucial difference between the way children and adults sleep. Infants' sleep patterns gradually develop into circadian rhythms by the time they reach the age of 2–3 months. As a result, they tend to sleep for more extended periods during the night and stay awake for more extended periods during the day. By 2 months of age, they usually shift to sleeping predominantly at night. At 3 months of age, the onset of sleep with NREM occurs due to a diurnal pattern of melatonin and cortisol cycling. At this stage of the sleep cycle, REM sleep decreases and progresses toward later stages of sleep. Notably, the typical NREM and REM sleep cycle lasts around 50 minutes, shorter than the 90-minute cycle observed in adults. When infants are 12 months old, they typically sleep about 14–15 hours daily.[5]

Toddlers (Age 1–3 Years) and Children (Age 3–9 Years) (Table 2)

Children aged 2–5 years sleep for 11 to 13 hours. At this stage, they spend significantly longer time in stage N3 than adolescents due to their longer REM sleep latencies.[6,7]

Adolescents (Age 10–18 Years) and Adults (18+ Years) (Table 2)

Teenagers get an average of 9–10 hours of sleep per night. Puberty brings hormonal changes that decrease slow-wave sleep and sleep latency while time spent in stage N2 increases. During mid-puberty, there is an increase in daytime sleepiness compared to earlier stages of puberty.[8]

FUNCTIONS OF SLEEP[9,10]

- The suprachiasmatic nucleus controls the circadian rhythm, which regulates the release of adrenocorticotropic hormone (ACTH), prolactin, melatonin, and norepinephrine.
- Developing neural abilities, i.e., learning, memory, cognition
- Helps in desirable synapse formation.

CLASSIFICATION OF SLEEP DISORDERS (BOX 1)

The third edition of the International Classification of Sleep Disorders (ICSD-3) is the recent classification for sleep disorders. Pediatric diagnoses are not differentiated from adult diagnoses, except for pediatric Obstructive sleep apnea (OSA), in ICSD-2. The ICSD-3 uses the American Academy of Sleep Medicine's Manual for the Scoring of Sleep and Associated Events to define specific findings on a polysomnogram (PSG), such as respiratory episodes or movement abnormalities.[11]

Insomnia

Insomnia disorders have been classified based on their length and assumed pathogenesis in the past. However, with the introduction of sleep-wake disorders, most diagnostic frameworks now differentiate between acute and chronic insomnia. The ICSD-3 task committee decided to group all diagnoses of insomnia (both "comorbid" and "primary") into a single category of chronic insomnia disorder. The fact that a choice has been made does not negate the existence of significant differences in the pathophysiology of the various types of chronic insomnia. Instead, we cannot consistently distinguish or utilize these differences to develop personalized therapeutic methods. According to the ICSD-3, duration criterion for chronic insomnia disorder is 3 months. The diagnosis of insomnia according to ICSD-3 is listed in **Box 2**.

Chronic Insomnia Disorder

In order to conduct a thorough evaluation of sleep-related concerns, it is crucial to take into account three essential elements:
1. Difficulties in initiating or maintaining sleep
2. Appropriateness of the sleep setting
3. Any impact on daily functioning.

All these problems should last for 3 months and at least three times/week.

It is important to note that experiencing trouble sleeping does not necessarily mean someone has insomnia. Some people may have occasional poor sleep without noticing any major impact on their daily life or mentioning it as a concern. Sleeplessness is often a symptom of various medical and mental issues. However, diagnosis of chronic insomnia is only made when it is severe, persistent, and requires professional attention and treatment.

Parents must teach their children sleep-promoting behaviors and sleep hygiene, including maintaining regular sleep and wake times, limiting play before bed, observing at least 1 hour of screen-free time before bed, using blue light-blocking apps on electronic devices in the evening, encouraging independent sleep, avoiding clock watching, and practicing relaxation techniques.[12]

The US Food and Drug Administration has not authorized any drugs for treating insomnia in children. Moreover, the available literature needs more information about the effectiveness of such treatments. However, melatonin, melatonin receptor agonists, adrenergic agonist, benzodiazepine, and nonbenzodiazepine receptor agonists may be used.[11]

Sleep-related Breathing Disorders

Sleep-related breathing disorders are categorized into four groups:
1. Obstructive sleep apnea
2. Complex sleep apnea (CSA) syndromes
3. Sleep-related hypoventilation disorders
4. Sleep-related hypoxemia disorders.

Obstructive Sleep Apnea

Obstructive sleep apnea often manifests in 1-5% of children aged 2-6 years. OSA affects 21.5-39.5% of obese children, with a higher prevalence in those who meet the criteria for morbid obesity.[13] Mechanical obstruction and decreased upper airway patency cause upper airway collapsibility. Tonsil and adenoid hypertrophy reduce airway size, increasing blockage risk as pharyngeal muscle tone decreases during sleep. Allergic rhinitis can increase the risk of OSA by causing nasal blockage and upper airway resistance.[14] OSA is common in individuals with various medical conditions, including Down syndrome, neuromuscular problems, epilepsy, cerebral palsy, obesity, Chiari malformations, headaches, attention deficit hyperactivity disorder, Prader–Willi syndrome, and Pierre Robin sequence.[12] Anatomical factors such as midface hypoplasia, high narrow arched palate, micrognathia, and neurological problems impairing the tone of the upper airway may also increase the chance of OSA. Hypoxemia or hypercapnia resulting from obstructive respiratory episodes can cause repeated awakenings, leading to fragmented sleep. OSA can be identified through symptoms such as snoring, apneas, labored breathing, sweating during sleep, headaches, restless sleep, dry mouth, enuresis, fatigue, and exhaustion. OSA has been linked to negative effects on executive function, memory, learning, school performance, intelligence quotient (IQ), behavior, and emotion control.[15] OSA is linked to several negative health effects in children, including high blood pressure, impaired endothelial function, and insulin sensitivity.[16]

Children showing symptoms of OSA should undergo a polysomnogram at a sleep laboratory or be referred to a pediatric sleep specialist for clinical evaluation. Due to their subtle symptoms, keeping the threshold for children to get a polysomnogram is important. Diagnosis of OSA requires an obstructive apnea-hypopnea index (AHI) of 1 event per hour or more, but other criteria for obstructive hypoventilation patterns also exist.[17] These diagnostic criteria for pediatric OSA have been adapted from the ICSD-3. The OSA is considered mild if the number of apnea and hypopnea events per hour (AHI) is between 1.0 and 4.9. If it is between 5.0 and 9.9, it is classified as moderate; if it is 10.0 or higher, it is considered severe. Apneas in children are scored based on >90% drop in airflow for more than two breath cycles. Depending on whether the effort is maintained, they are classified as central or obstructive. Hypopneas are scored if there is a ≥30% drop in airflow signal linked with cortical arousals or a ≥3% oxygen desaturation. Hypopnea is considered obstructive if they cause snoring, increased effort, or another obstructive pattern. If OSA is present, a central apnea index of 5 or above must prompt immediate evaluation of neurologic or cardiac conditions. Teenagers aged 13–18 years can use either adult or pediatric scoring criteria due to a lack of evidence on the ideal age for adult criteria and airway dynamics not directly related to sexual maturity (Tanner staging).

The severity of OSA, symptoms, and medical comorbidities influences the therapy option. Adenotonsillectomy is recommended as the initial treatment if adenotonsillar hypertrophy is present.[18] If adenotonsillectomy does not resolve OSA, continuous positive airway pressure may be considered.[19] Estimates for residual OSA after adenotonsillectomy vary widely, ranging from 31 to 73% for any severity and 13 to 22% for moderate-to-severe OSA.[20] A postoperative polysomnogram after adenotonsillectomy is recommended, especially for patients with moderate-to-severe OSA, asthma, or overweight.[21] Positive airway pressure, whether continuous or bilevel, has been proven effective in treating juvenile OSA. However, adherence may be suboptimal. Other therapies include intranasal corticosteroids, which significantly lower AHI in children with mild OSA.[22] The efficacy of oral montelukast in reducing OSA severity in children has been established by a randomized 16-week study.[23] For children with maxillary constriction and dental malocclusion, rapid maxillary expansion is an effective treatment for OSA.[24] This innovative technique involves using an appliance to progressively increase the transverse diameter of the hard palate. A study has been conducted involving adolescents with Down syndrome. The study involves implanting a hypoglossal nerve stimulator to help with sleep apnea. The pilot study results were promising, with a 56–85% reduction in AHI and four out of six adolescents achieving mild or no OSA with less than five events per hour.[25]

Disorders of Central Hypersomnolence

The conditions are defined by excessive daytime sleepiness (known as hypersomnolence). It is crucial to note that this condition must not be caused by any other sleep disorder, particularly those that interrupt sleep, such as breathing issues during sleep (e.g., sleep-related breathing disorder) or disruptions in the body's natural sleep–wake cycle. While other factors, such as illnesses or medications, may play a role in causing hypersomnolence, the primary cause of central disorders of hypersomnolence is intrinsic defects in the central nervous system's ability to regulate sleep and wakefulness. Insufficient sleep caused by behavior also falls under this category of disorders. **Box 3** provides a comprehensive list of specific diagnoses. Detailed descriptions are covered later in this chapter.

Excessive sleepiness is a common symptom of these illnesses. The ICSD-3 defines it as "daily episodes of

BOX 3: Disorders of central hypersomnolence.
- Narcolepsy type-1
- Narcolepsy type-2
- Idiopathic hypersomnia
- Kleine–Levin syndrome
- Hypersomnia due to a medical disorder
- Hypersomnia due to a medication or substance
- Hypersomnia associated with a psychiatric disorder
- Insufficient sleep syndrome

an uncontrollable urge to sleep or daytime sleepiness." In order to precisely measure objective sleepiness in individuals with conditions like Narcolepsy and idiopathic hypersomnia (IH), the multiple sleep latency test (MSLT) necessitates a sleep latency of <8 minutes.[26,27] Physicians must differentiate between individuals experiencing extreme sleepiness and those perceived as "typical" yet suffering from sleep deprivation. Doctors must be cautious when working with individuals with prolonged sleep needs who are susceptible to sleep deprivation. This is important because it may lead to incorrect results during diagnosing central hypersomnolence through MSLT.[28] It is advisable to keep track of sleep records and use actigraphy for at least a week before undergoing MSLT to eliminate the possibility of insufficient sleep or abnormal sleep patterns as potential factors for unusual MSLT results.

Narcolepsy

In the past, narcolepsy was classified into two types: (1) Narcolepsy with cataplexy and (2) narcolepsy without cataplexy. The term "with cataplexy" is no longer accurate, as hypocretin deficiency has been determined to be the root cause of the disorder.[29] Studies have documented that while some individuals with hypocretin deficiency eventually develop cataplexy, others do not. However, it is important to note that this is a less common occurrence.[30] It is important to understand that after establishing that hypocretin is the root cause of Narcolepsy, it requires a distinct and precise classification method. That is why the ICSD-3 has established "narcolepsy type 1" and "narcolepsy type 2" as definitive categories. Diagnosis of narcolepsy type 1 often relies on cataplexy detection due to the limited availability of hypocretin tests. Narcolepsy type 1 can be diagnosed if an individual experiences excessive daytime sleepiness and has low CSF fluid hypocretin-1 levels (<110 pg/mL or less than one third of the normal values based on the same standardized test) or mean latency <8 min in MSLT with evidence of ≥2 sleep-onset REM periods (SOREMPs) and clear cataplexy.

For diagnosing narcolepsy type 2, following predefined criteria during the MSLT test is crucial. This includes an average latency of <8 minutes and at least two SOREMPs (or one SOREMP on PSG and one or more on MSLT). It is also important to ensure that the CSF fluid hypocretin-1 levels do not meet the criteria for narcolepsy type 1 and that no cataplexy is present.

Treatment of narcolepsy: Children with narcolepsy must ensure they get enough sleep. Additionally, scheduling planned naps may be beneficial. Wakefulness-promoting agents such as modafinil, armodafinil, amphetamine, and methylphenidate derivatives can help combat drowsiness in many children with narcolepsy. However, none of these drugs are Food and Drug Administration (FDA) approved for narcolepsy.

Sodium oxybate is another option that acts both on excessive sleepiness and cataplexy. It acts through the $GABA_B$ receptor, promotes REM sleep, and reduces sleep fragmentation. The observed side effects include vomiting, headaches, loss of appetite, dizziness, and two unfavorable side effects: acute psychoses and suicidal thoughts. Sodium oxybate is FDA-approved medication for narcolepsy in patients older than 7 years. The FDA has recently approved selective dopamine and norepinephrine reuptake inhibitors in adults. However, pediatric experience is still lacking.

Idiopathic Hypersomnia

The criterion for *idiopathic hypersomnia* is a diagnosis of exclusion that needs there are subjective complaints of excessive daytime sleepiness along with MSLT of <8 minutes with fewer than two SOREMPs (including any SOREMP on the PSG from the preceding night), absence of cataplexy and low CSF hypocretin and no other identifiable cause. Only *excessive sleep* can be the initial symptom of IH in certain individuals. Those who fail to satisfy the MSLT criteria for sleepiness must undergo either a 24-hour PSG or a 1-week actigraphy/sleep diary with sound sleep.

Kleine–Levin Syndrome

Kleine–Levin syndrome is a cyclical disorder of hyperphagia and somnolence; each episode lasts for 2 days to 5 weeks and is associated with cognitive dysfunction and behavioral disorders; the patient has a normal function in between; hypersomina, confusion, apathy, and derealization are the four most common symptoms of Kleine–Levin syndrome.[17] Onset usually occurs during puberty; the estimated prevalence is 2.3 cases per million people. There is no definitive test for Kleine–Levin syndrome. Around 85% of cases eventually resolve, while 15% have long-term symptoms. Lithium, amantadine, and IV steroids are among the most promising treatments.

Parasomnia

Parasomnias are unwanted experiences or events related to sleep. Parasomnia can occur in any stage of sleep. During sleep, 75–80% of the time is spent in nonrapid eye movement (NREM) sleep. It ranges from drowsiness to the deepest slow-wave (N3) sleep. Parasomnia is common during non-REM sleep due to its length and diverse physiology. Parasomnia is broadly classified as non-REM and REM parasomnia. The detailed classification of parasomnia is given in **Box 4**.

Nonrapid Eye Movement Parasomnia

The ICSD-3 version recognizes NREM parasomnias as arousal disorders.[31] It comprises confusional arousals, sleepwalking, sleep terrors, and sleep-related eating disorders. Even though these conditions display varying symptoms, they share some important characteristics that are:

- Multiple episodes of partial arousal
- During the episode, the person has a lack of response or responds inappropriately.
- The individual has no recollection of the event.

BOX 4: Classification of parasomnia.

NREM-related parasomnias:
- Confusional arousals
- Sleepwalking
- Sleep terrors
- Sleep-related eating disorder

REM-related parasomnias:
- REM sleep behavior disorder
- Recurrent isolated sleep paralysis
- Nightmare disorder

Other parasomnias:
- Exploding head syndrome
- Sleep-related hallucinations
- Sleep enuresis
- Parasomnia due to a medical disorder
- Parasomnia due to a medication or substance
- Parasomnia, unspecified

(NREM: nonrapid eye movement; REM: rapid eye movement)

Usually, NREM parasomnia episodes occur during the first one third of the night, when deep/slow-wave sleep is more common.[32] Children with parasomnias experience rapid changes in the amplitude of slow bursts during slow-wave sleep.[33] NREM parasomnia is common during childhood and usually resolves with age. Sleep terrors are seen in 1–6% children, maximum at 1.5 years of age, while sleepwalking has a prevalence of 4–40%, peaking at age 10.[34-36] Confusional arousals are more common than other arousal disorders, with an occurrence rate of up to 17.3%.[36]

It is worth mentioning that parasomnias have predispositions to different factors, including family history, lack of sleep, youthfulness, certain medication intake (such as sedative-hypnotics, antihistamines, stimulants, and neuroleptics), and the presence of fever or illness.[37] Sleep disorders such as restless leg syndrome (RLS), periodic limb movement disorder (PLMD), and OSA can mimic or trigger parasomnia attacks.[37]

Types of NREM parasomnia
- *Sleepwalking:* It is characterised by sitting up in bed while asleep and staring blankly while engaging in repetitive and automatic actions, such as pulling at own's clothes or bed sheets, before eventually getting up and walking around.[32] Sometimes, children may wander freely around the house, entering different rooms, and even leaving the house. Young individuals tend to have reduced awareness and attentiveness toward their surroundings during a sleepwalking episode. This can make them less coordinated and more prone to tripping, falling downstairs, or even accidentally going through a window.[32] Sometimes, individuals may perform complex activities such as cooking, driving, or eating during sleepwalking. Sleepwalking usually lasts around 15 minutes but can last longer for some people. If parents attempt to wake a sleepwalking child, it may not be effective and can even lead to the child becoming upset or aggressive.
- *Sleep terror:* A typical episode of sleep terror is characterized by abruptly sitting up, screaming, appearing frightened appearance, and the child may lose control. This condition often involves physiological signs of autonomic arousal, such as rapid breathing, increased heart rate, sweating, dilated pupils, and heightened muscle tone.[36] Sometimes, when parents try to wake up their children during the episode, resulting in an ineffective effort, the children may appear disoriented and confused. Sleep terror episodes typically last between 30 seconds to 3 minutes. Children often go back to sleep afterward without recalling the incident the following day.
- *Confusional arousal:* Confusional arousals are identified by confused or sluggish thinking, disorientation, and inappropriate reactivity to external stimuli. Children may engage in instinctive behaviors such as kicking or thrashing, picking at clothing or bedclothes, or improperly using things. During these episodes, people may make sounds such as groaning, wailing, or sitting up, but they usually do not show signs of distress or move around. These episodes are not associated with fear or sleepwalking. Sometimes, attempting to wake up the child may lead to agitation. Confusional arousals typically last between 5 and 15 minutes, and the child will not remember them afterward.[36]
- *Sleep-related eating disorder:* Sleep-related eating disorder (SRED) is defined as an episode of unconscious consumption of food or drink while partially awake from sleep. This eating behavior is often disorganized, rapid, and uncontrolled.[38] During the episodes, people with SRED often eat foods high in calories and carbohydrates and sometimes consume non-nutritive substances.[36] The memory of the event is usually vivid in the morning.

Evaluation: Before beginning treatment, it is important to conduct a comprehensive assessment to accurately diagnose the condition and eliminate the possibility of nocturnal seizures, OSA, RLS, or other medical sleep disorders such as PLMD. When assessing incidents involving young children, parental or caregiver reports are frequently relied upon as the children may not recall. However, a thorough investigation must be conducted into the timing, duration, and nature of the events, including detailed descriptions of the child's movements and behaviors and reviewing the child's sleep history. This is crucial in ensuring that a comprehensive and accurate assessment is made. To supplement the explanations given by parents, home videos could be beneficial. While it may not capture parasomnia events, a polysomnography test may be required to eliminate the possibility of a medical sleep disorder. If there is a suspicion of nocturnal seizures, an electroencephalogram (EEG) is recommended.

Treatment of NREM parasomnia: Parents must avoid waking their child during parasomnia episodes to prevent the experience from becoming more intense or prolonged. Additionally, parents should be careful not to discuss the occurrence with their child the next day to prevent unnecessary worry or shame. In order to ensure safety while dealing with NREM parasomnias, it is important to take certain precautions. Clear any obstructions from the bedroom, secure doors, and windows, place the mattress on the ground, and consider adding locks and alarms to doors and windows. It is important to address and minimize triggers to treat the issue effectively. For individuals with a lack of sleep, improving sleep quality is crucial. Additionally, it is important to inform parents about appropriate sleep for their child's age.

Rapid Eye Movement Parasomnia

Sleep disorders such as nightmares, REM-sleep behavior disorder, and hypnagogic/hypnopompic hallucination, can occur during REM sleep. It is worth noting that the first REM cycle starts approximately 90 minutes after one has fallen asleep, and subsequent cycles occur every 90 minutes. As the night progresses, the duration of each REM cycle increases.

- *REM sleep behavior disorder (RBD)* is predominantly observed in older men, with the onset of symptoms typically occurring between the ages of 50 and 60 years. It is worth noting that some individuals may experience a subclinical prodromal condition, which can persist for many years. People with RBD experience a disruption in the normal process that typically causes muscle relaxation during REM sleep, causing them to act out their dreams physically. This may be due to malformations and lesions in the brain stem, which prevent the necessary muscle atonia during REM sleep.[39] In addition, people with RBD often have aggressive and violent dreams. They may exhibit physical movements like leg and body jerking, punching, kicking, yelling, shouting, swearing, springing out of bed, colliding with walls or furniture, and even unintentionally harming their bed partner.[32] There is a significant connection between RBD and neurodegenerative diseases such as Lewy body dementia, multiple systems atrophy, and Parkinson's disease.[40] More than half of the patients who had complaint of RBD ultimately developed parkinsonism. Acute RBD is often associated with the use and withdrawal of drugs such as benzodiazepines and barbiturates. Additionally, alcohol withdrawal can also contribute to this condition. Certain antidepressants, cholinergic drugs, and monoamine oxidase inhibitors have also been linked to a higher risk of developing acute RBD.[41] Antidepressants affect the quality of sleep by reducing the duration of REM sleep and increasing sleep latency. However, it is not yet clear how they cause RBD in the short term.

It is crucial to prioritize environmental safety when dealing with individuals with RBD, just as with any other sleep disorder. Educating patients and their partners on effective strategies to prevent injury is an absolute must. Clonazepam has been proven to successfully treat RBD in patients with dosages ranging from 0.5 to 1 mg at bedtime. This highly effective treatment has been known to reduce problematic behaviors and dangerous dreams in up to 90% of patients. While some may require higher dosages, developing a tolerance is rare. Additionally, melatonin is a useful supplement when taken alone or with clonazepam. Doses of 3-12 mg are helpful.[42] Levodopa, certain tricyclic antidepressants, and dopamine agonists are also used successfully.[43,44]

Nightmare

Nightmares are scary dreams or unsettling mental experiences that often cause individuals to wake up from their REM sleep. Dreams often involve themes of danger, such as being chased or attacked. Nightmares are commonly associated with feelings of fear and anxiety but can also include emotions such as sadness, anger, and unhappiness. Unlike sleep terrors, nightmares are not associated with confusion or disorientation, and the subject can relate dream content and accompanying fear and anxiety upon awakening. Sleep terrors may lead to sleepwalking, whereas dreams never do. Nightmares typically do not involve motor activity such as sitting up, hitting, thrashing, speaking, or walking, unlike REM-sleep behavior disorder. Nightmares can be caused or worsened by withdrawing from REM-suppressing drugs such as selective serotonin reuptake inhibitors, tricyclic antidepressants, hypnotics, and alcohol. Beta-blockers and dopaminergic agonists may also contribute to this.[45] There are several ways to treat nightmares, including psychotherapy, stress reduction, and avoiding medications that can trigger them. Establishing a regular sleep–wake cycle can also help reduce the frequency and intensity of nightmares, especially for those with poor sleep hygiene.[45,46] Medications such as prazosin (5–10 mg) and cyproheptadine (4–16 mg) can also be used to treat nightmares.[47]

Recurrent Isolated Sleep Paralysis

Sleep paralysis is characterized by the persistence of REM atonia into wakefulness, leading to the inability to perform voluntary movement at the onset of sleep (hypnagogic paralysis) or upon waking up (hypnopompic paralysis).[48] The respiratory and ocular muscles are spared during these episodes. Sleep paralysis is a cardinal feature of narcolepsy, but when it occurs spontaneously and recurrently (at least two episodes in 6 months of duration) is called recurrent isolated sleep paralysis (RISP). These episodes typically last around 6 minutes but can range from a few seconds to 20 minutes. The patients may experience intense fear during the episode as the consciousness remains intact.[49] Hallucinations may occur during a RISP episode and contribute to the patient's discomfort. Typically, onset occurs in adolescence, with a greater prevalence among females than males.[50] Factors such as insufficient sleep and an inconsistent sleep pattern can lead to RISP episodes. Tricyclic antidepressants or selective serotonin reuptake inhibitors treat RISP.[50]

Restless Leg Syndrome

Restless leg syndrome presents with leg pain that intensifies during nighttime and subsides with physical activity. Periodic limb movement disorder is diagnosed in children who exhibit high PLM indices and experience daytime symptoms such as sleepiness and does not fulfill the criteria of RLS. Restless sleep disorder is a newly identified condition where children experience restless sleep and daytime sleepiness but do not meet the criteria for periodic limb movement disorder (PLMD) or RLS. The prevalence of RLS is 2% in a few studies. Children with RLS often exhibit elevated periodic limb movement levels, characterized as >5 PLMs per hour on a polysomnogram. In contrast, typical levels for children are <5/h. According to epidemiological research, over 70% of children diagnosed with RLS have at least one parent with similar complaints.

Although family inheritance patterns suggest autosomal dominant inheritance with varying penetrance, causal genetic alterations are yet to be discovered. RLS can be caused by iron deficiency and dysfunction in the dopaminergic system. 83% of children with RLS had serum ferritin levels of 50 ng/mL, while 55% of those with serum levels of 50 ng/mL had RLS. Iron deficiency is common in children with RLS, and those with iron deficiency often have RLS. Iron therapy is considered when iron deficiency is detected. If serum ferritin levels are below 50 ng/mL in children, the International Restless Legs Syndrome Study Group recommends oral iron treatment. According to an extensive trial, children who took oral iron supplements in long-term experienced improvements in their RLS symptoms, PLM index, and blood ferritin levels.[12]

CONCLUSION

Diagnosing and treating sleep–wake disorders in children and adolescents can greatly improve their quality of life. Unfortunately, limited access to sleep experts and diagnostic facilities is a major obstacle. To tackle this issue, it is important to enhance the sleep-related education and training of pediatric postgraduates. Additionally, setting universal technical standards for pediatric nocturnal polysomnography and developing evidence-based protocols for diagnosing and treating specific diseases would be beneficial. Ongoing research on narcolepsy, circadian rhythm disorders, RLS, and sleep apnea genetics, as well as the connection between sleep and behavior, is in progress. In addition, hypocretin analogs are being developed with the goal of treating narcolepsy. This interdisciplinary field seeks to combine different clinical and fundamental research areas.[51]

REFERENCES

1. Bruni O, Novelli L. Sleep disorders in children. BMJ Clin Evid. 2010;2010:2304.
2. Gottesmann C. GABA mechanisms and sleep. Neuroscience. 2002;111(2):231-9.
3. Murillo-Rodríguez E, Arias-Carrión O, Sanguino-Rodríguez K, González-Arias M, Haro R. Mechanisms of sleep-wake cycle modulation. CNS Neurol Disord Drug Targets. 2009;8(4):245-53.
4. Watson CJ, Baghdoyan HA, Lydic R. Neuropharmacology of sleep and wakefulness. Sleep Med Clin. 2010;5(4):513-28.
5. Vazquez J, Baghdoyan HA. Basal forebrain acetylcholine release during REM sleep is significantly greater than during waking. Am J Physiol Regul Integr Comp Physiol. 2001;280(2):R598-601.
6. Carskadon MA, Acebo C, Jenni OG. Regulation of adolescent sleep: implications for behavior. Ann N Y Acad Sci. 2004;1021:276-91.
7. Gaudreau H, Carrier J, Montplaisir J. Age-related modifications of NREM sleep EEG: from childhood to middle age. J Sleep Res. 2001;10(3):165-72.
8. George NM, Davis JE. Assessing sleep in adolescents through a better understanding of sleep physiology. Am J Nurs. 2013;113(6):26-31; quiz 44, 32.

9. Zajac A, Skowronek-Bała B, Wesołowska E, Kaciński M. Sleep paroxysmal events in children in video/polysomnography. Przegl Lek. 2010;67(9):762-9.
10. Frank MG, Heller HC. The function(s) of sleep. Handb Exp Pharmacol. 2019;253:3-34.
11. Berry RB, Gamaldo CE, Harding SM, Brooks R, Lloyd RM, Vaughn BV, et al. AASM Scoring Manual Version 2.2 Updates: New chapters for scoring infant sleep staging and home sleep apnea testing. J Clin Sleep Med JCSM Off Publ Am Acad Sleep Med. 2015;11(11):1253-4.
12. Licis A. Sleep-wake disorders in childhood. Contin Minneap Minn. 2020;26(4):1034-69.
13. Brockmann PE, Urschitz MS, Schlaud M, Poets CF. Primary snoring in school children: prevalence and neurocognitive impairments. Sleep Breath Schlaf Atm. 2012;16(1):23-9.
14. Cao Y, Wu S, Zhang L, Yang Y, Cao S, Li Q. Association of allergic rhinitis with obstructive sleep apnea: a meta-analysis. Medicine (Baltimore). 2018;97(51):e13783.
15. Quan SF, Archbold K, Gevins AS, Goodwin JL. Long-term neurophysiologic impact of childhood sleep disordered breathing on neurocognitive performance. Southwest J Pulm Crit Care. 2013;7(3):165-75.
16. Tan H-L, Gozal D, Kheirandish-Gozal L. Obstructive sleep apnea in children: a critical update. Nat Sci Sleep. 2013;5:109-23.
17. American Academy of Sleep Medicine. International classification of sleep disorders. 3rd edition. Darien, IL: American Academy of Sleep Medicine; 2014.
18. Brodsky L, Moore L, Stanievich JF. A comparison of tonsillar size and oropharyngeal dimensions in children with obstructive adenotonsillar hypertrophy. Int J Pediatr Otorhinolaryngol. 1987;13(2):149-56.
19. Marcus CL, Brooks LJ, Draper KA, Gozal D, Halbower AC, Jones J, et al. Diagnosis and management of childhood obstructive sleep apnea syndrome. Pediatrics. 2012;130(3):576-84.
20. Bhattacharjee R, Kheirandish-Gozal L, Spruyt K, Mitchell RB, Promchiarak J, Simakajornboon N, et al. Adenotonsillectomy outcomes in treatment of obstructive sleep apnea in children: a multicenter retrospective study. Am J Respir Crit Care Med. 2010;182(5):676-83.
21. Schwab RJ, Kim C, Bagchi S, Keenan BT, Comyn FL, Wang S, et al. Understanding the anatomic basis for obstructive sleep apnea syndrome in adolescents. Am J Respir Crit Care Med. 2015;191(11):1295-309.
22. Chan CK, Au CT, Lam HS, Lee DLY, Wing YK, Li AM. Intranasal corticosteroids for mild childhood obstructive sleep apnea—a randomized, placebo-controlled study. Sleep Med. 2015;16(3):358-63.
23. Kheirandish-Gozal L, Bandla HPR, Gozal D. Montelukast for children with obstructive sleep apnea: results of a double-blind, randomized, placebo-controlled trial. Ann Am Thorac Soc. 2016;13(10):1736-41.
24. Pirelli P, Saponara M, Guilleminault C. Rapid maxillary expansion in children with obstructive sleep apnea syndrome. Sleep. 2004;27(4):761-6.
25. Diercks GR, Wentland C, Keamy D, Kinane TB, Skotko B, de Guzman V, et al. Hypoglossal nerve stimulation in adolescents with down syndrome and obstructive sleep apnea. JAMA Otolaryngol—Head Neck Surg. 2018;144(1):37-42.
26. Littner MR, Kushida C, Wise M, Davila DG, Morgenthaler T, Lee-Chiong T, et al. Practice parameters for clinical use of the multiple sleep latency test and the maintenance of wakefulness test. Sleep. 2005;28(1):113-21.
27. Arand D, Bonnet M, Hurwitz T, Mitler M, Rosa R, Sangal RB. The clinical use of the MSLT and MWT. Sleep. 2005;28(1):123-44.
28. Dinges DF, Pack F, Williams K, Gillen KA, Powell JW, Ott GE, et al. Cumulative sleepiness, mood disturbance, and psychomotor vigilance performance decrements during a week of sleep restricted to 4-5 hours per night. Sleep. 1997;20(4):267-77.
29. Nishino S, Ripley B, Overeem S, Lammers GJ, Mignot E. Hypocretin (orexin) deficiency in human narcolepsy. The Lancet. 2000;355(9197):39-40.
30. Andlauer O, Moore H, Hong SC, Dauvilliers Y, Kanbayashi T, Nishino S, et al. Predictors of hypocretin (Orexin) deficiency in narcolepsy without cataplexy. Sleep. 2012;35(9):1247-55.
31. Sateia MJ. International Classification of Sleep Disorders-Third Edition. Chest. 2014;146(5):1387-94.
32. Markov D, Jaffe F, Doghramji K. Update on parasomnias. Psychiatry Edgmont. 2006;3(7):69-76.
33. Bruni O, Ferri R, Novelli L, Finotti E, Miano S, Guilleminault C. NREM sleep instability in children with sleep terrors: The role of slow wave activity interruptions. Clin Neurophysiol. 2008;119(5):985-92.
34. Klackenberg G. Incidence of parasomnias in children in a general population. In: Guilleminault C (Ed). Sleep and its disorders. New York: Raven; 1987. pp. 99-113.
35. Ozgun N, Sonmez FM, Topbas M, Can G, Goker Z. Insomnia, parasomnia, and predisposing factors in Turkish school children. Pediatr Int. 2016;58(10):1014-22.
36. Mason TBA, Pack AI. Pediatric parasomnias. Sleep. 2007;30(2):141-51.
37. Petit D, Pennestri MH, Paquet J, Desautels A, Zadra A, Vitaro F, et al. Childhood sleepwalking and sleep terrors: a longitudinal study of prevalence and familial aggregation. JAMA Pediatr. 2015;169(7):653-8.
38. Winkelman JW, Herzog DB, Fava M. The prevalence of sleep-related eating disorder in psychiatric and non-psychiatric populations. Psychol Med. 1999;29(6):1461-6.
39. Ohayon MM, Caulet M, Priest RG. Violent behavior during sleep. J Clin Psychiatry. 1997;58(8):369-76; quiz 377.

40. Comella CL, Tanner CM, Ristanovic RK. Polysomnographic sleep measures in Parkinson's disease patients with treatment-induced hallucinations. Ann Neurol. 1993;34(5):710-4.
41. Schenck CH, Mahowald MW, Kim SW, O'Connor KA, Hurwitz TD. Prominent eye movements during NREM sleep and REM sleep behavior disorder associated with fluoxetine treatment of depression and obsessive-compulsive disorder. Sleep. 1992;15(3):226-35.
42. Schenck CH, Mahowald MW. REM sleep behavior disorder: clinical, developmental, and neuroscience perspectives 16 years after its formal identification in SLEEP. Sleep. 2002;25(2):120-38.
43. Fantini ML, Gagnon JF, Filipini D, Montplaisir J. The effects of pramipexole in REM sleep behavior disorder. Neurology. 2003;61(10):1418-20.
44. Takeuchi N, Uchimura N, Hashizume Y, Mukai M, Etoh Y, Yamamoto K, et al. Melatonin therapy for REM sleep behavior disorder. Psychiatry Clin Neurosci. 2001;55(3):267-9.
45. Schenck CH, Mahowald MW. REM sleep parasomnias. Neurol Clin. 1996;14(4):697-720.
46. Chokroverty S. Sleep disorders medicine: Basic science, technical considerations and clinical aspects, 4th edition. New Delhi: Springer; 2017.
47. Raskind MA, Peskind ER, Kanter ED, Petrie EC, Radant A, Thompson CE, et al. Reduction of nightmares and other PTSD symptoms in combat veterans by prazosin: a placebo-controlled study. Am J Psychiatry. 2003;160(2):371-3.
48. McCarty DE, Andrew L, Chesson J. A case of sleep paralysis with hypnopompic hallucinations. J Clin Sleep Med. 2009;5(1):83.
49. Sharpless BA, McCarthy KS, Chambless DL, Milrod BL, Khalsa SR, Barber JP. Isolated sleep paralysis and fearful isolated sleep paralysis in outpatients with panic attacks. J Clin Psychol. 2010;66(12):1292-306.
50. Sharpless BA. A clinician's guide to recurrent isolated sleep paralysis. Neuropsychiatr Dis Treat. 2016;12:1761-7.
51. Kotagal S, Pianosi P. Sleep disorders in children and adolescents. BMJ. 2006;332(7545):828-32.

Chapter 17

Learning Disorders in Children: Intellectual Disability and Specific Learning Disability

KS Multani

INTRODUCTION

Development and learning represent dynamic processes that result from the intricate interaction between a child's biological attributes and their surroundings. These elements mutually influence each other, ultimately shaping not only the child's present state but also their future growth trajectories. Learning is a lifelong process of acquiring new understanding, behavior, knowledge, and skills. However, we will restrict our discussion to learning issues seen in preschool and school-going children only which affect the cognitive development of the child (**Flowchart 1**). Learning disorders (LDs) encompass a diverse range of neurodevelopmental conditions marked by challenges in acquiring both social and academic skills, which can lead to hindered cognitive development.[1-3] It is important to note that "learning disorder" and "learning disability" are terms that denote the same neurodevelopmental conditions. However, there is a lack of consensus regarding their precise case definition. A vast majority of these may either present as poor scholastic performance (scholastic backwardness), behavior problems, or vague psychosomatic complaints. Most of these cases fall into either of the two categories: Intellectual disability (ID) or specific learning disability (SLD).

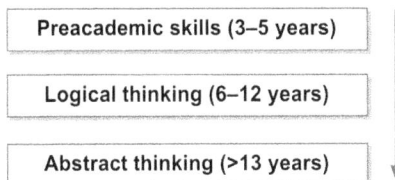

Flowchart 1: Stages of cognitive development in preschool and school-going children.

DEFINITION

Intellectual disability as per Diagnostic and Statistical Manual of Mental Disorders, Fifth Edition (DSM-5) is characterized by significant deficits in intellectual and adaptive functioning with onset in the early childhood period. The diagnosis of ID is usually used after 5 years of age, whereas global developmental delay (GDD) is the term used for a similar condition in children younger than 5 years of age. Based on intelligence quotient (IQ) levels, ID can be classified into mild (IQ 50-69), moderate (IQ 35-49), severe (IQ 20-34), and profound ID (IQ <20).[1-3]

Specific learning disability (SLD) refers to a subset of children with LDs who show significant deficits in language usage (reading and/or writing) and/or mathematics.[4-6] These include dyslexia (problems with reading), dysgraphia (problems with writing), and dyscalculia (problems with mathematics). A child can have one or more types of SLD. These skills significantly lag behind what is typically anticipated for children of the same chronological age and can disrupt the child's academic performance. These should be present for a period of at least 6 months before giving a label of SLD.

EPIDEMIOLOGY

The exact number of children with LDs is difficult to determine due to difference in definitions in various countries around the world and contrasting levels of severity. Also, many cases present with vague psychosomatic complaints and can easily be missed. As a rule, LDs are twice as common in children with chronic health conditions as compared to normal children. ID is seen in around 2.5% of children. SLD is seen in 3-10% of children.[7] Dyslexia and dysgraphia are the most common forms of LD.

In a study conducted at the population level, it was determined that the prevalence of reading disability among school-age children varied between 5 and 12%, depending on the criteria applied for its definition. These criteria included intelligence–achievement discrepancy and low achievement. Similarly, within the same population, the estimated prevalence of disorders related to written expression ranged from 7 to 15%. Additionally, in independent research efforts, the prevalence of dyscalculia, a condition related to math disability, was estimated to affect between 3 and 6% of the school-age population.[8,9]

ETIOPATHOGENESIS

Learning disorders arise from abnormalities in brain structure and function, which can be either present from birth or acquired later in life due to various factors such as illness, exposure to toxins, inadequate nutrition, medical treatments, sociocultural deprivation, or injury. The establishment of neural connections in the brain, which underpins all cognitive processes, communication, and learning, occurs most rapidly during fetal development and early childhood. While the processes of forming new neural connections and pruning unused ones continue throughout a person's life, they are most critical during the initial 3 years. Any harm inflicted on the developing brain during this period is likely to have enduring consequences. Genetic and neuropathologic factors are fundamental to LD, particularly in the case of reading disability. Nevertheless, the full manifestation of LD results from the interplay of these neuropathologic variances with other inherent and environmental factors influencing the learning process.

The list of conditions causing LDs is very large and varied. Few common conditions are listed in **Table 1**.

Environmental factors encompass a wide range of influences, including both school-related and home-related elements. School factors involve aspects such as the quality of student-teacher interactions, the suitability of the instruction pace, the student's prior exposure to learning opportunities within the school environment, the level of engagement facilitated by learning materials, and the physical arrangement of the classroom setting.

On the other hand, home factors pertain to the child's previous experiences with learning at home, the level of support provided by the family for reading and completing homework, and other related aspects of the home environment that can impact a child's learning journey.

TABLE 1: Conditions associated with learning disorders.

Category	Examples
Genetic conditions	Chromosomal disorders (Down syndrome, Turner syndrome, etc.), fragile X, tuberous sclerosis, neurofibromatosis 1, IEMs (phenylketonuria)
Antenatal conditions	Intrauterine growth retardation, intrauterine infection, fetal alcohol syndrome
Birth-related issues	Prematurity, birth asphyxia, hypoglycemia, sepsis, hyperbilirubinemia
Postnatal conditions	Meningitis, head injury, epilepsy
Environmental factors	Poor socioeconomic conditions, child neglect, child abuse
Idiopathic	–

(IEMs: inborn errors of metabolism)

CLINICAL FEATURES

Learning disorders can present as poor academic performance in school or as a medical or psychiatric condition. Some common presentations according to age are listed in **Table 2**. Few early markers seen in infancy are also listed.

A pediatrician needs to have a high index of suspicion as many children present with vague medical symptoms or behavior issues. These children often move from one doctor to another and thereby lose critical time of early formative years of school which is the most crucial and effective for early remediation methods.

DIAGNOSIS AND EVALUATION

A detailed history and physical examination along with vision and hearing evaluation is a must in all cases. *HEEADSSS* (home, education, eating habits, activities, depression, substance use, sexuality, and safety) is an essential tool for eliciting psychosocial history and finding the strengths and weaknesses of a child. Routine hemogram to look for underlying anemia and thyroid function tests to look for hypothyroidism are needed in all cases as conditions such as anemia can easily be treated by changing dietary habits and/or supplementation. Screening can be carried out by a teacher's feedback using *Rutter's child behavior questionnaire*. Intelligence testing should be carried out, especially to find the cases with borderline IQ. It can be done using standard tests of intelligence, e.g., Binet Kamat test of intelligence (BKT), Mallin's intelligence scale for Indian children (MISIC),

TABLE 2: Clinical presentation of learning disorders by age.

Early markers during infancy	Preschool symptoms	Early school symptoms	Mid-school symptoms
Feeding problems	Speech delay	Trouble making sentences	Poor comprehension
Excessive irritability	Problem with rhyming words	Trouble with mathematics—addition, subtraction, etc.	Difficulty in reading/writing/speaking
Poor sleep pattern	Problem with numbers	Poor pincer grasp	Poor organizational skills
Developmental delays	Poor peer interactions	Poor time management	Trouble following classroom work
Poor response to caregivers	Clumsy child	Poor self-help/care	Poor grasp of abstract concepts
	Psychosomatic complaints	Psychosomatic complaints	Psychosomatic complaints

Flowchart 2: Algorithmic approach to scholastic backwardness.

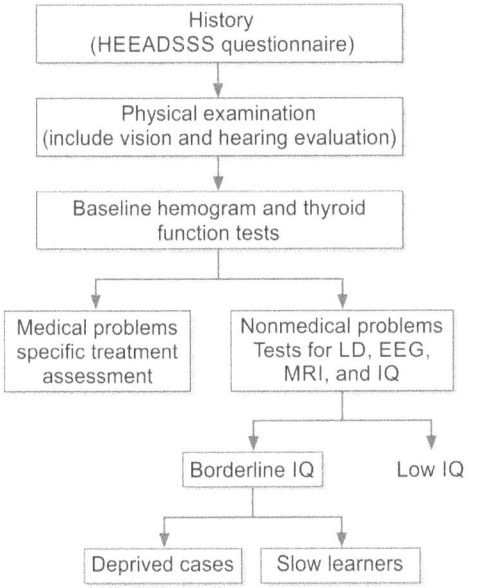

(EEG: electroencephalogram; HEEADSSS: home, education, eating habits, activities, depression, substance use, sexuality, and safety; IQ: intelligence quotient; LD: learning disability; MRI: magnetic resonance imaging)
Source: Adapted from Dalwai SH (Ed). IAP Handbook of Developmental and Behavioural Pediatrics, 1st edition. New Delhi: Jaypee Brothers Medical Publishers Pvt Ltd; 2021.

Wechsler's intelligence for children (WISC). Electroencephalogram (EEG), neuroimaging, and genetic testing should be carried out for clinical indications (dysmorphism, positive family history, history of seizures, etc.) **(Flowchart 2)**. Specific LD can be tested using curriculum-based assessment or National Institute of Mental Health and Neuro-Sciences (NIMHANS) SLD battery.

NEPSY-II (neuropsychological battery) is a comprehensive developmental neuropsychological assessment devised by Marit Korkman, Ursula Kirk, and Sally Kemp which can be used in children between 3 and 16 years of age to assess six functional domains: (1) Sensorimotor, (2) language, (3) visuospatial processing, (4) memory and learning, (5) attention/executive functions, and (6) social cognition. Autism and ADHD screening can be carried out using standard tests.

DIFFERENTIAL DIAGNOSIS

Common conditions which can present with similar symptoms are as follows:
- Hearing impairment
- Vision impairment
- Developmental coordination disorder
- Attention deficit hyperactivity disorder (ADHD)
- Autism spectrum disorder (ASD)
- Psychiatric conditions, such as depression or anxiety
- Environmental factors (e.g., lack of opportunity, frequent school absences)
- Sleep problems
- Chronic infections [e.g., chronic suppurative otitis media (CSOM)]
- Epilepsy
- Child abuse/neglect
- Substance abuse.

TREATMENT

Neuropathologic causes of learning difficulties can be alleviated with tailored and specialized instruction, as well as a nurturing and supportive learning environment. Conversely, these challenges can worsen when the learning environment lacks the necessary support and accommodations. A child's strengths and weaknesses should be identified, and an individualized education program (IEP) should ideally be prepared for every case consisting of academic curriculum as well as extracurricular activities using the help of a special educator. A pediatrician has to judiciously select among various interventions (remedial education, occupational therapy, and counseling) to formulate a goal-oriented individualized education program for each child and monitor the child's progress and updates the IEP accordingly.

Based on the assessments, the remedial educator plans intervention sessions (i.e., twice or thrice weekly) to work on building the child's skills such as: (1) reading—phoneme awareness, (2) reading—phonics, (3) writing skills—basic principles, and (4) math—basic principles. Effective remedial educational interventions have demonstrated associations with notable changes in brain function, particularly in areas related to language processing. Both parents and the child should be kept informed of the plan, and regular follow-up should be carried out by the pediatrician. They should be made aware of the various provisions by the Central Board of Secondary Education (CBSE). The aim of management is "inclusive education" and the child should be kept in the mainstream school. Children with borderline IQ who find the mainstream school education too difficult or stressful should be given the option of National Institute of Open Schooling (NIOS). Only very rarely should the child be referred to a special school.

Medications have a little role in the management of poor scholastic performance. Iron supplements, thyroxine, antiepileptics, or stimulant medications for cases with ADHD may be used in diagnosed cases. One should look for features of anxiety and depression in these children as these may require referral to a child psychiatrist. Children with chronic medical/surgical conditions need condition-specific enhancements in the classroom environment for better performance.

Insufficient awareness about LDs often places parents under significant stress when they try to handle their child's academic challenges and come to terms with the diagnosis. Pediatricians play a vital role in helping to alleviate parental and student stress effectively by— (1) providing clear explanations about the nature of the disability, (2) explanation of the rationale of evaluations and provisions for children with LD, (3) gradual preparation of parents to accept that LD is a lifelong condition, (4) empowerment of parents to guide their child in selecting an appropriate career, and (5) effective peer sensitization.

FOLLOW-UP

There is limited available data regarding the long-term persistence of LDs.[10] For instance, when it comes to reading disability, diagnostic stability rates range widely, from 28 to 78%, depending on the study. These variations in estimates can be attributed to several factors, including differences in the criteria used to define reading disability, the age at which the initial diagnosis was made, and the effects of treatment.

It is noteworthy that diagnostic stability tends to be lower among younger children, such as those in kindergarten and grade 1. This suggests that reading difficulties in younger children may stem from a variety of causes, some of which may be more responsive to intervention than others. In contrast, among older children, like those in grade 3 and higher, reading disability tends to persist over time. Even though reading skills may improve, measures of reading decoding and reading fluency skills typically remain below the normal range. The variability in how reading disability manifests over time poses challenges for consistent measurement and identification.

PREVENTION

The importance of the first 1,000 days needs to be emphasized again and again. Good nutrition during the antenatal period, institutional delivery, and care of girl child have far-reaching effects. When adults exhibit sensitivity and respond to an infant's babbling, crying, or gestures, they play a vital role in fostering the formation of neural connections that serve as the building blocks for a child's communication and social abilities, including self-regulation. These interactive exchanges, often referred to as "serve and return" interactions, actively shape the architecture of the brain. Right from birth, children are active learners who continuously absorb and organize information, creating meaning through their relationships, interactions with their environment, and overall life experiences.

The process of development and learning is propelled when children are encouraged to reach slightly beyond their current level of mastery, and when they are provided with ample opportunities to reflect upon and practice newly acquired skills. Thus, early identification of "at-risk" cases and early diagnosis has a large impact on the outcome of the case.

CONCLUSION

To summarize, early recognition and remediation of LDs is essential as delays can result in a negative lifelong impact on the child and family. Pediatricians should have a high index of suspicion of LDs in children presenting with vague, recurrent symptoms in the absence of any significant physical findings. Judicious use of the accommodations to the child that are offered by the CBSE/state boards, vocational training, and innovative ways of teaching using technology and multisensory methods will go a long way in helping these children perform better.

"Tell me and I forget. Teach me and I remember. Involve me and I learn."

—Benjamin Franklin

REFERENCES

1. National Consultation Meeting for developing Indian Academy of Pediatrics (IAP), Guidelines on Neurodevelopmental Disorders under the aegis of IAP Childhood Disability Group and the Committee on Child Development and Neurodevelopmental Disorders; Nair MKC, Prasad C, Unni J, Bhattacharya A, Kamath SS, Dalwai S. Consensus statement of IAP on evaluation and management of learning disability. Indian Pediatr. 2017;54:574-81.
2. Nair MKC, George B, Vinod SS, Verma S, Lukose R. Intellectual disability. In: Nair MKC (Ed). Developmental Pediatrics, 2nd edition. New Delhi: Noble Publishers; 2022. pp. 183-98.
3. Kamath SS, Multani KS. Scholastic backwardness. In: Dalwai SH (Ed). IAP Handbook of Developmental and Behavioral Pediatrics, 1st edition. New Delhi: Jaypee Brothers Medical Publishers Pvt Ltd; 2022. pp. 239-42.
4. Verma S, Lukose R, Kumar SV, Nair MKC. Specific learning disability. In: Nair MKC (Ed). Developmental Pediatrics, 2nd edition. New Delhi: Noble Publishers; 2022. pp. 199-209.
5. Dalwai S. Specific learning disability. In: Dalwai SH (Ed). IAP Handbook of Developmental and Behavioral Pediatrics, 1st edition. New Delhi: Jaypee Brothers Medical Publishers; 2022. pp. 248-52.
6. Shah HR, Sagar JKV, Somaiya MP, Nagpal JK. Clinical Practice Guidelines on Assessment and Management of Specific Learning Disorders. Indian J Psychiatry. 2019;61:211-25.
7. Joseph JK, Devu BK. Prevalence and pattern of learning disability in India: A systematic review and meta-analysis. Indian J Psy Nsg. 2022;19:152-62.
8. Chordia SL, Thandapani K, Arunagirinathan A. Children 'at risk' of developing specific learning disability in primary schools. Indian J Pediatr. 2020;87:94-8.
9. Shaywitz SE, Escobar MD, Shaywitz BA, Fletcher JM, Makuch R. Evidence that dyslexia may represent the lower tail of a normal distribution of reading ability. N Engl J Med. 1992;326(3):145-50.
10. Wilson AM, Lesaux NK. Persistence of phonological processing deficits in college students with dyslexia who have age-appropriate reading skills. J Learn Disabil. 2001;34(5):394-400.

Chapter 18: Fluency Disorders

S Sitaraman

INTRODUCTION

One of the frequent conditions, which is seen in pediatric OPD is the problem of speech. Fluency disorders are commonly associated with great deal of anxiety among parents. Fluency of speech is established as the child starts to speak and acquires a significant vocabulary. Stammering or stuttering is often seen in young children. The DSM-5 (Diagnostic and Statistical Manual of Mental Disorders, Fifth Edition) has changed the terminology of stammering to childhood-onset fluency disorder, but for the sake of general understanding, the old terminology will be continued in this article.

Fluency disorder is an interruption in the flow of speaking characterized by atypical rate, rhythm, and disfluencies (e.g., repetitions of sounds, syllables, words, and phrases; sound prolongations; and blocks), which may also be accompanied by excessive tension, speaking avoidance, struggle behaviors, and secondary mannerisms. The most common problem is *Stuttering*.[1]

- Stuttering or childhood-onset fluency disorder is a condition characterized by disturbances in the normal fluency and time patterning of speech that is inappropriate for the individual's age and language skills, and persists over time.

There are two types recognizable:
1. Developmental stuttering starts between 2 and 5 years (occasionally even at 18 months): Frequently some children become disfluent when they start to speak but, it gets resolved **(Table 1)**.
2. Neurogenic stuttering is associated with neurologic disease or trauma.

The incidence of stuttering in children is the range of 5–8%, with a male:female ratio of 4:1, but in preschool, both genders are equally effected.[2,3] Studies have reported higher incidence rates in preschool children.[4] Increased incidence of stuttering has been noted among those with a first-degree relative (e.g., parent, sibling) who stutters and an even greater likelihood if that relative is an identical twin.

The onset of symptoms is usually in the early childhood and may present as any of the following:
- Repetition of a word, syllable or sound (e.g., go go out)
- Word prolongation
- Body may get tense while speaking or accompanied with facial grimaces, eye twitching body movements (e.g., head nodding, leg tapping, fist clenching)
- Finds it difficult to utter the word or just lisps the word
- There are pauses while talking
- Due to inability to communicate effectively, they develop a lot of anxiety
- There may be prolongation of consonants (e.g., sssssssssome, etc.); earlier, it was also called hesitancy of speech. This is sometimes present when children are learning to speak.

TABLE 1: Characteristics of "typical disfluency" and "stuttering."

Typical disfluency	Stuttering
Speech characteristics:	*Speech characteristics:*
• Multisyllabic whole-word and phrase repetitions	• Sound or syllable repetitions
• Interjections	• Prolongations
• Revisions	• Blocks
Other behaviors:	*Other behaviors:*
• No physical tension or struggle	• Associated physical tension or struggle
• No secondary behaviors	• Secondary behaviors (e.g., eye blinks, facial grimacing, changes in pitch or loudness)
• No negative reaction or frustration	• Negative reaction or frustration
• No family history of stuttering	• Avoidance behaviors (e.g., reduced verbal output or word/situational avoidances)
	• Family history of stuttering

- There may be "word drops" in sentences when child either has difficulty in uttering the word, or sometimes just lisps the word.
- Over a period of time, they develop lot of movements like head jerks, body twists, or guttural sounds in an effort to clear the throat.

Some children use escape behaviors like adding fillers "um" or Ah' in the speech or avoid speaking complicated words. They would not be diagnosed early, and are classified as *covert stuttering*. Criteria for diagnosis have now changed in new DSM, notably, the removal of saying "ums", "ahs", and "you knows" and other interjections as a requirement for diagnosis. Child may have interjections as part of their speech but it need not be considered as stuttering.

Some children present with what is known as *Typical Disfluencies* which are transient in **Table 1** describes some characteristics of "typical disfluency" and "stuttering" (Adapted from Coleman, 2013).[5]

Stuttering may be worse when the person is excited, tired or under stress, or when feeling self-conscious, hurried, or pressured. Situations such as speaking in front of a group or talking on the phone can be particularly difficult for people who stutter (APA 2013). The children may make avoidance behaviors to mask the stuttering.

Persistent stuttering causes problems in communication, anxiety, poor interaction with peer group, being bullied or teased leading to low self-esteem, and disinterest in school activities requiring verbal interaction. Stuttering may be seen in association with other disorders such as attention-deficit hyperactivity disorder (ADHD), autism spectrum disorder (ASD), intellectual disability (ID), learning disability (LD), and anxiety disorders.[6] They would have problems in school, work place, social and emotional dysfunction.

PATHOPHYSIOLOGY

Causes are multifactorial, which include genetic as well as neurophysiological causes. There is no clear genetic association, but the disorder is seen more in identical twins and also in close family relatives (60% may have problems), giving us cue to its causation. Drayna and Kang found that gene mutations were present in close to 10% of cases of familial stuttering.[7] Current studies have reported few genetic abnormalities in these children involving genes, *GRIN 1* and *GRIN 2*, but these genetic abnormalities are also associated with other neurological disorders.

The brain structure of children with persistent stammering has shown changes in white matter and reduced gray matter in left hemisphere and also decreased blood supply to Broca's area, but these are not being consistently reported to give these findings a diagnostic utility.[8,9]

The stuttering occurring in early childhood tends to disappear in 70–80% cases by age of 5–6 years, but in some, it may persist. Risk factors such as male predominance, family history, late onset (after 3–4 years), and stuttering lasting for >6 months, are commonly associated in cases with persistence of stuttering.

Cluttering is another form of fluency disorder characterized by a perceived rapid and/or irregular speech rate, atypical pauses, maze behaviors, pragmatic issues, decreased awareness of fluency problems or moments of disfluency, excessive disfluencies, collapsing or omitting syllables, and language formulation issues, which result in breakdowns in speech clarity and/or fluency.[10,11] Individuals may exhibit pure cluttering or cluttering with stuttering. Cluttering may be found in 1.1–1.25% of children.[12]

Cluttering is characterized by improper syntax, dropping of words, rapid speech, and atypical pauses.[11] There may be deletion of syllables, e.g., instead of saying I want to watch television—he would say "I wan wat vision". The child would shift from one topic to another within a sentence, and would have excessive interjections or omission of words. Child is unaware of his inability because of poor pragmatic communication skills, hence makes no effort to correct it, but despite an ineffective social interaction, these are not diagnosed till adolescence or later.[13,14]

Children with stuttering, in addition can have cluttering too. There is no documented recovery from this disorder, although the fluency occasionally shows improvement when the child is asked to speak slowly.

The speech characteristics of cluttering are:
- Rapid rate
- Deletion of syllables
- Collapsing of syllables
- Omission of word endings
- Disfluencies
- Unusual prosody due to unexpected pauses.

The WHO-ICF (World Health Organization–International Classification of Functioning, Disability and Health)

framework can be used to describe the following comprehensive set of assessment features for fluency:[15]
- Impairment in body function
- Assessment related to measuring speech fluency and the severity of observed disfluencies.

Examples of specific assessment areas include:
- Determining speech efficiency and spontaneity in communication
- Measuring the frequency and severity of disfluencies
- Assessing physical concomitant behaviors and learned escape/avoidance behaviors
- Assessing tension and effort in communication (during both fluent and disfluent speech)
- Activity limitations and participation restrictions.

Assessment related to measuring the adverse impact of stuttering or cluttering on the speaker's life include evaluating functional communication abilities, cross situations and determining if the speaker is able to communicate.

Specific assessment includes:
- Ability of the speaker to communicate effectively
- Ability to achieve his educational objectives
- Impact of cluttering on QOL (Quality of life)
- Spontaneity in effective communication

Assessment related to coping reactions on the part of speaker:
- Own emotional responses to stuttering/cluttering, like frustration, shame or fear while speaking
- Level of self-confidence
- Self-appreciation as effective speaker
- Able to understand his/her limitations and able to interact with others

Few environmental factors are also important:
- Family, school, or workplace support groups
- Peer group interaction
- Exposure to bullying and teasing
- Response to any therapeutic intervention and influence on problem-solving skills.

When to refer to speech and language pathologist (SLP)?
- If stuttering lasts for >6 months/becomes more frequent as the child grows older
- It is associated with other speech or language problems
- It is associated with lot of motor movements and visible difficulty in speaking
- Child experiences difficulty in communicating in school or in social functions
- Due to anxiety, child develops fear and avoids situations requiring verbal interaction.

REMEDIAL MEASURES AND TREATMENT PLAN (TABLE 2)

For child: Speech therapist can make significant difference, and prevent secondary complications, if started early. The SLP has individual-centered approach and aims at enhancing the readiness of the individual and motivates also. He would also interact with the family and friends to give a conducive environment to the child. Some children may require psychotherapy to overcome their anxiety and overcome their fears, and feelings of embarrassment. The use of cognitive behavioral therapy (CBT) has proven useful.

The basic management would involve:
- Practice of vowel's utterances
- Slow the rate of speech
- If pitch is high, that is modulated since it leads to lot of physical tension.

For parents: (Seven tips for talking with child who stutters. Adapted from "Stuttering foundation USA")
1. *Reduce the pace:* Speak with your child in an unhurried way, pausing frequently. Wait a few seconds after your child finishes before you begin to speak.
2. *Full listening:* Try to increase those times that you give your child your undivided attention and are really listening.
3. *Asking questions:* Asking questions is a normal part of life—but try to resist asking one after the other. Sometimes, it is more helpful to comment on what your child has said and wait.
4. *Turn taking:* Help all members of the family take turns talking and listening. Children find it much easier to talk when there are fewer interruptions.
5. *Building confidence:* Use descriptive praise to build confidence. Praise strengths unrelated to talking as well such as athletic skills, being organized, independent, or careful.
6. *Special times:* Set aside a few minutes at a regular time each day when you can give your undivided attention to your child. This quiet calm time—no TV, iPad or phones!!!
7. *Normal rules apply:* Discipline the child who stutters just as you do your other children and just as you would if he didn't stutter.

TABLE 2: Physician's checklist for referral.			
	The child with normal disfluencies (Age of onset: 1½ to 7 years of age)	**The child with mild stuttering** (Age of onset: 1½ to 7 years of age)	**The child with severe stuttering** (Age of onset: 1½ to 7 years of age)
Speech behavior you may see or hear	Occasional (not more than once in every 10 sentences), brief, (typical 1/2 second or shorter) repetitions of sounds, syllables or short words, e.g., li-li-like this	Frequent (3% or more of speech), long (1/2 to 1 second) repetitions of sounds, syllables, or short words, e.g., li-li-li-like this. Occasional prolongations of sounds	Very frequent (10% or more of speech), and often very long (1 second or longer) repetitions of sounds, syllables or short words. Frequent sound prolongations and blockages
Other behavior you may see or hear	Occasional pauses, hesitations in speech or fillers such as "uh", "er", or "um", changing of words or thoughts	Repetitions and prolongations begin to be associated with eyelid closing and blinking, looking to the side, and some physical tension in and around the lips	Similar-to-mild stutterers only more frequent and noticeable; some rise in pitch of voice during stuttering. Extra sounds or words used as "starters"
When problems most noticeable	Tends to come and go when child is—tired, excited, talking about complex/new topics, asking or answering questions or talking to unresponsive listeners	Tends to come and go in similar situations, but is more often present than absent	Tends to be present in most speaking situations; far more consistent and non-fluctuating
Child reaction	None apparent	Some show little concern, some will be frustrated and embarrassed	Most are embarrassed and some are also fearful of speaking
Parent reaction	None to a great deal	Most concerned, but concern may be minimal	All have some degree of concern
Referral decision	Refer only if parents moderately to overly concerned	Refer if continues for 6–8 weeks or if parental concern justifies it	Refer as soon as possible

This chart may be photocopied and distributed without permission of the publisher.
www.stutteringhelp.org • www.tartamudez.org
STUTTERING FOUNDATION OF AMERICA
1-800-992-9392

Feedback devices alter the way the child hears own voice. They include:
- *Delayed auditory feedback (DAF):* These play own voice back to the child a fraction of a second after speaking
- *Frequency-shifted auditory feedback (FSAF):* These play voice back to the child at a lower or higher frequency
- *Combined DAF/FSAF devices:* These use a combination of both methods mentioned above.

These devices are often fitted inside or around the ear, similar to a hearing aid, and can help improve the fluency of some people's speech. There are also apps for smartphones and computers that work in a similar way.

PHARMACOLOGICAL MANAGEMENT

No drug is currently approved for the treatment of stuttering, but in view of its similarity with Tourette syndrome, trials of dopamine antagonist (haloperidol, olanzapine, and risperidone) have been done which have shown to improve fluency, but their use is limited on account of side effects, when given on long-term basis.

CONCLUSION

Fluency disorders are fairly common in children which can lead to other psychobehavioral disorders in child such as anxiety, depression, aggression, excessive emotional lability and so on, owing to the frustration associated with it. Along with the child, it affects the parents as well, so management involves child as well as parents; the burden of providing easing environment to the child rests on the parents which helps child to overcome this problem. Speech therapy and CBT are the mainstay of management and pharmacological agents have minimal role to play. Best results are achieved when the treatment starts early, i.e., in preschool years. The Derner School of Psychology has successfully employed virtual reality self-modeling (VRSM) using 360-degree virtual reality videos to remediate severe stuttering and potentially revolutionize the treatment of stuttering; innovations like this may prove to be of prime use in upcoming years.

REFERENCES

1. American Speech-Language-Hearing Association. (1993). Definitions of communication disorders and variations. [online] Available from: https://www.asha.org/policy/rp1993-00208/#:~:text=A%20communication%20disorder%20is%20an,severity%20from%20mild%20to%20profound. [Last accessed October, 2023].
2. Mansson H. Childhood stuttering: Incidence and development. J Fluency Disord. 2000;25(1):47-57.
3. Yairi E, Ambrose N. Epidemiology of stuttering: 21st century advances. J Fluency Disord. 2013;38(2):66-87.
4. Reilly S, Onslow M, Packman A, Cini E, Conway L, Ukoumunne O, et al. Natural history of stuttering to 4 years of age: A prospective community-based study. Pediatrics. 2013;132(3):460-7.
5. Coleman C. (2013). How can you tell if childhood stuttering is the real deal? [online] Available from: http://blog.asha.org/2013/09/26/how-can-you-tell-if-childhood-stuttering-is-the-real-deal/. [Last accessed October, 2023].
6. Briley PM, Ellis C Jr. The coexistence of disabling conditions in children who stutter: Evidence from the National Health Interview Survey. J Speech Lang Hear Res. 2018; 61(12):2895-905.
7. Drayna D, Kang C. Genetic approaches to understanding the causes of stuttering. J Neurodev Disord. 2011;3(4): 374-80.
8. Chang SE, Zhu DC, Choo AL, Angstadt M. White matter neuroanatomical differences in young children who stutter. Brain. 2015;138(3):694-711.
9. Desai J, Huo Y, Wang Z, Bansal R, Williams SC, Lythgoe D, et al. Reduced perfusion in Broca's area in developmental stuttering. Hum Brain Mapp. 2017;38(4):1865-74.
10. St Louis KO, Schulte K. 2011. Defining cluttering: The lowest common denominator. In: Ward D, KS Scott (Eds). Cluttering: Research, Intervention and Education. United Kingdom: Psychology Press; 2011. pp. 233-53.
11. Van Zaalen Y, Reichel IK. Cluttering treatment: Theoretical considerations and intervention planning. Perspect Glob Issues Commun Sci Related Disord. 2014;4(2):57-62.
12. Van Zaalen Y, Reichel I. Prevalence of cluttering in two European countries: a pilot study. Perspect ASHA SIGs. 2017;2(17):42-9.
13. Teigland A. A study of pragmatic skills of clutterers and normal speakers. J Fluency Disord. 1996;21(3-4): 201-14.
14. Ward D, Scaler SK. Cluttering: A Handbook of Research, Intervention and Education. United Kingdom: Psychology Press; 2011.
15. Coleman C, Scott YJ. A comprehensive view of stuttering: Implications for assessment and treatment. Perspec School-Based Issues. 2014;15(2):75-80.

FURTHER READING

1. American Speech-Language-Hearing Association. [online] Available from: https://www.asha.org/practice-portal/clinical-topics/fluency-disorders. [Last accessed October, 2023].
2. Guitar B, Conture EG. Child Who Stutters to the Pediatrician, 6th edition. USA: Stuttering Foundation of America; 2015.
3. Smith A, Weber C. How stuttering develops: The multifactorial dynamic pathways theory. J Speech Lang Hear Res. 2017;60(9):2483-505.

Chapter 19: Habit Disorders in Children

Anil Kumar Arora, BD Gupta

INTRODUCTION

Habit can be defined as a regularly repeated behavior that requires little or no thought; it is learned rather than innate. The word habit is pulled from the Latin words *habere*, which means "have, consist of," and *habitus*, which means "condition, or state of being". Habits are context–behavior associations in one's memory that develop as people repeatedly experience rewards for a given action in a given context. Thus, it can be a part of any activity, ranging from eating or sleeping to thinking or reacting, and is developed through reinforcement and repetition. Different types of habits can include motor habits, intellectual habits, and habits of character. Motor habits are related to physical activity such as walking, standing, and running. Bad habits are often just a coping strategy; children may fall back on these behaviors when they are stressed, bored, frustrated, unhappy, insecure, or tired. Many of these "bad habits" are calming and soothing to the child.

"Habit disorders" are a broad class of disorders characterized by repetitive, unwanted behaviors that are distressing and disturbing, and often result in significant functional impairment. Habit disorders are linked together by the presence of repetitive and relatively stable behaviors that seem to occur without awareness of the person performing the behavior such as nose picking, hair pulling, nail biting, and head banging. Psychosocial distress in habit disorders can be considerable and usually involves secondary phobias, depression, social anxieties, low self-esteem, and disturbance in daily activities as well as quality of life.

CLASSIFICATION

There are two primary classes of habit disorders:
1. Tic disorders
2. Body focused repetitive behaviors (BFRBs)

Tic disorders are defined by the presence of one or motor and/or vocal tics, while the BFRB categorization involves a broadly defined set of self-focused repetitive behaviors that can cause physical harm, if left untreated. Both tic disorders and BFRBs commonly begin in childhood.[1]

TOURETTE SYNDROME AND CHILDHOOD TIC DISORDERS

Movement disorders that cause abnormal, unwanted movements usually unrelated to weakness or spasticity are central nervous system disorders. These disorders in children often involve the frontal cortex and basal ganglia dysfunction.[2] These disorders are divided into two categories as follows:
1. *Hyperkinetic movement disorders* are disorders with excess of movements such as tics, stereotypies, myoclonus, and tremors. Hyperkinetic movement disorders, particularly tic disorders, are relatively common in pediatric population.
2. *Hypokinetic movement disorders* such as bradykinesia, akinesia, and rigidity are characterized by paucity of movements.[3]

Tics are classified as "sudden, rapid, recurrent, non-rhythmic, stereotyped motor movements or vocalizations". They are meaningless and serve no purpose. Tics are involuntary contractions of functionally related groups of skeletal muscles in one or more parts of the body. They may be simple or complex **(Table 1)**.

Simple tics are brief vocalizations or movements that typically have no social significance and mainly confined to the upper body, particularly eyes, head, shoulders, and face. Tics can also be vocal and include throat clearing, etc. Some recurrent involuntary somatic sensations are classified as sensory tics; however, these are rare and present as warm or tingling sensations and are often

TABLE 1: Classification of tics.		
Tics	Motor	Vocal
Simple	• Blinking, wrinkling, eye rolling, wide eye-opening, eyebrow raising, lip movement, jaw movement • Grimacing, turning up nose mouth opening • Head jerking, head-shaking, turning, twitching, nodding • Shoulder shrugging, hand movements, legs and foot movements	• Grunting or barking, coughing, rasping • Sniffing or snorting, snuffling • Shouting, whistling, humming • Throat clearing, making animal noises, spitting
Complex	• Combinations of simple tics (e.g., head turning plus shoulder shrugging), hopping, jumping, finger tapping, clapping • Foot stamping, dystonic tics, writing tics • *Copropraxia:* Using sexual or obscene gestures • *Echopraxia:* Imitating someone's movements • Palipraxia (rare)	• Blocking speech, stuttering • *Coprolalia:* Saying obscene words • Uttering socially inappropriate words (e.g., obscenities, ethnic slurs) • *Echolalia:* Repeating one's own or another's sounds or words • Palilalia (involuntary repetition of one's own spoken words)

muscle focused which cause muscles to be tensed or released as a relief.

Tics are characterized as complex when there is a contraction in more than one muscle group and can take the form of self-inflicted repetitive motions. Simple tics can be combined with complex tics, which extends their duration and gives them the appearance of intentionality. Complex vocal tics manifest themselves as repeated phrases or swear words. Tics do not signify improper behavior and are not voluntary. Stress and exhaustion can make tics worse, but they are typically more noticeable when the body is at ease and may go away when patients are working on something. Even though severe tics can be physically dangerous and/or socially awkward, they rarely interfere with motor coordination and rarely cause problems.

Since tics in elementary-aged children are frequently mild, momentary, and cause no impairment, they cannot be referred to as a disease. Their correct diagnosis is important so as to avoid inadequate treatments and to take preventive action against prejudice and teasing. Even presently, it frequently takes 5–10 years before a patient is diagnosed.[4]

Types of Tics

Tics can be identified and grouped in children as follows:
- *Motor tics:* Simple motor tics, by definition, affect only a small number of muscle groups and involve short-lasting circumscribed movements, most often seen in the face and head, with ocular tics being particularly common. In contrast, complex motor tics are defined as those that involve multiple muscle groups and/or seem to fulfil a purpose.
- *Vocal tics:* The most prevalent vocal tics are throat clearing and sniffing; exclamations and shouts are much less common. Tics are frequently misdiagnosed in children as an airway disease such as asthma.
- *Tourette syndrome:* This neuropsychiatric condition is characterized by combined vocal and motor tics, with at least two types of motor and at least one type of vocal tics. It usually develops in childhood. Although there may be symptom-free stretches of time lasting several months, the diagnostic criteria call for the illness to have started in childhood or adolescence, to have lasted for at least 1 year, and to have fluctuated over time. No specific level of severity is necessary. About 80–90% of Tourette syndrome patients also experience psychiatric symptoms in addition to tics.
- *Chronic motor tic disorder:* This condition only differs from Tourette syndrome in that it lacks vocal tics. The comorbidities are generally rarer and less severe, and the motor tics are typically milder than those observed in patients with Tourette syndrome.
- *Chronic vocal tic disorder:* It is a rare condition. It is distinguished by the recurring, exclusive occurrence of vocal tics. Comorbidities are just as common as in Tourette syndrome.
- *Transient tic disorder:* This condition is only seen in children and is indicated by tics that go away after a year. Children might not even notice these typically mild, simple motor tics **(Table 2)**.

Epidemiology and Clinical Course

It is estimated that 1% of people worldwide have Tourette syndrome.[5] Epidemiological studies have shown that tic disorders are actually quite common and that the

TABLE 2: ICD-10 classification of primary tic disorders.

F 95.0	Transient tic disorder (duration <12 months)
F 95.1	Chronic motor or vocal tic disorder (duration >1 year, no remission for longer than 2 months, only motor or only vocal tics; first tics before age 18 years)
F 95.2	Combined tic disorder, at least one vocal and at least two motor tics (Gilles de la Tourette syndrome)
F 95.8	Other tic disorders
F 95.9	Tic disorder, unspecified

TABLE 3: Nongenetic risk factors.

Prenatal	Perinatal	Postnatal
• Smoking during pregnancy • Psychosocial stress during pregnancy • Excessive nausea and vomiting • Inadequate weight gain • Intrauterine growth • Retardation, low birth weight • Alcohol and cannabis use	Premature birth Perinatal hypoxia	• Infection, especially Group A β-hemolytic streptococci (GABHS) with PANDAS (pediatric autoimmune neuropsychiatric disorders associated streptococcal infections). It is unclear whether the temporal association reflects causation or coincidence • Psychosocial stress (often worsens tics)

diagnosis is frequently delayed, despite the fact that it was previously believed to be an extremely rare condition (an "orphan disease").[4] It is estimated that up to 10–15% of elementary school students have brief simple motor tics. About four times as many boys and men are affected as girls and women.[5,6]

Tics usually appear with gradually increasing intensity between the ages of 6 and 8 years.[7] Others reported that tics typically begin at approximately 5-7 years of age, peak in early adolescence, and then gradually decline with a waxing and waning course.[8] There is no relation between age of onset and severity of the tics.[6] Motor tics appear 2–3 years earlier than vocal tics typically involving face and head initially. The tics are most severe between the ages of 10 and 12 years.[9] About 90% patients have spontaneous improvement after the tics reach their peak; however, there is still a debate regarding disappearance of tics. Most patients say that tics become more frequent under emotional stress[10,11] and less common with relaxation or concentration.

Etiology

Developmentally related abnormal functional brain connectivity and impaired function of the cortical–striatal–thalamic–cortical circuits, as well as aberrant associated neurotransmitter function, including dopamine, serotonin, and gamma-aminobutyric acid (GABA), are involved in the pathophysiology of tic disorders.[12,13] Multiple factors, including polygenic and nongenetic ones like environmental factors and immune-mediated mechanisms, play a role in the multifactorial etiology of tic disorders and help to explain the heterogeneous clinical phenotype.[14]

Environmental Elements

It has been difficult to pinpoint the precise environmental factors that affect the onset of tic disorders. Numerous studies have assessed and looked into prenatal and perinatal epigenetic influences. As prenatal risk factors for chronic tic disorder, tics have been linked to maternal life stress during pregnancy **(Table 3)**.[15-18]

Genetic Influences

Georges Gilles de la Tourette suggested possible genetic influences in 1885.[19] Tourette syndrome and other tic disorders are currently thought to be polygenic inherited diseases caused by multiple genes **(Table 4)**.

Immune System Components

One significant underlying cause of tics has been suggested to be an abnormal immune response to antigens. Such immune-mediated mechanisms have been supported by studies. This includes a reduced ability of the innate immune system to respond, particularly to bacterial infection;[20] an increase in interleukin-12 and tumor necrosis factor;[21] a deficiency in T-cell regulation;[22] a rise in the levels of adhesion molecules,[23] which serve as markers of a systemic inflammatory response; a change in the immunoglobulin profile;[24] the presence of oligoclonal bands in the central spinal fluid;[25] microglial involvement; and overactivity of systemic immune responses.[26]

TABLE 4: Susceptibility genes associated with tic disorders.

Gene	Tic disorders
SLITRK1 gene	SLIT and NTRK proteins play a role in the development of corticostriatal–thalamocortical circuitry
Histidine decarboxylase (HDC) gene	The enzyme HDC catalyzes the formation of histamine
IMMP2L (mitochondrial inner membrane protease subunit 2) gene	The mutated protein leads to functional impairment of the cytochrome 1c protein and thereby activates apoptosis
NLGN4X gene	The protein neuroligin-4 plays a role in synaptogenesis
CNTNAP2 (contactin-associated protein 2) genes	The protein product of this gene influences the distribution of calcium channels in the central nervous system

Some cases of Tourette syndrome may represent a central nervous system autoimmune disorder following infection as evidenced by a significant elevation of antistreptolysin O (ASO) titers in children with tics, and a positive correlation between ASO titers and tic severity.[27] The most common basal ganglia-binding antigen was similar to the antigen detected in Sydenham's chorea.[28] Thus, an autoimmune process caused by the cross-reaction of streptococcal bacterial antigens and brain antineuronal antibodies has been suggested as a pathophysiological mechanism of Tourette syndrome.

Children who develop tics or obsessive-compulsive disorder (OCD) suddenly after contracting a streptococcal infection may have pediatric autoimmune neuropsychiatric disorders associated with streptococcal infections (PANDAS).[29] It is hypothesized that the pathophysiology of PANDAS is connected to immunoglobulin G (IgG) antineuronal autoantibodies, which cross the blood–brain barrier and may cause excessive dopamine release, neuronal signal transduction, and host-group A *Streptococcus* molecular mimicry.[30]

Diagnosis

Clinical diagnoses for tic disorders are made based on a thorough history, a neurological examination, and a psychiatric examination. Rarely is further diagnostic testing necessary. If symptoms are unusual, a secondary tic disorder may be present.[31] Only hyperkinesia and sound productions that satisfy the established diagnostic criteria should be referred to as "tics." Movement disorders of unknown origin and conversion disorders with tic-like movements should not be classified as tics.

The hyperkinetic movement disorders chorea, dyskinesia, hemifacial spasm, restless legs syndrome, and focal epileptic seizures can all be distinguished from tics with relative ease. However, it can be challenging to differentiate tic disorders from the following:
- Dissociative disorders of movement
- Obsessive habits
- Widespread hyperactivity
- Manners
- Stereotypes
- Myoclonus and dystonia.

Tics can be a manifestation of other diseases rarely like Wilson's disease, neuroacanthocytosis, fragile X syndrome, Sydenham's chorea, and Huntington's disease. Additionally, medications such as carbamazepine, phenytoin, lamotrigine, amphetamines, dopaminergic drugs, or cocaine can cause tics. Rare side effects of using neuroleptics include tardive tics.[32]

Comorbidities

Among all ages, 50–90% patients also suffer from attention-deficit/hyperactivity disorder (ADHD), obsessive-compulsive behavior and anxiety, impulsive-control disorders, emotional dysregulation, disorders of social behavior, autism spectrum disorders (ASDs), etc.[33]

Treatment

It is not uncommon that patients and their attendants feel stressed; hence, it is always important for parents of child, teachers, and other family members to understand the nature of the condition. Thorough patient education should include information about the cause as well as prognosis of the disease. Parental counseling should be done on social issues such as compensatory aids, certification of disabled person, the issue of vehicle driving, and the choice of occupation.

Since there is no causal therapy, tics cannot be cured. Even symptomatic treatment poses challenges because there is medication that can treat all Tourette syndrome symptoms. Anytime there is significant physical and/or psychosocial impairment, tics should be treated symptomatically. The course of this disorder is unaffected by any of the available treatments. Treatment of tic disorders includes comprehensive behavioral intervention, alpha-adrenergic agonists or antipsychotics, and treatment of comorbidities, but a proper assessment of the severity of the condition is mandatory.

The first stage of therapy should always be psychoeducation **(Flowchart 1)**.[34] The natural history of tics should be understood by kids, their parents, and school staff. Consideration should be given to comprehensive behavioral intervention for tics (CBIT), a type of behavioral therapy that may be able to help some older children control or lessen the frequency or intensity of their tics. It consists of cognitive-behavioral therapy, which includes relaxation techniques, information about tics, and habit reversal (learning a new behavior to replace the tic). Sometimes, the natural peaks and valleys of tics give the impression that a certain treatment is working.

Tics have been treated with a variety of dietary or nutritional supplements, such as fish oil, calcium, magnesium, and vitamins B, C, D, and E. There have also been experiments with complementary and alternative treatments such as prayer, massage, meditation, diet, yoga, acupuncture, hypnosis, and homeopathy.[35,36] For a brief period, acupuncture may be helpful in treating tics, but the evidence is scant. It is difficult to not know specific benefits beyond any placebo effect without randomized controlled studies to establish dosing, safety, and efficacy.[36] If a patient has used complementary and alternative therapies, the treating physician must ask about them.[35]

Medications

Tic suppressants and behavioral therapy should be considered when tics cause physical, emotional, or social impairment (e.g., musculoskeletal injury, peer relation difficulty such as bullying, low self-esteem, or difficulty in physical or academic activities). The goal of treatment is to lessen the severity of the tics to improve the patient's quality of life. Oral alpha-adrenergic agonist drugs clonidine and guanfacine are usually used for mild symptoms and also helpful for treatment of ADHD. Clonidine is started with 0.05 mg at bedtime and gradually increased up to 0.1–0.4 mg/day in two divided doses. Alternatively, Guanfacine is started with 0.025 mg at bedtime and gradually increased up to 4 mg/day in two divided doses. Other drugs that can help to control tics and associated comorbidities are listed below[5] **(Table 5)**.

In order to make tics manageable, the lowest dose of each medication is prescribed, and doses are increased as tics subside. The use of these antipsychotics may be restricted by the infrequent but serious side effects of dysphoria, Parkinsonism, akathisia, and tardive dyskinesia; however, using lower daytime doses and higher bedtime doses may lessen side effects. Drug tolerance can emerge and impede the ability to continue treatment.[34]

Treatment of Comorbidities

Comorbidities must be treated with low doses of stimulants that help to control ADHD without exacerbating tics, but an alternative medication, such as atomoxetine, may be preferred. A selective serotonin reuptake inhibitor (SSRI) may be helpful if obsessive or compulsive behaviors are bothersome. Children who struggle in school and have tics should also be tested for learning disorders and given support, if necessary.

Conclusion

Many patients with Tourette syndrome and chronic tic disorders have mild tics that do not need to be treated. To avoid stigmatization, it is crucial that the patient, his or her family, and other people who regularly interact with the patient receive psychoeducation. The therapeutic

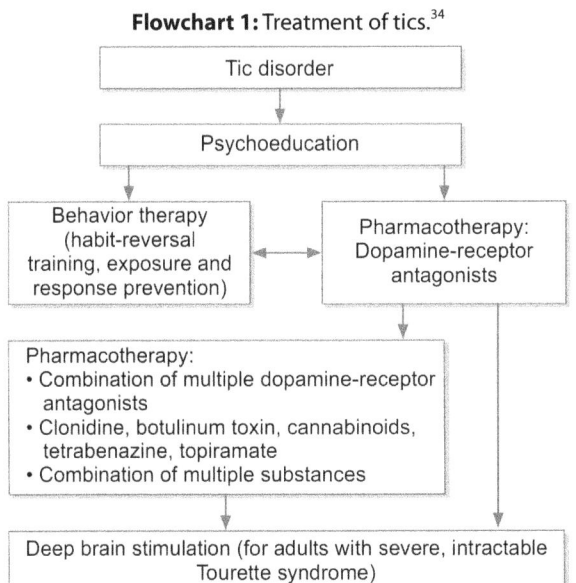

Flowchart 1: Treatment of tics.[34]

TABLE 5: Pharmacological agents used for tic disorders.[5]

Drug	Initial dose (mg) and dosage	Recommended dose (mg)	Maximum approved dose (mg)	Remarks
Tiapride	50–100 mg 2–3 times/day	600–800 mg	1,200 mg	Drug of first choice
Risperidone	0.5–1 mg 2 times/day	4–8 mg	16 mg	Effective against aggression as well
Aripiprazole	2.5 mg Once daily	10–30 mg	30 mg	Often better tolerated than other neuroleptic drugs
Pimozide	0.5–1 mg Once daily in evening	8–12 mg	16 mg	Combination with macrolides and sertraline can lead to fatal QT_c prolongation
Haloperidol	0.5 mg 2–3 times/day	10–15 mg	100 mg	Highly effective but more severe side effects
Tetrabenazine	12.5 mg 3 times/day	75 mg	200 mg	Causes depression more commonly than neuroleptic drugs. Must not be combined with MAO inhibitors. Reserve drug suitable for single selected tic
Sulpiride	50–100 mg 2 times/day	800–1,200 mg	1,600 mg	OCD, also effective against depression

(MAO: monoamine oxidase; OCD: obsessive-compulsive disorder)

options that are currently available are still inadequate for tic disorders that are severe enough to require treatment. New strategies for the pharmacotherapy of tic disorders are anticipated to be based on genetic studies.

TRICHOTILOMANIA

The term "compulsive hair pulling", also used to describe the hair-pulling disorder trichotillomania (TTM), is a mental illness characterized by an urge to pull one's own hair out.[37] Aristotle first made reference to hair pulling in the 4th century BC, but it was not until 1885 that it was first discussed in the modern literature.[38] The French dermatologist Francois Henri Hallopeau first used the term "trichotillomania" in 1889.[37] OCD in children is more likely to cause it. Anxiety may cause episodes of hair pulling, which are then briefly followed by a positive feeling after the hairs are pulled out. The majority of hair-pulling attempts end in failure. Any part of body can have hair removed, but the head and the area around the eyes are the most popular areas. Hair loss and distress are the results of excessive hair pulling. People who pull their hair frequently admit it, and close inspection may reveal broken hairs. Similar symptoms are also present in body dysmorphic disorder, but in that condition, people remove their hairs to fix what they perceive to be a flaw in their appearance.

Epidemiology

Despite the fact that no population-based epidemiologic studies have been carried out as of 2009, it is estimated that 0.6-4.0% of the general population experiences TTM at some point in their lifetime.[37] TTM is a disorder that can affect people of any age. However, it typically starts in childhood or adolescence, with a mean onset age of 9-13 years old,[40] and a notable peak at 12-13 years old. The genders are equally represented among preschoolers, but there seems to be a female predominance among preadolescents and young adults (70% and 93%, respectively). Females typically outnumber the males by ratio 3:1.[41]

Symptomatology

The scalp is the most frequently pulled-at site, followed by the brows, eyelashes, face, arms, and legs. Less-frequently pulled-at sites include the pubic area, underarms, beard, and chest. The "Friar Tuck" form of vertex and crown alopecia is the traditional manifestation.[40] The likelihood that a child will pull something other than their scalp is lower. Hair-pulling episodes can last for hours at a time because they frequently only pull one hair at a time. Some people report feeling more content when they pull an "anagen phase hair", while the inner, gel-like root sheath is still present at the hair's base. Additionally, the condition can enter remission-like states in which the patient may not have any urge to "pull hair" for days, weeks, months, or even years.

Low self-esteem can also have psychological repercussions because of one's appearance and the attention one receives. Some children do not display symptoms when they are in low-stress environments, but these symptoms frequently return when they leave those environments, indicating that there is a significant stress-related component. TTM is a relatively minor issue that only manifests as frustration, but for some people it results in social isolation and significant emotional stress, which can lead to psychiatric disorders such as mood or anxiety disorders. Therefore, family members may seek professional assistance to deal with this issue.

Trichotillomaniacs have hairs of various lengths, including broken hairs with blunt ends, some new growth with tapered ends, and still more broken mid-shaft or uneven stubble. A hair-pull test is negative (the hair does not come out easily), there is no scaling on the scalp, and overall hair density is normal. Hairs are frequently removed in an erratic fashion, leaving an odd shape. Trichotillomaniacs may feel ashamed of their hair-pulling behavior.

Complications

Infection, permanent hair loss, repetitive stress injury, and gastrointestinal obstruction brought on by trichophagia are examples of medical complications. Trichophagia is the practice of eating the hair that trichotillomaniacs pull; in severe (and uncommon) cases, this can result in a hair ball (trichobezoar).[39] If misdiagnosed, Rapunzel syndrome, a severe form of trichobezoar in which the hair ball's "tail" extends into the intestines, can be fatal.[41-43]

Etiology

Precise cause(s) of TTM are unknown as of 2023; however, it may be brought on by a confluence of genetic and environmental factors. In those with TTM, anxiety, depression, and OCD are more common. There is significant overlap between TTM and post-traumatic stress disorder, and some cases may be brought on solely by stress.

According to the neurocognitive model, which holds that the frontal lobes are essential for suppressing or inhibiting such habits and that the basal ganglia play a significant role in habit formation, TTM is classified as a habit disorder.[39] According to several MRI studies, people with TTM have an average of more gray matter than those without the condition.

It is likely that a number of different genes work together to increase susceptibility to TTM. TTM has been linked to mutations in the *SLITRK1*,[44,45] *5HT2A*,[46] and *SAPAP3*[47] genes.

Diagnosis

Patients may actively try to hide symptoms that are not always immediately apparent or that have been concealed to avoid disclosure out of shame, which makes diagnosis challenging. Evaluation for alopecia areata, iron deficiency, hypothyroidism, tinea capitis, traction alopecia, alopecia mucinosa, thallium poisoning, and loose anagen syndrome are among the conditions for differential diagnosis. A hair-pull test comes back negative for TTM.

A biopsy may be beneficial and show damaged hair follicles with perifollicular bleeding, fragmented hair in the dermis, empty follicles, and malformed hair shafts. Shaving a portion of the affected area and watching for the growth of normal hairs is an alternative procedure to biopsy, especially for young patients.[48]

The following diagnostic standards are provided by the Diagnostic and Statistical Manual of Mental Disorders, Fifth Edition (DSM-5) for TTM:

- *Criteria A:* Consistent hair pulling that must cause hair loss.
- *Criteria B:* There must be proof that the individual has made an effort to stop their hair-pulling behavior.
- *Criteria C:* Hair pulling must first be ruled out for general medical conditions and other disorders that may cause it, and TTM can only be identified if the behavior is not a reaction to another disorder. Examples include body dysmorphic disorders or delusions.

Treatment

Treatment is typically with cognitive behavioral therapy. It is based on the age of preschool children, and most of them outgrow the condition if managed conservatively. In adolescents, raising awareness of the condition is an important reassurance for the family and patient.

Psychotherapy

The highest rate of success in treating TTM is achieved by habit reversal training (HRT) which has also been a successful adjunct to medication.[49] With HRT, the individual is trained to learn and recognize their impulse to pull and also teach them to redirect this impulse. When compared, cognitive behavioral therapy (including HRT) has shown significant improvement over medication alone. It has also proven its efficacy in treating children.

Medication

There are no drugs for the treatment of TTM that have received Food and Drug Administration (FDA) approval in the United States. Although there is conflicting evidence, some drugs have been used to treat TTM. Tricyclic antidepressant clomipramine treatment has been shown to improve symptoms,[50] but other studies on clomipramine for the treatment of TTM have produced inconsistent results. The drug naltrexone might work as a remedy. The effectiveness of fluoxetine and other SSRIs in treating TTM is constrained, and they can have serious side effects. When compared to fluoxetine, behavioral therapy has been found to be more effective.[51] Contrarily, some medications, depending on the person, may make people pull their hair out more.

THUMB-SUCKING

Humans, chimpanzees, ring-tailed lemurs, and other primates all engage in thumb-sucking. It is a self-soothing practice that provides stimulation and serves as an adaptive function. After 6 months of age, a baby's natural urge to suck typically lessens. Although many infants continue to suck their thumbs for an extended period of time, it can develop into a habit, especially in those who do so to calm themselves when they are uncomfortable or bored. The thumb, fingers, or toes that are within reach are typically put into the mouth and repeatedly sucked rhythmically for a considerable amount of time. It is thought to be calming for the individual. As a child develops this habit, he or she frequently sucks on a "favorite" finger.

A baby's reflexive sucking of any object placed in its mouth at birth is known as the "sucking reflex," and it is crucial for breastfeeding. This offers not only essential nutrition but also a great deal of enjoyment, coziness, and warmth. Over time, this behavior (whether from a mother, bottle, or pacifier) starts to be linked to a very potent, pleasurable oral sensation that is self-soothing. Children can continue to enjoy those pleasantly calming sensations as they get older by sucking their thumbs, fingers, or toes. Although this reflex goes away around the age of 4 months, thumb-sucking can last much longer because it is not an instinctive behavior. Thumb-sucking can start prior to birth, as early as 15 weeks after conception, according to ultrasound scans. However, it is unclear whether this behavior is intentional or the result of the fetus's irrational movements while in the womb.

Thumb-sucking typically ends by the age of 4 years, but some older kids still practice this bad habit that can harm their teeth. It has been demonstrated that as long as the habit is broken before the onset of permanent teeth, at around 5 years old, the damage is reversible, so most dentists would advise breaking the habit as early as possible.[52] Their jaws and teeth are not harmed until after the age of 6–8 years old, when the eruption of permanent teeth may have an impact on the dentition's or oral cavity's shape. Thumb-sucking causes the tongue to lower itself, which allows it to counterbalance the buccal group of muscles' forces for a longer period of time than usual. As a result, the upper arch narrows and a posterior cross bite develops. Because the thumb rests on the teeth while sucking, it can also cause the mandibular and maxillary central incisors to tip lingually and labially, respectively, leading to an anterior open bite malocclusion. As a result, mandibular incisor retrusion also happens along with maxillary incisor proclination. A posterior cross bite results from transverse maxillary deficiency and eventually causes a malocclusion.[53]

Treatment

There are two categories of techniques to break the habit of sucking: (1) Preventive therapy and (2) appliance therapy. Most dentists concur and advise taking the following corrective measures:

- Rather than chastising or punishing kids who suckle
- Praise them when they do not. If a child is sucking his/her thumb when feeling insecure or needing comfort, focus instead on correcting the cause of anxiety and provide comfort to your child.
- If a young child is thumb-sucking out of boredom, try to engage him/her in a fun activity.
- Allow older kids to choose a technique to stop thumb-sucking.
- A pediatric dentist can encourage the child and inform him or her of the potential consequences of continuing to suck.
- It is only if the previous suggestions fail that the child should be reminded of the behavior by wrapping the thumb in bandages or covering the hand with a sock or glove at night.

The Indian Academy of Pediatrics has issued guidelines to help thumb-suckers and their parents. Accordingly, parents and their child must be taken into confidence and they must be told about the problem as well as its solution. Various activities and games which use hands such as drawing, craft, and painting can be encouraged.[54]

Intervention should be preceded by 1-month moratorium on parental attention. Many times, it is successful. If it fails, the following steps of intervention are required:
- *Monitoring of the habit:* It allows parents and child to keep progress (or lag) and that provides the basis for delivery of motivational incentives. Make a chart of progress and record daily.
- *Motivation, rewards, and incentives:* Praise the child for substitute behavior.
- *Sensory feedback:* Application of noxious nail polish (on nails only), two to three times a day. The child must know about this application of polish. Most of the children improve in 2 weeks and do not require any further treatment.

Appliance Therapy

When the abovementioned interventions fail, we must take the opinion of a dentist or a pedodontist and think for appliance therapy. Two types of appliances are available:
- *Removable appliances:* A removable habit-correction appliance can be taken in and out of the mouth. It requires 100% compliance and will only be effective if worn by a willing patient, or otherwise appliance can be easily removed by patient himself/herself. Thus, such appliances have low success rates.
- *Fixed appliances:* A fixed habit-correction appliance cannot be readily removed from mouth at will and hence, suckers have to start the habit-breaking process. However, they can experience difficulties in adjusting to eating, speaking, and cleaning around the appliance. The devices are as follows:
  - The hay rake
  - Thumb crib
  - Bluegrass appliance.

However, fixed intraoral appliances create problems during eating, as children have a risk of breaking them while removing these appliances.[55]

Alternative Methods

- *Mechanical therapies:* These can be effective for mild thumb-sucking habits such as covering the finger or strapping the hand down, but some patients find a way to remove and free their thumbs. These may not be effective in long term.
- *Chemical therapy:* This includes the use of a spicy, bitter tasting or foul-smelling liquid applied to thumbs or fingers. Rather, the use of bitterants or piquants is not endorsed as they may cause discomfort or pain.[55]

TGuard

TGuard **(Fig. 1)** has been breaking the thumb-sucking habit for over 25 years. Since 1995, dental health professionals have recommended TGuards as the best advice to stop thumb-sucking. It breaks the thumb-sucking habit quickly, effectively, and at a much cheaper cost than intraoral appliances. According to clinical studies, devices such as TGuards can be 90% effective in helping people kick the thumb- or finger-sucking habit. TGuards end the habit by simply removing the suction that causes the feelings of nurturing and comfort.

TGuards are ventilated because of air vents that provide a consistently cool and moisture-free environment. They are flexible of ergonomic shape and ensure that the child stops thumb-sucking habit in the most comfortable way. Each kit contains 30 wrist lock bands of various colors so that the patient can choose a unique band each day. Instalocks not only simplify adjustment but also provide a peace of mind that the device is locked and cannot be removed. This device does not prevent thumb from going into the mouth, but prevents suction from forming as the air flows into the tube, so that there pleasure is no longer left in the habit. *Simple*: No suction, i.e., no pleasure.

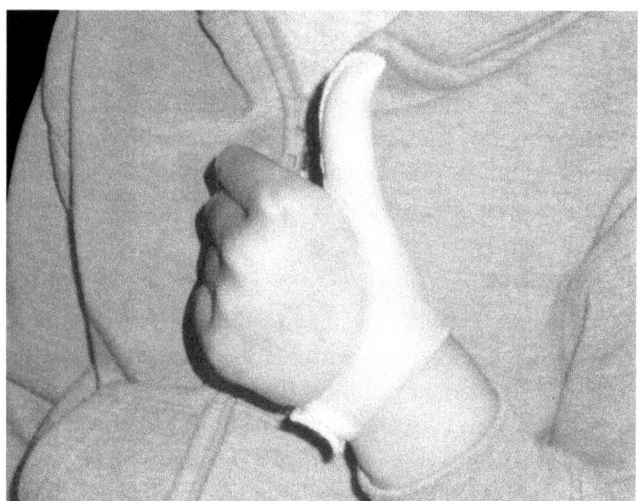

Fig. 1: TGuard appliance.

The children have no incentive to continue, and this makes the total treatment more effective in breaking the habit quickly and pain free.

There are various other devices, including fabric thumb guards, each with unique advantages and features based on the child's age, level of motivation, and willpower.

Conclusion

The effectiveness of clinical interventions to stop thumb-sucking was investigated through a review. When compared to no treatment, it was found that orthodontic appliances and psychological interventions (positive and negative reinforcement) were more effective at preventing thumb-sucking (short and long term). In repetitive behaviors that are body-focused, psychological interventions such as HRT and decoupling have been effective.

BRUXISM

Children are susceptible to various habit disorders that are conducted without consciousness, and among them, bruxism is one disorder that disturbs parents and they often seek medical consultation. Bruxism is derived from a Greek word "brychein," which means tooth grinding. The term bruxism was introduced in 1931 for involuntary excessive grinding, clenching, or rubbing of teeth during nonfunctional movements of the masticatory system. It describes jaw and tooth movements that go beyond those involved in speaking, chewing, and swallowing. In 2005, the International Classification of Sleep Disorders changed the classification of sleep bruxism from parasomnia to sleep-related movement disorder. Diurnal bruxism, or the grinding of the teeth without conscious awareness, is more common during stressful situations or when concentrating. Every time the child is made aware of the activity, it can be stopped or modified. On the other hand, it is impossible to stop sleep bruxism, which manifests as teeth grinding or clenching.

Prevalence

The prevalence of bruxism in children is difficult to determine because estimates are generally based on parental reporting or clinical findings of tooth wear. Its occurrence may be variable over the time. Moreover, tooth wear is not necessarily indicative of current tooth grinding. Its prevalence in children varies between 7 and 88%. About 14–20% children under 11 years are of age most commonly affected.[54] In healthy infants, sleep bruxism usually begins around the age of 1 year, shortly after the eruption of the primary incisors. An estimated 13% of people between the ages of 18 and 29 years exhibit bruxism, which then significantly declines with age.[55] The role of gender in this habit disorder is not definitive; however, some authors have reported that girls are more frequently affected.[54,56] It appears to be more common among individuals with developmental disabilities, particularly those with profound intellectual disabilities, ASD, and Down syndrome.[6,57]

Etiology

Although the etiology of bruxism is still debatable, consensus holds that it is multifactorial. According to recent research, pathophysiological and psychological factors, rather than morphological ones, control sleep bruxism in the center.[58]

Pathophysiological Factors

Smoking, alcohol, illegal drugs, trauma, and other pathophysiological factors can cause adolescents to grind their teeth. Many times, teeth grinding causes a change in sleep stage, usually toward lighter sleep or awakening. Non-rapid eye movement (NREM) or light sleep stages 1 and 2 account for more than 80% of sleep bruxism episodes in young adults, while REM (deep sleep stages) accounts for 5–10%.[59] Sleep bruxism can be brought on by issues with sleeping as well as sleep disturbances such as noise in the room, sleeping for fewer than 8 hours every night, and sleeping with a light on.[60]

A number of pediatric conditions, such as basal ganglia infarction, cerebral palsy, Down syndrome, epilepsy, Leigh disease, meningococcal septicemia, multiple system atrophy, gastroesophageal reflux, and Rett syndrome have also been linked to bruxing in these patients. Given that there is increased cortical and autonomic cardiac activity prior to bruxing, there seems to be a connection with the autonomic nervous system. It appears at various levels of consciousness and vanishes when consciousness has significantly increased. The dopaminergic system may be involved in sleep bruxism because certain medications, such as antidepressants and SSRIs, may have an adverse effect on the dopaminergic system. When handling these children, this needs to be taken into account. The amphetamines used to treat ADHD can also cause bruxism. Hyperactivity is also linked to teeth grinding.

Psychological Influences

The causes of bruxism have been linked to factors such as stress and personality. Stress and anxiety are linked to clenching or grinding during sleep, but the precise mechanism by which these and other psychological factors contribute to the etiology is still unknown. However, those who have bruxism have higher catecholamine levels in their urine.[61] Many authors have agreed with the idea that psychologic factors do have an impact on bruxism.[62-64]

Respiratory Factors

Regular snoring and teeth grinding have a lot in common. Children who mouth breathe frequently complain of sleep bruxism. According to one theory, obstructive sleep apnea causes sleep bruxism and that there is a connection between the two. It seems to occur more frequently while supine sleeping, which is consistent with the potential for airway obstruction. Adenotonsillectomy surgery has also been shown to help some children with their bruxism.[65] Additionally, allergic conditions such as asthma or infections of the respiratory airways may be to blame.[66]

Genetics

Uncertain is the genetic component of bruxism. However, it has been noted that there is a link between parental and child bruxism, and 20-50% of sleep bruxism patients have immediate family members who did not grind their teeth as children.[59] Additionally, a parasomnia called sleep talking and bruxing share a genetic background.[61] However, the precise genetic mechanism underlying the etiology of bruxism is unknown; only one allele has been linked to the condition.[63]

The evaluation of these children's symptoms is fraught with methodological issues; for instance, tooth wear may be noticeable but not necessarily indicate a current bruxing habit. As a result, there is not a consensus among authors regarding the best way to record this parafunction. It can be challenging to distinguish between wear in children's primary dentition caused solely by bruxism and wear caused by other factors such as diet or endogenous factors. Although studies have shown a link between bruxing and the signs and symptoms of temporomandibular disorders (TMDs) in children and adolescents, the connection between TMD and bruxism is also debatable and unclear.[56]

Treatment

Bruxism is so common in children that it is often considered as a normal behavior. It only becomes pathological when a child has severe tooth damage and reports pain, or sleep is interrupted, or the noise is enough to disturb parents. Others contend that even at the start of the mixed dentition, bruxism cannot be regarded as normal.[65] Additionally, there is insufficient evidence in the literature to support using a rigid occlusal splint for primary dentition, a common treatment for bruxism in older patients, to treat it in children. Avoiding chewing gum, sleeping without a pillow, wet heat, and no television before bedtime are some local therapies for children who grind their teeth. Treatment is not advised for children with the condition because they typically outgrow it.

Patients with severe psychological issues or upper airway obstructions, however, should be referred to the appropriate specialists. Other options should be discussed with the patient's primary care provider in children or adolescents who are taking medications for conditions that could lead to bruxism. Additionally, it might be even harder to treat bruxism in children with developmental disabilities. This population may be approached using prosthodontics, oral surgery, behavior modification, music therapy, massage, or botulinum A-toxin injections. However, Lang et al. concluded that the evidence base is incredibly thin, so it is impossible to make a firm determination about the effectiveness of treatment.[60]

Conclusion

Despite the prevalence of bruxism in children, there is a dearth of research on its diagnosis and treatment, making it difficult to develop evidence-based clinical practice guidelines. The treatment will continue to be anecdotal until the cause of bruxism is understood. It is obvious that well-designed studies on the causes and treatment of bruxism in children are urgently needed. Treatment is not advised in the current environment because most children outgrow the condition.

REFERENCES

1. Himle MB, Flessner CA, Bonow JT, Woods DW. In: Diagnostic and Statistical Manual of Mental Disorders, 4th edition. American Psychiatric Association, Washington, DC: University of Wisconsin; 2000. pp. 1-33.
2. Mink JW. The basal ganglia and involuntary movements: Impaired inhibition of competing motor patterns. Arch Neurol. 2003;60:1365-8.

3. Fahn S, Jankovir J, Hallet M. Principles and Practice of Movement Disorders. Amsterdam: Elsevier Health Sciences; 2011. pp. 350-79.
4. Mol Debes NM, Hjalgrim H, Skov L. Limited knowledge of Tourette syndrome causes delay in diagnosis. Neuropediatrics. 2008;39:101-5.
5. Ludolph AG, Roessner V, Munchau A, Muller-Vahl K. Tourette syndrome and other tic disorders in childhood. Dtsch Arztebh Int. 2012;109(48):821.
6. Leckman JF, Zhang H, Vitale A, Lahnin F, Lynch K, Bondi C, et al. Course of tic severity in Tourette syndrome: the first two decades. Pediatrics. 1998;102:14-9.
7. Freeman RD, Fast DK, Burd L, Kerbeshian J, Robertson NM, Sandor P. An international perspective on Tourette syndrome: selected findings from 3500 individuals in 22 countries. Dev Med Child Neurol. 2000;42:439-47.
8. Leckman JF, King RA, Cohen DJ. Tics and tic disorders. In: Leckman JF and Cohen DJ (Eds). Tourette Syndrome: Tics, Obsessions, Compulsions: Developmental Psychopathology and Clinical Care. New York: Wiley; 1999. pp. 23-42.
9. Khalifa N, Von Knorring AL. Prevalence of tic disorders and Tourette syndrome in a Swedish school population. Dev Med Child Neurol. 2003;45:315-9.
10. Hockstra PJ, Steenhwis MP, Kallenberg CG, Minderaa Rb. Association of the small events with self-reports of tic severity in pediatric and adult tic disorder patients: a prospective longitudinal study. J Clin Psychiatry. 2004;65:426-31.
11. Lin H, Yeh CB, Peterson BS, Scahil L, Grantez H, Finalley DB, et al. Assessment of symptom exacerbation in a longitudinal study of children with Tourette's syndrome or obsessive compulsive disorder. J Am Acad Child Adolesc Psychiatry. 2002;41:1070-7.
12. Yael D, Vinner E, Bar Gad I. Pathophysiology of tic disorders. Mov Disord. 2015;30:1171-8.
13. Robertson MM, Eapen V, Singer HS, Martino D, Scharf JM, Paschon P, et al. Gilles de la Tourette syndrome. Nat Rev Dis Primers. 2017;3:16097.
14. Veda K, Black KJ. J Clin Med. 2021;10(11):2479.
15. Leckman JF, Dolnansky ES, Hartin MT, Clubb M, Walkup JT, Stevenson J, et al. Prenatal factors in the expression of Tourette's syndrome. An explanatory study. J Am Acad Child Adolesc Psychiatry. 1990;29:220-6.
16. Chao TK, Hu J, Pringsheim T. Prenatal risk factors for Tourette disorder. A systematic review. BMC Pregnancy Childbirth. 2014;14:53.
17. Ayubi E, Mansori K, Doostitravs A. Effect of maternal smoking during pregnancy on Tourette syndrome and chronic disorders among offspring: A systematic review and meta- analysis. Obstet Gynecol Sci. 2021;64:1-12.
18. Mahews CA, Scharf JM, Miller LC, Macdonald-Wallis C, Lawlor DA, Ben-Shhamo Y. Association between pre- and perinatal exposures and Tourette syndrome or chronic tic disorder in the AKSPAC Cohort. Br J Psychiatry. 2014;204:40-5.
19. Pauls DL, Fernandez TV, Mathews CA, State MW, Scharf JM. The inheritance of Tourette disorder: A review. J Obsessive Compuls Relat Disord. 2014;3:380-5.
20. Weidinger E, Krause D, Wildenauer A, Meyer S, Gruber R, Schwarz MJ, et al. Impaired activation of the innate immune response to bacterial challenge in Tourette syndrome. World J Biol Psychiatry. 2014;15:453-8.
21. Leckman JF, Katsovich L, Kawikova J, Lin GH, Zhang H, Kronig V, et al. Increased serum levels of interleukin 12 and tumor necrosis factor-alpha in Tourette syndrome. Biol Psychiatry. 2005;57:667-3.
22. Kawikova I, Leckman JF, Kronig H, Katsovich L, Bessen DE, Ghebremichael M, et al. Decreased numbers of regulatory T cells suggest impaired immune tolerance in children with Tourette syndrome: A preliminary study. Biol Psychiatry. 2007;61:273-8.
23. Martino D, Church AJ, Defazio G, Dek RC, Quinn NP, Robertson MM, et al. Soluble adhesion molecules in Gilles de la Tourette syndrome. J Neurol Sci. 2005;234:79-85.
24. Bos-Veneman NG, Oleiman R, Tobiasova Z, Hoekstra PJ, Katsovich L, Bothwell AL, et al. Altered immunoglobulin profiles in children with Tourette syndrome. Brain Behav Immun. 2011;26:532-8.
25. Martino D, Zis P, Buttiglione M. The role of immune mechanisms in Tourette syndrome. Brain Res. 2015;1617:126-43.
26. Kondo K, Kabasarwa T. Improvement in Gilles de la Tourette syndrome after corticosteroid therapy. Ann Neurol. 1978;4:387.
27. Cordona F, Orefici G. Group A streptococcal infections and tic disorders in an Italian population. J Pediatr. 2001;138:71-5.
28. Church AJ, Dale RC, Lees AJ, Giovannoni G, Robertson MM. Tourette's syndrome: A cross sectional study to examine the PANDAS hypothesis. J Neurol Neurosurg Psychiatry. 2003;74:602-7.
29. Swedo SE, Leonard HL, Rapoport JL. The pediatric autoimmune neuropsychiatric disorders associated with streptococcal infection (PANDAS) subgroup: Separating fact from fiction. Pediatrics. 2004;113:907-11.
30. Cunningham MV. Molecular mimicry, autoimmunity and infection: The cross reactive antigens of Group A Streptococci and their sequelae. Microbiol Spectr. 2019;7;10.1128/microbiolspec.GPP3-0045-2018.
31. Cath DC, Hadderly T, Ludolph AG, Stern JS, Murphy T, Hartmann A, et al. European clinical guidelines for Tourette syndrome and other tic disorders. Part I assessment. Eur Child Adolesc Psychiatry. 2011;45:155-71.
32. Khalifa N, Von Knorring AL. Psychopathology in a Swedish population of school children with tic disorders J Am Acad Child Adolesc Psychiatry. 2006;45:1346-53.
33. Leckman JF. Tourette's syndrome. Lancet. 2002;360: 1577-86.
34. Roessner V, Plessen KJ, Rothenberger A, Ludolph AG, Rizzo R, Skov L, et al. European clinical guidelines for Tourette syndrome and other tic disorders. Part II:

pharmacological treatment. Eur Child Adolesc Psychiatry. 2011;20:173-96.
35. Kompoliti K, Fan W, Leurgans S. Complementary and alternative medicine use in Gilles de la Tourette syndrome. Mov Disord. 2009;24:2015-9.
36. Kumar A, Duda L, Mainali G, Asghar S, Byler D. A comprehensive review of Tourette syndrome and complementary alternative medicine. Curr Dev Disord Rep. 2018;5:95-100.
37. Huynh M, Gavino AC, Magid M. Trichotillomania. Semin Cutan Med Surg. 2013;32 (2):88-94.
38. Salaam K, Carr J, Grewal H, Sholevar E, Baron D. Untreated trichotillomania and trichophagia: surgical emergency in a teenage girl. Psychosomatics. 2005;46(4):362-6.
39. James W, Berger TE, Elston D. Andrews' Diseases of the Skin: Clinical Dermatology, 10th edition. Philadelphia; Saunders; 2005. p. 62.
40. Chamberlain SR, Menzies L, Sahakian BJ, Fineberg NA. Lifting the veil on trichotillomania. Am J Psychiatry. 2007;164(4):568-74.
41. Christenson GA, Mackenzie TB, Mitchell JE. Characteristics of 60 adult chronic hair pullers. Am J Psychiatry. 1991; 148(3):365-70.
42. Ventura DE, Herbella FA, Schettini ST, Delmonte C. Rapunzel syndrome with a fatal outcome in a neglected child. J Pediatr Surg. 2005;40(10):1665-7.
43. Pul N, Pul M. The Rapunzel syndrome (trichobezoar) causing gastric perforation in a child: a case report. Eur J Pediatrics. 1996;155(1):18-9.
44. Matejů E, Duchanová S, Kovac P, Moravanský N, Spitz DJ. Fatal case of Rapunzel syndrome in neglected child. Forensic Sci Int. 2009;190(1-3):e5-e7.
45. Zuchner S, Cuccaro ML, Tran-Viet KN, Cope H, Krishnan RR, Pericak-Vance MA, et al. SL1TRK 1 mutations in trichotillomania. Mol Psychiatry. 2006;11(10):887-9.
46. Hemmings SM, Kinnear CJ, Lochner C, Seedat S, Corfield VA, Moolman-Smook JC, et al. Genetic correlates in trichotillomania: A case-control association study in the South African Caucasian population. Isr J Psychiatry Relat Sci. 2006;43(2):93-101.
47. Züchner S, Wendland JR, Ashley-Koch AE, Collins AL, Tran-Viet KN, Quinn K, et al. Multiple rare SAPAP3 missense variants in trichotillomania and OCD. Mol Psychiatry. 2009;14(1):6-9.
48. James W, Berger T, Elston D. Andrews' Diseases of the Skin: Clinical Dermatology, 10th edition. Philadelphia: Saunders; 2005. p. 63.
49. Woods DW, Wetterneck CT, Flessner CA. A controlled evaluation of acceptance and commitment therapy plus habit reversal for trichotillomania. Behav Res Ther. 2006;44(5):639-56.
50. Swedo SE, Leonard HL, Rapoport JL, Lenane MC, Goldberger EL, Cheslow DL. A double-blind comparison of clomipramine and desipramine in the treatment of trichotillomania (hair pulling). New Engl J Med. 1989;321(8):497-501.
51. Christenson GA, Mackenzie TB, Mitchell JE, Callies AL. A placebo-controlled, double-blind crossover study of fluoxetine in trichotillomania. Am J Psychiatry. 1991; 148(11):1566-71.
52. Friman PC, McPherson KM, Warzak WJ, Evans J. Influence of thumb sucking on peer social acceptance in first-grade children. Pediatrics. 1993;91(4):784-6.
53. Shetty RM, Shetty M, Shetty NS, Deoghare A. Three-alarm system: revisited to treat thumb-sucking habit. Int J Clin Pediatr Dent. 2015;8(1):82-6.
54. Singh D, Manglik AK, Khatri PC, Shah SR. (2021). Thumb sucking, Temper Tantrums, and PICA. [online] Available from: https://iapindia.org/pdf/IAP-Parental-Guideline-Thumb-sucking-Temper-Tantrums-and-PICA.pdf [Last accessed October, 2023].
55. Jesse McGuire. (2019). What is a thumb sucking appliance? [online] Available from: https://prosmilesortho.com/what-is-a-thumb-sucking-appliance/ [Last accessed October, 2023].
56. Stop Thumb sucking with Aerothumb. [online] Available from: https://tguard.com/ [Last accessed October, 2023].
57. Cheifetz AT, Osganian SK, Allred EN, Needleman HL. Prevalence of bruxism and associated correlates in children as reported by parents. J Dent Child (Chic). 2005;72(2):67-73.
58. Macedo CR, Silva AB, Machado MA, Saconato H, Prado GF. Occlusal splints for treating sleep bruxism (tooth grinding). Cochrane Database Syst Rev. 2007;4:CD005514.
59. Barbosa Tde S, Miyakoda LS, Pocztaruk Rde L, Rocha CP, Gavião MB. Temporomandibular disorders and bruxism in childhood and adolescence: review of the literature. Int J Pediatr Otorhinolaryngol. 2008;72(3):299-314.
60. Lang R, White PJ, Machalicek W, Mandy R, Kang S, et al. Treatment of bruxism in individuals with developmental disabilities: a systematic review. Res Dev Disabil. 2009;30(5):809-18.
61. Yap AU, Chua AP. Sleep bruxism: current knowledge and contemporary management. J Conserv Dent. 2016;19(5):383-9.
62. Lavigne GJ, Khoury S, Abe S, Yamaguchi T, Raphael K. Bruxism physiology and pathology: an overview for clinicians. J Oral Rehabil. 2008;35(7):476-94.
63. Vanderas AP, Menenakou M, Kouimtzis T, Papagiannoulis L. Urinary catecholamine levels and bruxism in children. J Oral Rehabil. 1999;6(2):103-10.
64. Restrepo CC, Alvarez E, Jaramillo C, Velez C, Valencia I. Effects of psychological techniques on bruxism in children with primary teeth. J Oral Rehabil. 2001;28(4):354-60.
65. DiFrancesco RC, Junqueira PA, Trezza PM, de Faria ME, Frizzarini R, Zerati FE. Improvement of bruxism after T & A surgery. Int J Pediatr Otorhinolaryngol. 2004;68(4):441-5.
66. Grechi TH, Trawitzki LVV, de Felício CM, Valera FCP, Alnselmo-Lima WT. Bruxism in children with nasal obstruction. Int J Pediatr Otorhinolaryngol. 2008;72(3):391-6.

Chapter 20

Aggressive Behavior

Pramod Sharma

INTRODUCTION

Aggressive behavior denotes harming others by physical or verbal means. It is neither competitiveness nor anger. Competitiveness is an attitude; anger is an emotion whereas aggression is a behavior. However, both competitiveness and anger may contribute to aggression.

DEFINITION

Aggressive behavior is a disruptive behavior/symptom in which the affected child has improper self-control of emotions and/or behaviors. The cardinal feature of this syndrome is that the affected child violates the rights of the other child and thereby tries to defy social norms.[1] Harm done to others unintentionally or accidentally must be excluded.[1] The child reacts in a hostile way toward peers, siblings, or adults which can include verbal and physical aggression.[2]

Temper tantrums, physical aggression such as hitting or biting other children, stealing other children's possessions, and defiance of authority are distressing to all those who come in contact with the child (families, school staff, society, etc.). The child may have verbal or physical outbursts aimed at peers and parents alike.

Since few episodes of temper tantrums in children aged 1–3 years and rebellion during adolescent years may be considered normal for that age but when these episodes are frequent and persistent they must be taken seriously and considered psychiatric disorders. The chances of reversal without intervention are bleak.

INCIDENCE

Statistics indicate that approximately 3–7% of children and adolescents exhibit signs of aggression. Disease is much more common in boys and comparatively less common in girls. Physical aggressiveness is much more common in boys whereas interpersonal coercive behavior (relational bullying), especially in peer relationships is more common in girls.[2] These disorders usually have their onset in childhood or adolescence.[3]

TYPES

Many conditions such as intermittent explosive disorder (IED), oppositional defiant disorder (ODD), conduct disorder (CD), antisocial personality disorder (ASPD), kleptomania, etc., may be grouped under this head. The diagnosis should be made only when other psychiatric/mental disorders have been ruled out.

Intermittent Explosive Disorder

As per DSM-5 (The Diagnostic and Statistical Manual of Mental Disorders, Fifth Edition) criteria,[3] the affected child has recurrent behavioral outbursts representing a failure to control aggressive impulses as manifested by either verbal aggression such as temper tantrums, tirades, verbal arguments, or fights.

The aggressiveness expressed is grossly out of proportion to the provocation or to any precipitating psychosocial stressors and the outbursts are impulsive and/or anger based not done to achieve some tangible objects (money, power, intimidation). Such outbursts may have financial or legal consequences. Attacks are neither premeditated nor instrumental.

Oppositional Defiant Disorder

As per DSM-5 criteria,[3] there is a pattern of angry/irritable mood, argumentative/defiant behavior, or vindictiveness lasting at least 6 months as evidenced by at least four symptoms from any of the following categories exhibited during interaction with at least one individual who is not a sibling.

Angry/irritable mood:
1. Often loses temper
2. Is often touchy or easily annoyed
3. Is often angry and resentful

Argumentative/defiant behavior:
4. Often argues with authority figures or, for children and adolescents, with adults
5. Often actively defies or refuses to comply with requests from authority figures or with rules
6. Often deliberately annoys others
7. Often blames others for his or her mistakes or misbehavior

Vindictiveness:
8. Has been spiteful or vindictive at least twice within the past 6 months.

The cardinal feature of ODD is a frequent and persistent pattern of angry/irritable mood, argumentative/defiant behavior, or vindictiveness. The affected child deliberately annoys others and puts blame on others for his deeds. Usually, the episodes occur at one place (usually home) but may occur at multiple sites.

Conduct Disorders

When the symptoms of children having ODD become persistent or increase, they are put in this category. As per DSM-5 criteria, it is defined as—"A repetitive and persistent pattern of behavior in which the basic rights of others or major age-appropriate societal norms or rules are violated".[3]

Conduct disorders have been discussed in detail in Chapter 11 of this book.

Antisocial Personality Disorder[4]

As per DSM-5 criteria,[3] it is defined as a pervasive pattern of disregard for, and violation of, the rights of others occurring since 15 years of age and continues in adulthood **(Table 1)**. For diagnosis, the child must be 18 years of age with evidence of CD (onset <15 years) and he/she must have three or more of the following points:
1. Failure to conform to social norms with respect to lawful behaviors, as indicated by repeatedly performing acts that are grounds for arrest.
    - Deceitfulness, as indicated by repeated lying, use of aliases, or conning others for personal profit or pleasure.
    - Impulsivity or failure to plan ahead
    - Irritability and aggressiveness, as indicated by repeated physical fights or assaults.
    - Reckless disregard for safety of self or others
    - Consistent irresponsibility, as indicated by repeated failure to sustain consistent work behavior or honor financial obligations.
    - Lack of remorse, as indicated by being indifferent to or rationalizing having hurt, mistreated, or stolen from another.
2. The individual is at least 18 years of age
3. There is evidence of conduct disorder with onset <15 years of age
4. The occurrence of antisocial behavior is not exclusively during the course of schizophrenia or bipolar disorder.

EPIDEMIOLOGY/RISK FACTORS

The various factors that may influence or precipitate the syndrome are:
- *Genetic:* There is often a family history of psychiatric illnesses or aggressive behavior, indicating some genetic trait.
- *Poor family environment:* Poor parental relationships, poor child–parent/caretaker relationships, denying emotional attachment to child, domestic violence, rejection/belittling of the child are important precipitating factors. Such factors are said to act as a role model for the child to develop aggression as the child is not able to develop appropriate behavior regulation skills. Severe physical punishment, incarceration, etc., may pave the children to use aggressive behavior as a solution to the problem.
- *Mass media:* The incidence of child developing aggression due to impact of violent content on TV/Internet/social media is on rise and at times, difficult to treat. The actors in the films, etc., doing violence become role model for the child. Since parents usually do not keep an eye on what their children are watching or following facilitates development of such behaviors.
- *Socioeconomic factors:* Persistent joblessness, community violence put the child in depression vis-a-vis aggression.
- The role of child neglect and physical/sexual abuse is profound in development of aggressive behavior.
- *Peer effect:* If the children live in company of children having such behaviors, they too may adopt the same. Living in an area of criminals also imparts similar

TABLE 1: Showing comparison of types of aggressive behaviors.[5]

	Oppositional defiant disorder (ODD)	Conduct disorder (CD)	Antisocial personality disorder (ASPD)	Intermittent explosive disorder (IED)
Onset	Usually <8 years of age, no later than early adolescence	• Child onset <10 years • Adolescent onset after 10 years but rarely after 16 years of age	Since 15 years or adulthood	Usually 6 years or equal developmental level
Symptoms	Trouble with authority, breaks school rules, always seems angry, argumentative, easily annoyed, noncompliant	Significant aggression towards others, cruel to animals, destruction of property, theft/stealing, setting fires, serious violation of rules, law breaker, substance abuse, poor scholastic performance	Disregard for others, criminal offences, substance abuse and poor school performance	• Verbal or physical aggression • Onset is rapid and episode lasts for <30 minutes and usually occur on minor provocation by a close intimate or associate. They are usually not premeditated or instrumental • Rapid onset • Episode last for <30 minutes
Attack rate for diagnosis	On most days for at least 6 months (for children <5 years). For >5 years once per week episode for at least 6 months	3+ incidents within the last 12 months with at least one in past 6 months	Pervasive pattern since age of 15 years	• Behavioral outbursts twice-a-week for 3 months • Physical aggression (destruction of property, cruelty to animals or other individuals (at least 3 episodes within 1 year)
Associated features	• Distress in individual or peers or persons in contact – ADHD and CD • Increased risk for suicidal attempts	Misreading of other's intention, suspiciousness, insensitive to punishment, and substance misuse (especially in girls)	Lacks empathy, is callous, cynical and contemptuous of the feelings, rights and suffering of others[4]	Depression, anxiety and substance use disorders
Special worse in features	In mild cases confined to single settings whereas in moderate-to-severe cases, symptoms exhibited at multiple sites	They behave very aggressively and often bully others physically or by internet media	Irresponsible and exploitative in sexual relationships	Disturbance in levels of neurotransmitters (serotonin), especially in the limbic system have been said to be causative factor
	Affected child considers himself normal and justifies his/her behavior as a result of prevailing circumstances	• They may be cruel to animals • Involve themselves in stealing, snatching • Run away from home	Irresponsible parenthood (children have poor hygiene and are taken care by other relatives or neighbors)	Onset rare in adulthood
Course	Many children may subsequently develop conduct disorders, anxiety or depression disorders, poor peer relationships, etc.	Variable. Prognosis is worse in childhood onset type	Chronic	• Episodic • Recurrent episodes over many years

effect. Peer rejection is an another important provoking factor.
- Neuropsychiatric disorders such as ADHD, anxiety, depression, mood disorders etc have a high association with the aggressive behaviors. Aggression due to these disorders is more common in girls.
- *Parental psychiatric illness:* Parents dealing with mental health issues might find it challenging to provide adequate emotional support and guidance to their children.
- *Maternal factors:* Maternal alcoholism, smoking during pregnancy, and teen age pregnancy can increase the risk of antisocial behavior.
- *Lead neurotoxicity:* Higher blood lead levels are said to be associated with such disorders; however, the prevalence is decreasing.
- History of head injury and abnormal electroencephalogram (EEG) are also associated with increased incidence though exact cause is not known.
- *Other factors:* History of moving schools, mistreating animals or weaker children, and witnessing criminal behavior and substance abuse within their families.

ETIOPATHOGENESIS[6]

Exact pathogenesis is not known, however, following theories have been put forward:
- *Freudian theory:* This theory links aggression to oral phase of development and links it to early experiences and relationships.
- *Humanistic theory:* Aggression is viewed as a product of frustration, stemming from the obstruction of life goals and desires.
- *Social learning theory:* Aggression is not innate but acquired through experience. It is considered a learned behavior reinforced by the circumstances.
- *Hormonal theory:* Androgens have been blamed as males generally display higher levels of aggression than females.
- *Neurotransmitter theory:* Disturbance in levels of serotonin and/or GABA, specifically in areas of the limbic system (anterior cingulate and orbitofrontal cortex), has been seen in individuals with IED.

Different forms of aggression:
- *Accidental aggression:* It is just an accident in which a child hurts another child without trying.
- *Expressive aggression:* It is committing an aggressive act because the act feels good for the child.
- *Hostile aggression:* It is aggression done on purpose to hurt someone physically or psychologically. Affected children experience satisfaction from seeing others hurt and feel powerful (bullying). Often children who exhibit hostile aggression are unpredictable, unprovoked, and illogical. Being provoked, however, is a different type of aggression called reactive aggression.
- *Instrumental aggression:* The children fight over objects, territory, or rights, and in the process, someone gets hurt. Most aggression exhibited by children of 2-6 years is instrumental, with the majority of outbursts happening in fights over materials and toys.[7]
- *Cyber bullying:* This is particularly common in adolescents. The affected child uses social media platforms to harass the target child.[2]
- Aggressive behavior can be either impulsive (reacting to a trigger) or proactive (premeditated).

Assessment

Managing aggressive behavior in children necessitates a thorough examination/assessment of various dimensions, encompassing biological, psychological, social, and cultural aspects. This multifaceted assessment aims to provide a comprehensive understanding of the underlying factors contributing to the behavior.
- *Detailed behavioral history:* Gathering a comprehensive history (including understanding the frequency, intensity, triggers, and context of aggressive episodes) of the child's behavior is pivotal.
- *Clinical interviews:* Conducting clinical interviews with both the child and caregivers helps uncover relevant information about the child's behavior and potential contributing factors.
- *Biopsychosocial factors:* This involves understanding genetic predispositions, past experiences, family dynamics, and cultural influences.
- *Historical data review:* Examining school reports and previous assessments, provides insights into the child's behavior over time.
- *Observations:* Observing the child's behavior in different settings can offer valuable information about triggers, patterns, and the severity of aggressive episodes.
- *Psychological testing:* Utilizing psychological tests can help uncover underlying emotional, cognitive,

or developmental issues that might contribute to aggressive behavior.
- *Questionnaires:* Collecting input from both parents and teachers through questionnaires provides a broader perspective on the child's behavior. Tools such as the Strength and Difficulties Questionnaire (SDQ) or the Achenbach System Of Empirically Based Assessment (ASEBA) can aid in identifying coexisting issues.[1]
- *Peer and caretaker interviews:* Interviews with peers and caregivers provide additional insights into the child's behavior.
- *School perspective:* Collaborating with teachers can shed light on behavior patterns and triggers within the educational environment.

DIFFERENTIAL DIAGNOSIS

- *Attention-deficit hyperactivity disorder:* Any of the three core symptoms of impulsivity, inattention, and motor overactivity can be misconstrued as antisocial.
- *Mood disorders:* Depression can present with irritability and oppositional symptoms but unlike typical ODD/CD, mood is usually clearly low and there are often vegetative features. Aggression is not premeditated or committed to achieve a tangible objective. Lying and stealing are also absent.[1]
- Early bipolar disorder should not be diagnosed without clear evidence of manic features such as racing thoughts, increased activity or energy, and expansive mood.[1]
- *Adjustment disorder:* Onset occurs soon after exposure to an identifiable psychosocial stress factor such as divorce, bereavement, trauma, abuse, or adoption. The onset should be either 1 month (ICD-10 criteria) or 3 months (DSM-5 criteria) and symptoms should not persist for more than 6 months after the cessation of the stress or its sequelae.[1]
- *Autistic spectrum disorders (ASD):* Marked tantrums or destructiveness are usually associated with ASD. Enquiring about other symptoms of ASDs should reveal their presence.[1]
- *Subcultural deviance:* Many children defy social norms and indulge in activities such as shop lifting, recreational drug use but do not express aggressive or defiant behavior. Drug and alcohol usage should always be asked about, but often this will fall short of a diagnosable dependence syndrome, both in terms of symptoms and major impairment.[1]

COMPLICATIONS[8]

The various complications are:
- *Impaired relationships:* Aggressive behavior can strain relationships with peers, family members, teachers and other caregivers leading to social isolation, rejection, and difficulties in having healthy communications.
- *Academic challenges:* Inability to focus and engage in learning leads to poor scholastic performance, disciplinary actions, and long-term educational setbacks.
- *Emotional distress:* Both the aggressive child and those on the receiving end of their behavior can experience emotional distress. Aggressive children might struggle with emotional regulation and empathy, while their peers might experience fear, anxiety, and low self-esteem.
- *Mental health disorders:* These children may have anxiety and depression.
- *Legal issues:* Severe aggression that results in physical harm or destruction of property, stealing/theft, vandalism, rape, murder, etc., can have legal implications, leading to legal actions against the child and potentially affecting their future opportunities.
- *Continuity of aggressive behavior:* If left untreated, aggressive behavior in childhood can persist into adolescence and adulthood, resulting in a more ingrained pattern of aggressive conduct that can be difficult to modify.
- *Peer rejection:* Aggressive behavior can lead to rejection by peers, making it challenging for children to establish healthy social networks and develop crucial interpersonal skills.
- *Low self-esteem:* Such behaviors can lead to negative consequences and strained relationships, children might develop low self-esteem and negative self-perceptions.
- *Substance abuse:* Over time, untreated aggressive behavior might increase the risk of engaging in risky behaviors, such as substance abuse, as a coping mechanism.
- *Increased risk of injury:* Aggressive behavior can lead to physical altercations, increasing the risk of injury to both the aggressive child and those around them.
- *Long-term behavioral patterns:* Without intervention, aggressive behavior in childhood can set the stage for long-term behavioral patterns that affect social, academic, and professional success.

- *Community effect:* Sometimes such children may pave way for community unrest, fear and poor intercommunity relationships eroding the social fabric.
- *Economic impact:* Loss of productivity, increased healthcare costs, and loss due to damaged infrastructure do have an economic impact.
- *Suicide:* Suicide rates are high in children who have been bullied by some aggressive child.[2]

TREATMENT

No specific treatment is available. Only psychotherapy, motivation, and guarded use of drugs can be of help. A multidisciplinary team is likely to give better results. Family members/teachers/caretakers must be involved in the treatment plan.

Aim of therapy is to:
- Reduce children's aggressive behavior such as shouting, pushing, and arguing.
- Increase prosocial interactions such as entering a group, starting a conversation, participating in group activities, sharing, cooperating, asking questions politely, listening, and negotiating.
- Correct the cognitive deficiencies, distortions and inaccurate self-evaluation.
- Ameliorate emotional regulation and self-control problems to reduce emotional lability, impulsivity and explosiveness, enabling the child to be more reflective and able to consider how best to respond in provoking situations.

All caretakers must follow following points:
- *Be a model of nonaggressive behavior:* Be calm when dealing with such children. Keep the voice level firm, your movements controlled, and have an eye contact with the child.
- Avoid sharp objects or weapons in house, even one should avoid purchasing of toy weapons for his/her ward.
- Manage materials to minimize potential frustration among children. If the children (especially young toddlers) have a conflict over a particular item like toy than parents must give them multiple items to avoid conflict.
- Praise children when their behavior is appropriate.
- Make it clear that aggression is unacceptable.
- *Personalizing the treatment plan:* The treatment plan should follow the assessment and fit the particular needs of the child and family. Intervention needs to be tailored according to the needs and strengths of the family and be reasonably congruent with their beliefs.
- *Parent training:* Most parenting programs target skills, such as promoting play and developing a positive parent–child relationship, using praise and rewards to increase desirable social behavior, giving clear directions and rules, using consistent and calm consequences for unwanted behavior, and reorganizing the child's day-to-day activities to prevent problems.
- *Interventions in school:* Teachers are taught techniques that they can apply to all children in their class, as well as to those exhibiting antisocial behavior. Typically, they target four areas of functioning. First, they promote positive behaviors such as compliance and following established classroom rules and procedures. Second, the interventions prevent problem behaviors such as talking at inappropriate times and fighting. Third, they teach social and emotional skills such as conflict resolution and problem-solving. Fourth, they prevent the escalation of angry and acting-out behavior.

Specific Skills for Handling Specific Aggression

- *Accidental aggression management:* Defuse the situation by identifying the wronged child's feelings and explaining that it was an accident.
- *Expressive aggression management:* In this situation, focus on allowing the aggressor to continue the pleasurable physical movement while changing the situation, so it becomes harmless. For example, if the child is breaking other children's toys or items, then he/she should be persuaded to do it on his/her own items.
- *Hostile aggression management:* Children must be told that hostile behavior will not be tolerated. Clear boundaries and consistent expectations must be given to children who use hostile aggression. There are many children who have poor peer relationships, they must be brought together and motivated to become friends and form a new group which is not as hostile as previously they were.
- *Instrumental aggression management:* Needs conflict mediation skills.

He should clarify child's perspective, and generate alternatives and making him agree on alternative plans or solution.[7]

DRUG THERAPY[5]

- *Stimulants (guanfacine, clonidine):* These drugs may reduce irritability in cases of impulsive aggression with underlying disorders such as ADHD.
- *Selective serotonin reuptake inhibitors (SSRIs):* They are useful where anxiety is root cause. Fluoxetine is most commonly used drugs; however, sertraline, citalopram, and escitalopram have also been tried.
- Mood stabilizers (valproic acid and lamotrigine) have also been tried.
- Atypical antipsychotics such as risperidone and aripiprazole have also been used with different success rates.

PROGNOSIS

The prognosis for individuals exhibiting aggressive behavior depends on a variety of factors, including the underlying causes, the severity of the behavior, the effectiveness of interventions, and the support systems available. While each case is unique, understanding certain general trends can provide insight into the potential trajectory and outcomes of aggressive behavior:

Factors predicting poor outcome:
- *Onset:* Early onset of severe problems, before the age of 8 years.
- *Phenomenology:* Antisocial acts which are severe, frequent, and varied; physical aggression and premeditated acts.
- *Comorbidity:* Hyperactivity and attention problems; callous-unemotional traits.
- *Intelligence:* Lower IQ
- *Family history:* Possibly maternal anxiety during pregnancy, smoking, and alcoholism, poor parenting, disturbed child–parent/caretaker relationships, and presence of interparental violence are all poor prognostic indicators.

Prognosis can be better if:
- Early intervention
- *Addressing underlying causes/factors or comorbidity* such as mental health issues, family dynamics, or environmental stressors.
- *Severity:* Mild-to-moderate cases might respond well to interventions, while severe and persistent aggression might require more intensive and prolonged treatment.
- *Consistency of treatment:* The consistency and continuity of interventions, therapies, and support systems are crucial for long-term improvement. Regular therapy sessions, behavioral interventions, and skill-building programs contribute to better outcomes.
- *Family and social support:* A strong support system, including family, peers, educators, and mental health professionals, can positively influence the prognosis. A supportive environment fosters better emotional regulation and interpersonal relationships.
- *Response to interventions:* Individuals who respond positively to interventions and show progress in managing their aggression tend to have a more favorable prognosis.
- *Adolescent development:* Adolescence is a critical phase for prognosis. While aggressive behavior might persist for some, others may naturally develop better emotional regulation and social skills as they mature.
- *Motivation and willingness:* The individual's motivation and willingness to participate in treatment and work towards behavioral change also impact prognosis.
- *Long-term strategies:* Developing and implementing long-term strategies for managing triggers and stressors can contribute to sustained improvements in behavior.

It is important to note that individual responses vary, and prognosis is not set in stone. Some individuals might continue to exhibit aggressive tendencies despite interventions, while others may overcome them entirely. With the right combination of early intervention, consistent support, appropriate treatment, and a conducive environment, individuals with aggressive behavior can navigate a path toward healthier emotional expression, improved interpersonal interactions, and a brighter future.

KLEPTOMANIA[9]

It is a mental illness that creates a strong urge to steal that somebody cannot control. As per DSM-5 criteria, the diagnostic points are:
- Recurrent failure to resist impulses to steal objects that are not needed for personal use or for their monetary value.
- Increasing sense of tension immediately before committing the theft.
- Pleasure, gratification, or relief at the time of committing the theft.
- The stealing is not committed to express anger or vengeance and is not in response to a delusion or a hallucination.

- The stealing is not better explained by conduct disorder, a manic episode, or antisocial personality disorder.

Incidence varies from study to study. Onset is usually during adolescence (may occur since childhood or during adulthood). The act is usually unplanned and is usually done without help of some associate. Low levels of neurotransmitters such as serotonin and opioid systems have been blamed behind the disorder.

BREATH-HOLDING SPELLS[10,11]

Breath-holding spells (BHS) are common nonepileptic paroxysmal events affecting 4–5% of pediatric population. They are brief periods when young children stop breathing for <1 minute. These spells are most commonly observed between 6 and 18 months of age and peculiarly attacks disappear after 5 years of age. They are three times more common in male children.

Etiology

Exact etiology is unknown, however, it may be due to following factors:
- *Emotional factors:* These factors seem probable as the spell is preceded by emotional triggers such as crying, anger, or frustration. The whole attack appears to be a sort of emotional blackmailing by the child to get the desired thing done. This is obvious as it is commonly seen in overprotective child, children with disturbed child–parent relationships and children of overanxious parents.
- There is some evidence that children with anemia (especially iron deficiency) are more prone to BHS.
- *Genetic:* A positive family history is seen in 20–30% cases suggesting some genetic involvement (possibly an autosomal dominant trait with reduced penetrance).

Clinical Features

The attack occurs in a sequence. Firstly, there is a provocative stimulus which leads to apnea and color change, followed by limpness and abnormal posturing and stupor occurs in the last. The cerebral symptoms are mostly due to poor cerebral perfusion. The spells are either cyanotic (70–75%) or pallid or they may be mixed.

Cyanotic BHS are usually precipitated by anger or frustration **(Table 2)**. The child cries, holds breath, and the forced expiration leads to cyanosis and other typical symptoms (limpness etc.). The attack is followed by a long inspiration, disappearance of cyanosis, and the child

TABLE 2: Showing comparison between cyanotic and pallid breath-holding spell (BHS).

	Cyanotic BHS	Pallid BHS
Provocative factors	Usually anger leading to vigorous cry	Fright or pain or an unexpected event
Autonomous system involved	Sympathetic overactivity	Parasympathetic overactivity
Cerebral hypoperfusion	Yes	Yes
Cyanosis	Yes	No
Loss of consciousness	May or may not	Much more common

recovers. Some child may fall asleep for an hour or so. Child may have seizures if there is prolonged apnea.

Pallid BHS: A painful stimulus is the most common trigger factor. The child turns pale (as opposed to blue) and become unconscious with little if any crying. Recovery (alertness) occurs within a minute or so.

The attack rate may be once-a-day to many attacks a day. Duration of attack is 10–60 seconds and if the attack is prolonged (>1 minute), then the clinician must think of other diagnosis.

The episodes are without any postictal phase and no incontinence (as witnessed with seizures). EEGs are normal in these children. There is no neurological sequelae.

Diagnosis

The diagnosis is made clinically. A proper history with sequence of events (if possible parents be asked to show video recording of attack), no incontinence and no postictal phase, help to make an accurate diagnosis. ECG may be done to rule out cardiac arrhythmia as a cause.

Differential Diagnosis

The BHS must be differentiated from seizures/epilepsy as shown in **Table 3**. The other diseases to be included in differential diagnosis are pertussis, congenital laryngeal stridor, sepsis, stiff baby syndrome, and shuddering.

Treatment

Since parents are highly frightened although the episode is benign in nature, hence reassurance of parents is the crux of treatment. They must be convinced that this is just

TABLE 3: Breath-holding spell (BHS) and seizures.

	BHS	Seizures
Age	6–18 months. Rare after 5 years	All ages
Family history	Present in many cases	Same
Trigger factors	Present	Absent
Relation with sleep	No	Usual
Postictal changes	No	Usually present
Electroencephalogram (EEG)	Normal	Abnormal

an attention-seeking exercise and as the age advances, the child will outgrow it. Parents should be asked to pay attention to the triggers and should be warned not to give up. They must be told that it does not affect the IQ and future cerebral development of the child. The case has good prognosis without any sequelae.

Pharmacotherapy: No definite role but still following can be given—
- *Iron therapy:* Iron therapy should be given, irrespective of presence or absence of anemia. It has been found to decrease the incidence as well as severity of spells.
- Some studies have supported the use of piracetam (40 mg/kg/day).
- Atropine sulfate (0.01 mg/kg/24 h in divided doses with a maximum daily dose of 0.4 mg) to antagonize vagal hyperactivity has been used with good results in cases with prolonged asystole associated with frequent and severe pallid spells.
- Cardiac pacers may be required in refractory cases.

TEMPER TANTRUMS[11,12]

Temper tantrums are brief episodes of unpleasant, undesirable, disruptive behaviors, or emotional outbursts that are extreme and usually disproportionate to the situation.

These are usually in early childhood (18 months to 4 years) and signify the appearance of autonomy and simultaneously seeking parental/caretaker's attention. Tantrums usually show child's anger/frustration and at times are because the child may not have the vocabulary to express his/her feelings. Mostly, they are part of normal behavior; however, in some disorders such as autism, we may come across atypical tantrums as a feature of behavioral or developmental disorder.

Precipitating factors:
- Over protective child, and single child
- Parental disharmony and failure to set limits
- Unfulfilled demands, frustration, and anger
- Fatigue, hunger, fear (especially punishment), and illness
- Overstimulating environment
- Children with delayed speech, behavioral/developmental disorders have more frequent and aggressive tantrums.

Clinical Features

In response to a trigger, the child cries, turn around, undertakes head banging, screams and yells, may pound fists or feet, kick or bite, may hold breath and make themselves vomit. They may go limp, throw items, push others, and sometimes may turn into BHS. Episode usually lasts for 1–3 minutes; however, in atypical cases may last for >15 minutes. Attack rate too is usually once a day but rarely there may be even >5 attacks/per day. Physical examination is normal.

Management

- No laboratory tests are required.
- Rule out diseases such as neurocutaneous stigmata, dysmorphic facies, autism, vision and hearing impairment, iron deficiency anemia, and lead toxicity.
- Reassure the parents and convince them about its benign nature and also persuade them to leave the room and they should never give in to the child.
- Parents must stay calm as shouting and hitting the child will worsen the situation. They must avoid arguing with the child.
- Parents should try to distract the child and engage them in different activities.
- Keep child from getting hurting himself or others.
- Keep child in a safe place until they calm down.
- As far as possible ignore the tantrum—attention fuels their desire to act out.
- If they hold their breath, let them; they will breath naturally eventually as they cannot suffocate themselves.
- Reward the child when he behaves normally.
- After the episode is over, stay calm and express love to the child and address the trigger factor.
- Drugs usually do not have any role. Iron supplementation to be given if there is anemia or BHS.

- Low-dose antipsychotic agents, e.g., risperidone or aripiprazole for few weeks as an adjuvant to nonpharmacological management may be given to reduce severity, especially in children with associated developmental or psychiatric disorders.

CONCLUSION

To conclude, aggressive behavior represents a significant concern. It may manifest in many ways as described above but in any case, it is due to interplay of many factors, viz., biological, psychological, environmental factors, hormonal imbalances and neurological abnormalities. Addressing aggressive behavior in children requires a multifaceted approach that encompasses early intervention, family support, access to mental health services, and a commitment to fostering positive social and emotional development. Recognizing the complexity of the issue and tailoring interventions to the individual needs of each child is paramount in achieving positive outcomes and preventing long-term consequences.

REFERENCES

1. Scott S. Oppositional and conduct disorders. In: Thapar A, Pine DS, Leckman JF, Scott S, Snowling MJ, Taylor E (Eds). Rutter's Child and Adolescent Psychiatry, 6th edition. Hoboken, NJ: John Wiley & Sons, Inc.; 2015. pp. 966–80.
2. Moseley LR, Sinclair-McBride K, DeMaso DR, Walter HJ. Aggression. In: Kliegman RM, St. Geme JW, Blum NJ, Shah SS, Tasker RC, Wilson KM (Eds). Nelson Text book of Pediatrics, 21st edition. USA: Elsevier; 2020. pp. 242-3.
3. Disruptive, impulse-control, and conduct. Diagnostic and statistical manual of mental disorders DSM-5-TR. Washington, DC: American Psychiatric Association; 2022. pp. 522-37.
4. Cluster B Personality Disorders. In: Diagnostic and statistical manual of mental disorders DSM-5-TR. Washington, DC: American Psychiatric Association; 2022. pp. 749-52.
5. Zahrt DM, Melzer-Lange MD. Aggressive behavior in children and adolescents. Pediatr Rev. 2011;32(8):325-32.
6. Practical Psychology. (2023). Theories of aggression: Exploring psychological explanations. [online] Available from: https://practicalpie.com/theories-of-aggression/. [Last accessed October, 2023].
7. California Childcare Health Program. Aggressive behavior in young children. [online] Available from: https://cchp.ucsf.edu/sites/g/files/tkssra181/f/Aggressive_EN_new.pdf. [Last accessed October, 2023].
8. Marjorie K, Purcell SE, Debra SE, Nelson ME, Krumbach EM, Janet SH, et al. (2010). Helping children resolve conflict: Aggressive behavior of children G2016. [online] Available from: https://digitalcommons.unl.edu/cyfsfacpub/72. [Last accessed October, 2023].
9. Antisocial Personality Disorder. In: Diagnostic and statistical manual of mental disorders DSM-5-TR. Washington, DC: American Psychiatric Association; 2022. pp. 538-41.
10. Jayakumar C, Chakrabarty P, Muralidhar. Indian Academy of Pediatrics. Breath holding spells. Standard treatment Guidelines 2022. [online] Available from: https://iapindia.org/pdf/Ch-089-Breath-holding-Spell.pdf. [Last accessed October, 2023].
11. Moseley LR, Sinclair-McBride K, DeMaso DR, Walter HJ. Tantrums and Breath-Holding Spells. In: Kliegman RM, St. Geme JW, Blum NJ, Shah SS, Tasker RC, Wilson KM (Eds). Nelson Text book of Pediatrics, 21st edition. USA: Elsevier; 2020. pp. 240-1.
12. Chandra T, Hrishikesh, Gupta A (2022). Indian Academy of Pediatrics. Temper tantrums. Standard treatment guidelines. [online] Available from: https://iapindia.org/standard-treatment-guidelines-details.php?id=143. [Last accessed October, 2023].

Chapter 21

Rumination Disorder

Shivji Ram Choudhary, RK Maheshwari

INTRODUCTION

Rumination (Latin *"ruminare"* means "to chew the cud") is a behavioral disorder in which an effortless and painless regurgitation of undigested food occurs into the mouth soon after a meal.[1] The regurgitated food may be rechewed, reswallowed, or spit out. Regurgitation is typically frequent and daily and is absent during sleep.

As per Diagnostic and Statistical Manual of Mental Disorders, Fifth Edition (DSM-5) criteria, the disorder must be present for at least 1 month after a period of normal functioning and is not better explained by any gastrointestinal illness or psychiatric or medical conditions.[2]

EPIDEMIOLOGY

Rumination is a rare disorder manifesting mostly in infancy (commonly at 3–12 months of age) but at times, also seen in childhood or adolescence. Disease is more common in males and in those with intellectual disability.[3]

PATHOPHYSIOLOGY

The pathophysiology is not well understood. The disease is observed in infants who receive inadequate emotional interaction and have learned to soothe and may stimulate themselves through rumination and show signs of gaining considerable satisfaction from the activity. It involves a rise in intragastric pressure generated by either voluntary or unintentional contraction of the abdominal wall muscles causing movement of gastric contents back up into the esophagus. As a consequence, when food enters the stomach, the body has learned a new behavior involving contraction of the abdominal muscles putting pressure on the stomach and the food or fluid coming back up. After this event has gone away, the newly learnt behavior remains in place, almost similar to a "habit".

CAUSES

- Neglect of the child either due to disturbed relationship with primary caregivers or other factors
- Lack of an appropriately stimulating environment
- Stressful life situations
- Anxiety/depression, especially in adult patients
- Attention-seeking phenomenon.

CLINICAL FEATURES

Symptoms often begin with some "triggering" event like a viral infection, gastrointestinal disease, or stress happening in the patient's life. Infants may show a characteristic position of straining and arching the back with the head held back, making sucking movements with tongue. The child is usually irritable and hungry in between two episodes of rumination.

The affected child has bad breath, tooth decay, repeated stomach aches, and indigestion as well as raw and chapped lips. The child may have normal weight but many go into malnutrition.

Two criteria (ROME-IV and DSM-5) are available to label a child with this disease.

Rome IV Criteria

- *Neonate/Toddler* (all criteria to be met for at least 2 months):
  - Repetitive contractions of the abdominal muscles, diaphragm, and tongue
  - Effortless regurgitation of gastric contents, which are either expelled from the mouth or rechewed and reswallowed.

Minimum three of following:
1. Onset between 3 and 8 months
2. Does not respond to management for gastroesophageal reflux disease and regurgitation

3. Unaccompanied by signs of distress
4. It does not occur during sleep and when the infant is interacting with individuals in the environment.
- *Children/Adolescent* (all criteria to be met for at least 2 months):
    - Repeated regurgitation and rechewing or expulsion of food that begins soon after ingestion of a meal
    - It does not occur during sleep
    - Not preceded by retching.

DSM-5 Criteria

As per these criteria, there should be recurrent regurgitation of food (which may be spit out, rechewed, or reswallowed) for at least a month. All other gastrointestinal causes as well as diseases such as anorexia nervosa, binge-eating disorder, or bulimia nervosa should be ruled out.

COMPLICATIONS

Progressive malnutrition, dehydration, and poor immunity are common complications which may result in delayed growth and poor learning potential. Mortality is rare but may occur in severe cases.

LABORATORY EXAMINATION

There is no specific laboratory test to diagnose this disease. In very severe cases, laboratory measures of serum electrolytes and a hematologic workup should be done to determine need for medical intervention.[3] Invasive investigations may be required to exclude conditions which can mimic rumination disorders. High-resolution esophageal manometry with concurrent impedance may be useful in confirming the diagnosis and also in differentiating primary and secondary rumination disorder.

DIFFERENTIAL DIAGNOSIS

The rumination must not be confused with vomiting or belching. They must be differentiated as shown in **Table 1**.

It also needs to be differentiated from congenital gastrointestinal system anomalies, hypertrophic pyloric stenosis, gastroparesis, hiatal hernia, Sandifer syndrome, raised intracranial pressure, diencephalic tumors, inborn errors of metabolism, adrenal insufficiency, anorexia nervosa, and bulimia nervosa.[1]

TREATMENT

The treatment requires a multidisciplinary approach which consists of psychotherapy, nutritional intervention, behavioral techniques, and drug therapy for anxiety/depression, if present.

- Habit reversal (or behavioral interventions) may compel child to adopt alternative behavior and skip the previous behavior which used to cause rumination/regurgitation.
- Squirting lemon juice into child's mouth after the episode has been tried in the past to relieve the symptoms (Aversive behavioral interventions). However, now a days stress is on habit-reversal techniques.
- Psychotherapy should be given to child and his/her caretakers in case of neglected child.
- Hiatal hernia, if present, should be treated accordingly.
- Adolescent patients may benefit from diaphragmatic breathing and paradoxical intention.[4]

TABLE 1: Differential diagnosis.

	Rumination	Vomiting	Belching
Definition	Painless regurgitation effortless and of undigested food occurs into the mouth soon after a meal	The forcible voluntary or involuntary emptying of stomach contents through the mouth or, less often, the nose	Its body's way of expelling excess air from your upper digestive tract
Cause	Behavioral disorder	Both peripheral and central	Physiological—to remove excessive gas from upper gastrointestinal tract (GIT)
Preceded by nausea	No	Usually yes	No
Gastric contents	Undigested or sometimes partially digested	Usually partially digested	No expulsion of gastric contents
Treatment	Behavioral therapy	As per the cause	No treatment required except proper feeding or burping

- Many drugs such as metoclopramide, cimetidine, and antipsychotics have been used with varied results
- Treatment of refractory cases includes Baclofen and Nissen's fundoplication. Baclofen works by increasing the resting tone of the lower esophageal sphincter (LES), thereby reducing the ease of reflux of gastric contents!

It can also be treated with Nissen's fundoplication in order to enhance the resting pressure of LES and to partially negate the intragastric propulsive force provided by contraction of anterior wall musculature by reducing concurrent L#S relaxation.

COURSE AND PROGNOSIS

Spontaneous remissions are quite common. Many-a-times, the disease may go undiagnosed. It may result in poor school attendance and may keep child away from sports or athletic activities. Habit reversal techniques may improve prognosis.

CONCLUSION

In conclusion, rumination disorder is a unique eating disorder characterized by the regurgitation and rechewing of food, leading to potential physical and psychological consequences. It is essential to seek professional help for a proper diagnosis and treatment plan. With the right interventions, individuals with rumination disorder can manage their symptoms and improve their overall quality of life.

REFERENCES

1. Samsel CB, Walter HJ, De Maso DR. Rumination disorder. In: Kliegman RM, St. Geme JW, Blum NJ, Shah SS, Tasker RC, Wilson KM (Eds). Nelson TextBook of Pediatrics, 21st edition. USA: Elsevier; 2020. pp. 204-5.
2. Call C, Walsh BT, Attia E. From DSM-IV to DSM-5: changes to eating disorder diagnoses. Curr Opin Psychiatry. 2013; 26(6):532-6.
3. Boland R, Verduin ML, Ruiz P. Neurodevelopmental disorders and other childhood disorders. Kalpan & Sadock's Synopsis of psychiatry, 12th edition. North America: Wolters Kluwer; 2022. pp. 164-6.
4. Murray HB, Zhang F, Call CC, Keshishian A, Hunt RA, Juarascio AS, et al. Comprehensive cognitive-behavioral interventions augment diaphragmatic breathing for Rumination syndrome: a proof-of-concept trial. Dig Dis Sci. 2021;66:3461-9.

Chapter 22

Enuresis and Encopresis

DR Dabi, Harshna Aseri

ENURESIS

INTRODUCTION

The problem of enuresis is quite common and prevalent all across the globe. It affects socioemotional development of the child. Considerable stress on the child is the fear of it being detected by other classmates or other family members.[1] In our country, parents often consider it as an age-related issue and they hope that the child would outgrow it as he gets older.

DEFINITION

The word enuresis is derived from a Greek word (*Enourein*) that means "to void urine." It is defined as normal, nearly complete evacuation of the bladder at a wrong place and time at least twice a month after 5 years of age.[2] More than 85% children attain complete diurnal and nocturnal control of the bladder by 5 years of age.

PREVALENCE

The occurrence of enuresis in children aged 6–12 years globally ranges from 1.4 to 28%.[3] Diurnal enuresis is more common in girls and rarely occurs after the age of 9 years. Overall, 25% of children have diurnal enuresis.[4] However, data specific to the incidence and prevalence of enuresis in India is quite limited. It is estimated to be from 7.61 to 16.3%.[5-7] The prevalence of the enuresis decreases from 15 to 20% in <5 years to 1–2% in adolescence.[6] Bedwetting can often be inherited also. Bedwetting gene is strong among families. If one parent wets the bed as a child, the child has a 25% chance of bedwetting. If both parents were bedwetters as children, their child's chances increases to about 75%.

CLASSIFICATION

- *Primary enuresis:* It is labeled when the child has never gained continence for >6 months. Nearly 80% cases fall in this category.
- *Secondary enuresis:* It is labeled when symptoms reappear after the child had gained continence for at least 6 months[8] **(Box 1)**.

It may be further classified as:
- *Monosymptomatic nocturnal enuresis:* When the incontinence is only during sleep **(Flowchart 1)**
- *Nonmonosymptomatic enuresis:* When there is day time enuresis and the affected child also has urgency, voiding difficulties and/or abnormally low or high day time voiding frequency.

However, as per the International Children's Continence Society (ICCS), it can be classified as depicted in **Table 1**:

BOX 1: Common causes of secondary enuresis.

- Idiopathic
- Urge syndrome and dysfunctional voiding
- Cystitis
- Constipation
- Psychological stress
- Acquired neurogenic bladder
- Seizure disorder
- Obstructive sleep apnea
- Diabetes mellitus
- Acquired diabetes insipidus
- Acquired urethral obstruction
- Heart block
- Hyperthyroidism
- *Drugs:* Selective serotonin reuptake inhibitors, valproic acid, clozapine

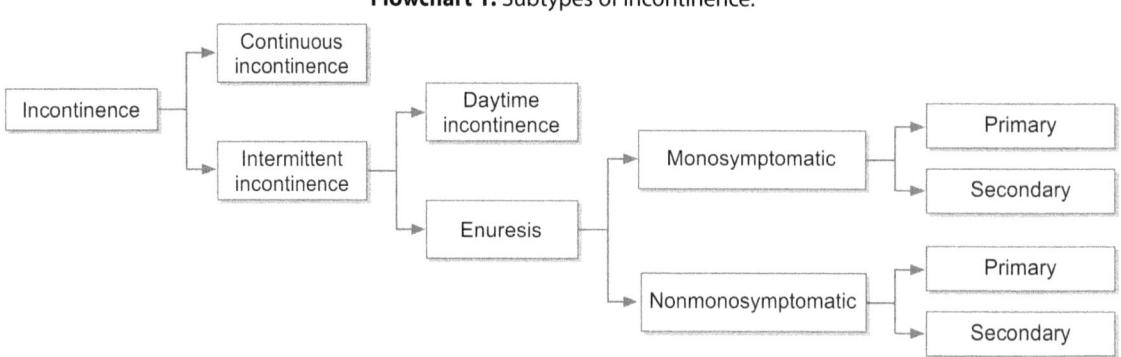

Flowchart 1: Subtypes of incontinence.

TABLE 1: Classification of nighttime wetting according to the International Children's Continence Society (ICCS).

	Longest period of dryness <6 months	Longest period of dryness >6 months
General	Primary nocturnal enuresis (PNE)	Secondary nocturnal enuresis (SNE)
No daytime bladder dysfunction	Primary monosymptomatic nocturnal enuresis (PMNE)	Secondary monosymptomatic nocturnal enuresis (SMNE)
With daytime bladder dysfunction	Primary nonmonosymptomatic nocturnal enuresis (PNMNE)	Secondary nonmonosymptomatic nocturnal enuresis (SNMNE)

RISK FACTORS

- *Genetic:* Common among siblings
- *Sex:* More common in male children
- *Family causes:* More common in children living with single parent or step parents. Parental disharmony, poor parent–child relationships, ill parents, punitive behavior of parents, and poor scholastic performance all contribute or increases chances of having this disorder.
- Diseases such as attention deficit hyperactivity disorder (ADHD) and sleep apnea also have high incidence of enuresis[9]
- Urinary tract anomalies are commonly associated with nocturnal or diurnal enuresis.

PATHOPHYSIOLOGY

The precise reasons and mechanisms behind enuresis are still not fully understood. Pathophysiology of nocturnal enuresis rests on three main factors: (1) Excessive urine production during sleep, (2) abnormal bladder function, and (3) inability to awaken to the signals of a full urinary bladder. In primary enuresis, an altered antidiuretic hormone profile, arousal failure, and delayed bladder maturation are the main pathological factors.[10-12] Central nervous system disorders may also contribute to the same.[13-15] The increased production of urine at night may be a result of abnormalities in the circadian rhythm and the impaired release of vasopressin. Children with overactive bladders often experience symptoms during the day, such as urgency, frequency, and incontinence. Furthermore, the *ENUR1* gene is believed to be involved in the underlying cause of enuresis.[16]

DIAGNOSIS

The DSM-5 criteria to diagnose the disease are as follows:[17]
- Whether involuntary or intentional, repeated voiding of urine into bed or clothes.
- The behavior should be clinically significant, with either:
  - Frequency of at least two times a week for at least 3 months consecutively
  - Clinically significant distress
  - Academic (occupational), social, or other areas of functioning are impaired.
- Chronological age of at least 5-year or equivalent developmental level is required.
- The behavior is not attributable to another medical condition (seizure disorder, diabetes, urinary tract infection, spina bifida, neurogenic bladder, etc.) or substance (diuretic, antipsychotic, etc.).

History

Taking a comprehensive and thorough patient history is extremely important. One must record:
- Age of onset, its duration, and severity
- Whether had continence in past, if yes duration of continence
- Ask about history of other urinary tract symptoms like urgency, dysuria, etc.
- History of taking any treatment about any urinary illness
- Enquire about constipation
- Enquire about family issues described as risk factors
- Record total fluid intake, urine output, etc.
- *Maintain a voiding diary:* Record dry as well as wet days or night

Clinical Examinations

- *Ear, nose, throat (ENT) checkup:* Looks for adenotonsillar hypertrophy, etc., to rule out obstructive sleep apnea
- Per abdominal examination to see for enlarged bladder, fecoliths, spina bifida, or other vertebral malformation
- *Genital examination:* To look for hypospadias/epispadias, meatal stenosis, ectopic ureter and labial adhesions and also see if there are any signs of sexual abuse
- *Rectal (PR) examination:* To see for perianal and perineal sensation, tone of rectal sphincter, perianal excoriations and also see for vulvovaginitis
- *Neurological examination:* Abnormal tendon reflexes in lower limbs, abnormal gait

Laboratory Investigations

Although there are no laboratory tests to confirm enuresis, but clinician may be required to go for following tests to rule out other disorders:
- *Urine examination:* If glucose/ketones are present, then one must rule out diabetes. If there are pus cells, then one may go for urine culture. Low specific gravity of urine may indicate diabetes insipidus.
- Renal function tests may be prescribed to rule out renal disorders.
- *Thyroid function tests:* To rule out thyroid disorders
- *Hemoglobin (Hb) electrophoresis:* To diagnose sickle cell disease

Imaging Studies
- USG or voiding cystourethrography to see for any structural abnormality, to see for vesicoureteral reflux, and measurement of residual urine
- *Cystometry:* To evaluate bladder dysfunctions
- Magnetic resonance imaging (MRI) or plain X-ray of lumbosacral spine to see for anatomic vertebral disorders.

MANAGEMENT

Urotherapy

Urotherapy includes all nonpharmacological and nonsurgical approaches used to resolve lower urinary tract symptoms. The affected child (especially those who are 5–7-year-old) must be given behavioral therapy. Fluids, beverages, and caffeine drinks should be restricted after evening hours. The child must be trained to urinate before going to bed and again just before falling asleep (double voiding). In daytime, he/she must void urine every 2 hours.

Alarm Therapy

Alarm therapy is generally recommended in children >6 years old.

Bed devices: The urine alarm features a moisture-sensitive switching system which, when closed by contact with urine seeped into pajamas or bedding, completes a small voltage electrical circuit, and activates a stimulus theoretically strong enough to cause waking (e.g., buzzer, bell, light, or vibrator). The device is placed on the bed. The child turns off the alarm and follows steps such as using the bathroom, changing clothes, and returning to bed. Sometimes, parents are alerted by the alarm first and they guide the child through the steps.

Pajama devices are simpler versions of alarms. The alarm is either placed in a pocket or pinned to the child's pajamas. Two wires are attached near the pajama bottoms. When the child wets, urine absorption completes an electrical circuit and activates the alarm. Different stimuli such as buzzing, ringing, vibrating, or lighting can be used with these devices.

Reward Therapy

Positive reinforcement, like using star charts, has been found to be more effective than negative punishment. The star chart involves placing a star on the calendar for every dry night as a reward. No punishment is given for wet nights. A streak of consecutive stars, such as 7, may earn a treat. However, for this to work, the child should already be having a good number of dry nights.

Pharmacotherapy

Pharmacotherapy for nocturnal enuresis is second-line treatment.[18]

Desmopressin (DDAVP), an analog of antidiuretic hormone, is given orally in tablet form in the dose of 0.2–0.4 mg/day 60 minutes prior to bedtime. Desmopressin is also available as a mouth-dissolving tablet (Meltab), which is given in the dose of 120–240 µg. Response rate is better with the use of tablet. Unfortunately, the relapse rate is high when drugs are discontinued.

It is also available in the form of a nasal spray pump, which is convenient to use and is given in the dose of 10 µg/0.1 mL spray (1 spray per nostril) given at nighttime and dose can be increased up to 40 µg. The use of nasal spray can be affected by stuffy nose from cold/allergies. Sublingual tablets are superior to nasal sprays and are used more frequently. This is because nasal sprays have a risk of not being absorbed properly and need to be used frequently, which can lead to a risk of hyponatremia and may result in seizures. Fluid intake should be restricted to 250 mL. If the child responds (60–70% cases), then the drug may be continued for 3–6 months, and after that, it may be stopped without tapering. The drug may also be stopped if the child does not regain control after 4 weeks of therapy. Usually, the drug is well tolerated but sometimes, it may cause hyponatremia and rarely seizures.

Tricyclic antidepressants (Imipramine) are not used routinely. They are preferred in adolescent boys with ADHD and persistent nocturnal enuresis. For children aged 6–12 years, starting dose is 10 mg and after 1–2 weeks, it is gradually increased up to a maximum of 50 mg/day. For 12–18 years, it is started at the dose of 10 mg and after 1–2 weeks, it is increased, the maximum dose being 75 mg/day.

Anticholinergic drugs such as Oxybutynin improve bladder capacity by decreasing uninhibited bladder contractions and decreasing detrusor muscle tone as well as urgency and frequency. Oxybutynin is given above 6 years of age in the dose of 5 mg/day at bedtime. Better response can be there if it is combined with desmopressin.[19] End goals of therapy include reduction in frequency of wet nights, staying dry on specific occasions (such as sleepovers, night camps), positive impact on child and family and lack of recurrences.

ENCOPRESIS

DEFINITION

According to the DSM-5, these are the four features out of the following that must be present to support the diagnosis of encopresis:[20]

1. Repeated passage of feces into inappropriate places (e.g., clothing, floor), whether involuntary or intentional.
2. At least one such event occurs each month for at least 3 months.
3. Chronological age is at least 4 years (or equivalent developmental level).
4. The behavior is not attributable to the physiological effects of a substance (e.g., laxatives) or another medical condition, except through a mechanism involving constipation.
5. *Specify* whether:
   a. *With constipation and overflow incontinence:* There is evidence of constipation on physical examination or by history.
   b. *Without constipation and overflow incontinence:* There is no evidence of constipation on physical examination or by history.

CLASSIFICATION

Encopresis may be classified in two ways. It could be constipation-associated encopresis or overflow encopresis. Like enuresis, it may be primary (when continence has never been attained) or secondary (when incontinence returns after a period of normal continence).

Causes:[21]
- Constipation (psychological, poor training, thyroid disorders, etc.)
- Anorectal disorders, e.g., fissure-in-ano, anal excoriations, hemorrhoids
- Postsurgical Hirschsprung disease
- Spinal cord disorders such as spinal trauma, tumor
- Cerebral palsy
- Myopathies affecting pelvic floor or anal sphincter.

PATHOPHYSIOLOGY

Exact pathophysiology is not known, however, persistent constipation leads to hardening of feces in the rectosigmoid colon and ultimately feces leak between the solid mass and rectal wall. Depending on the severity, it may be diurnal or nocturnal.

RISK FACTORS

The various risk factors or factors precipitating the disease are:
- *Poor socioeconomic status:* Absence of toilet in house, dirty toilets, etc.
- Living in war-affected areas
- *Psychological factors:* Bullying at school, anxiety, depression, poor scholastic performance, disruptive behavior
- Hospitalization of child for another illness, especially if affecting mobility

EVALUATION

- *History:* Ask for age of onset, find out whether primary or secondary encopresis, toilet habits, toilet training, pain in defecation, whether stool mixed with blood (fresh/altered), frequency and time of leak (day/night). Also enquire about family issues (parental disharmony), presence or absence of toilet in house, psychological issues, death of a close relative, etc.
- *Physical examination:* Per abdominal examination should be done to look for fecoliths. Perianal area should be seen for anal excoriations, etc., and PR examination to rule out anorectal anomalies (piles, fissure, tone of anal sphincter, rectum empty or loaded, etc.).
- *Lumbosacral area* must be examined for spinal deformities.

INVESTIGATIONS

No specific test is available to diagnose the disease. However, following tests may be done:
- *X-ray abdomen:* To look for abdominal gas shadows
- *USG abdomen:* Especially look for any tumor, fecoliths, organomegaly, etc.
- *Ba-meal/enema:* Useful in diagnosing Hirschsprung disease
- *Anorectal manometry:* Sphincters loose tone in Hirschsprung disease

TREATMENT

- *Bowel cleaning:* Since the constipation is the main cause, every effort must be done to clear the gut. Hard stools or loaded colon must be evacuated by enemas or drugs such as polyethylene glycol (PEG) in a dose of 1.5 g/kg/day orally. One can also use Lactulose (1–3 mL/kg/day). Mineral oils and irritant laxatives (e.g., Senna and Bisacodyl) should be avoided, especially in infants. Suppositories may also be used, especially in infants.[22] Drug may be given for long periods to prevent re-impaction. High-fiber diet is also helpful to avoid constipation.
- *Psychotherapy* should be given when the cause is anxiety/depression or other psycho disorders.
- *Toilet training:* Child should be motivated to try to pass the stool. He should not be punished rather be rewarded when he/she cooperates.

CONCLUSION

Enuresis may be primary or secondary, physiological, or associated with organic disorders, and here comes the role of the healthcare provider to evaluate the condition, establish a cause, and rectify it accordingly. As the condition leads to low self-esteem in the child as well as worrisome for the parents, gentle reassurance and empathy from the pediatrician have a big role to play in the management.

REFERENCES

1. Warzak WJ. Psychosocial implications of nocturnal enuresis. Clin Pediatr (Phila). 1993;Spec No:38-40.
2. Nevéus T, von Gontard A, Hoebeke P, Hjälmås K, Bauer S, Bower W, et al. The standardization of terminology of lower urinary tract function in children and adolescents: Report from the Standardisation Committee of the International Children's Continence Society. J Urol. 2006;176(1):314-24.
3. Reddy NM, Malve H, Nerli R, Venkatesh P, Agarwal I, Rege V. Nocturnal Enuresis in India: Are We Diagnosing and Managing Correctly? Indian J Nephrol. 2017;27(6):417-26.
4. Meadow SR. Day wetting. Pediatr Nephrol. 1990;4:178-84.
5. De Sousa A, Kapoor H, Jagtap J, Sen M. Prevalence and factors affecting enuresis amongst primary school children. Indian J Urol. 2007;23:354-7.
6. Srivastava S, Srivastava KL, Shingla S. Prevalence of monosymptomatic nocturnal enuresis and its correlates in school going children of Lucknow. Indian J Pediatr. 2013;80:488-91.
7. Deivasigamani TR. Psychiatric morbidity in primary school children - An epidemiological study. Indian J Psychiatry. 1990;32(3): 235-40.
8. Ramakrishnan K. Evaluation and treatment of enuresis. Am Fam Physician. 2008;78:489-96.
9. Graham KM, Levy JB. Enuresis. Pediatr Rev. 2009;30:165-72.

10. HeRittig S, Knudsen UB, Nørgaard JP, Pedersen EB, Djurhuus JC. Abnormal diurnal rhythm of plasma Vasopressin and urinary output in patients with enuresis. Am J Physiol. 1989;256:F664e71.
11. Wolfish NM, Pivik RT, Busby KA. Elevated sleep arousal thresholds in enuretic boys: Clinical implications. Acta Pædiatrica. 1997;86:381e4.
12. Neveus T. The Pathogenesis of enuresis e towards a new understanding. Int J Urol. 2017;24(3):174e82.
13. Yu B, Sun H, Ma H, Peng M, Kong F, Meng F, et al. Aberrant whole-brain functional connectivity and intelligence structure in children with primary nocturnal enuresis. PloS One. 2013;8(1):e51924.
14. Lei D, Ma J, Shen G, Tian M, Li G. Altered brain activation during response inhibition in children with primary nocturnal enuresis: an fMRI study. Hum Brain Mapp. 2011;33(12):2913e9.
15. von Gontard A, Schmelzer D, Seifen S, Pukrop R. Central nervous system involvement in nocturnal enuresis: evidence of general neuromotor delay and specific brainstem dysfunction. J Urol. 2001;166(6):2448e51.
16. Arnell H, Hjälmås K, Jägervall M, Läckgren G, Stenberg A, Bengtsson B, et al. The genetics of primary nocturnal enuresis: inheritance and suggestion of a second major gene on chromosome 12q. J Med Genet. 1997;34(5):360-5.
17. Von Gontard A. Klassifikation der Enuresis/Enkopresis im DSM-5 [Classification of enuresis/encopresis according to DSM-5]. Zeitschrift fur Kinder- und Jugendpsychiatrie und Psychotherapie. 2014;42(2):109-13.
18. Neveus T, Fonseca E, Franco I, Kawauchi A, Kovacevic L, Nieuwhof-Leppink, et al. Management and treatment of nocturnal enuresis: an updated standardization document from the International Children's Continence Society. J Pediatr Urol. 2020;16(1):10-9.
19. Emily KR, DeMaso DR. Enuresis and Encopresis. In: Kleigman RM, Stanton RMD, St. Geme J, Schor NF, Behrman RE (Eds). Nelson Textbook of Paediatrics, 19th edition. US: Elsevier Publications; 2019. pp. 71-4.
20. American Psychiatric Association. Diagnostic and statistical manual of mental disorders, 5th edition. Arlington, VA: American Psychiatric Publishing, 2013.
21. Olaru C, Diaconescu S, Trandafir L, Gimiga N, Olaru RA, Stefanescu, et al. Chronic Functional Constipation and Encopresis in Children in Relationship with the Psychosocial Environment. Gastroenterol Res Pract. 2016;2016:7828576.
22. Bagga A, Sinha A, Shrivastava RN. Disorders of kidney and urinary tract. In: Vinod K Paul, Arvind Bagga (Eds). Ghai Essential Pediatrics, 9th edition. New Delhi, CBS Publishers and Distributors Pvt Ltd; 2019. pp. 279-80.

Chapter 23: Gratification Disorder in Children

Pankaj Agrawal

INTRODUCTION

Gratification or masturbatory behavior is very common and normal and benign phenomena in life of children. Lifetime prevalence of masturbatory behavior ranges between 90 and 94% in males and 50 and 60% in females. Discomfort and disability due to excess gratification behavior is known as gratification disorder, and it is rarely seen in young children. It is often misdiagnosed as a seizure or movement disorder resulting in unnecessary investigations and treatment. Although there are limited studies and literature available about these disorders, but we have tried to highlight the differentiating features between gratification disorders and seizure disorders.

Masturbatory or gratification behavior occurs as a normal part of psychosexual behavior and development. Although rarely seen in children, but excessive indulgence in masturbation resulting in discomfort and impairment, is referred to as a "gratification disorder." This condition is alternatively termed "benign idiopathic infantile dyskinesia" and it may present as different behavior patterns. These disorders have a tendency to form habit and comprise a group of self-stimulatory behaviors.[1]

EPIDEMIOLOGY

This phenomenon has been documented in approximately 90–94% of males and 50–60% of females at various points in their lifetimes. Onset typically occurs between 3 months and 3 years of age, with a second peak in incidence observed during adolescence.

Masturbatory activity in infants and young children is difficult to recognize because it often does not involve manual stimulation of the genitalia at all. It is often misinterpreted as epilepsy, abdominal pain, paroxysmal dystonia, or dyskinesia by a general pediatrician.[2]

ETIOLOGY AND PREDISPOSING FACTORS

The precise mechanism behind infantile masturbation remains inadequately comprehended, although it has been linked to factors such as self-soothing, monotony, heightened arousal, genital infections, and insufficient stimulation. There is an established connection between childhood gratification behavior and potential factors such as sexual abuse, genital irritation, family-related stress, emotional neglect, and absence of breastfeeding.[3]

RELATION OF SCREEN TIME AND GRATIFICATION DISORDERS

Excessive and prolonged media exposure can indeed have an impact on the brain and behavior. When individuals are constantly exposed to stimulating media, such as television, video games, or social media, the brain can become accustomed to a high level of sensory input and stimulation. The constant stimulation from media activates reward pathways in the brain, releasing neurotransmitters such as dopamine, which is associated with pleasure and motivation. When media exposure is abruptly reduced or discontinued, the brain may experience a decrease in dopamine levels, leading to feelings of restlessness, irritability, and dissatisfaction. To compensate for the loss of the stimulatory brain activity, individuals may engage in gratification behaviors. Case has been reported about association of sudden withdrawal of media exposure (web streaming) with gratification behavior in child.[4]

CLINICAL FEATURES

Some of the typical clinical features are as follows:[5]
- Beginning between 3 months and 3 years of age
- Consisting of repetitive episodes of varying durations
- Accompanied by vocalizations often characterized by quiet grunting

- Accompanied by facial flushing and sweating
- Involving pressure on the perineum and distinctive lower-extremity posturing
- Not leading to any changes in consciousness
- Coming to a halt upon distraction
- Yielding normal examination results and laboratory studies. Sometimes, on clinical examination, perineal irritation may be found due to recurrent and daily friction.

This clinical presentation often poses the risk of being misdiagnosed as seizures, paroxysmal nonepileptic movement disorders, or abdominal colic. Therefore, it necessitates a thorough physical and neurological assessment, including but not limited to magnetic resonance imaging, electroencephalogram (EEG), intravenous pyelography, small bowel biopsy, and gastrointestinal barium swallow, to arrive at an accurate diagnosis.

DISTINCTION BETWEEN SEIZURE AND GRATIFICATION DISORDER

Children displaying gratification disorder often exhibit an altered state of consciousness characterized by a distant, unfocused gaze. Importantly, this condition can be distinguished from seizures by its voluntary nature, as it can be interrupted through distraction. When interrupted, children may express irritation. Furthermore, it is worth noting that torsional postures and rocking motions are not typical features of seizures in this context. Misdiagnosis becomes more likely when there is no direct genital stimulation with the hands and the behavior primarily involves repeated thigh adduction. Additionally, when parents describe their child during the episode as having a fixed gaze, trembling, and exhibiting twitching or movement in one or more limbs for an extended period, the potential for misdiagnosis increases. Differentiation between gratification disorders and seizure disorder has been shown in **Table 1**.

DIAGNOSIS

Meticulous history-taking and careful evaluation of video clips in presence of parents are the key to diagnosis of childhood gratification disorders. Clinician should make a habit to request the parent make a video recording of neurological events. Sometimes, it can be diagnosed by direct observation of the act. Unnecessary investigations should be avoided.

One of the most important symptoms is that the child may be stopped during gratification if distracted and also shows anger and annoyance when interrupted.

MANAGEMENT

Behavioral Therapy[7]

It is the mainstay of treatment in gratification disorders. It involves counseling and psychoeducation of both, parent and child.

TABLE 1: Distinctive features between seizures and gratification disorders.[6]

Clinical features	Seizure disorder	Gratification disorder
Age of onset and remission	Variable/Any age	Onset at 2–3 months and usually remits before 3 years
Onset	May initiate with aura	No aura
Association with sleep	More often in sleep	Never in sleep
Symptoms/features	Tonic, rhythmic clonic, or myoclonic motor phenomena, may have facial twitching	Facial flushing, grunting, diaphoresis, pressure on the perineum with posturing and rubbing of the lower limbs
Loss of consciousness	More often	Never
Cyanosis	May be present	Never
Duration	Few minutes	Usually long (up to 30 minutes)
Termination	Cannot be terminated by distraction	Can be terminated by interruption
Postevent	Postictal confusion, weakness, aphasia, or headache	Looks exhausted or falls asleep
Physical examination and EEG	Can be abnormal	Always normal

(EEG: electroencephalogram)

- *Psychoeducation and normalization*: Typically, the approach to addressing this issue involves counseling parents and providing them with education to help them recognize that it is a normal behavior in children and is not harmful. Parents are guided to understand that scolding, shaming, or threatening the child could inadvertently reinforce this behavior and lead to low self-esteem. Instead, they are encouraged to have gentle conversations with their child, emphasizing the importance of avoiding such behaviors, especially in public settings, and gradually, even in private.
- *Distraction techniques:* Parents are encouraged to explore alternative playful activities that can redirect their child's attention away from masturbatory behaviors.
- *Session with child:* Distraction activities and activity schedule of child can be remodeled according to their interests. Children who are able to express themselves, can be allowed to acknowledge, validate, universalize, and empathize with their concerns.
- *Sex education:* Older children can be informed about the harmless nature of masturbation but should be advised the importance of maintaining privacy when it comes to masturbation, emphasizing that engaging in such activities in public is considered inappropriate behavior.

Pharmacological Treatment

When cases of gratification disorder do not respond to behavioral management strategies, healthcare professionals may recommend the use of different psychopharmacological agents. These may include selective serotonin reuptake inhibitors (such as escitalopram) and antipsychotic medications (like risperidone and aripiprazole). It has been reported that the mechanism of action of these medications involves reduction in dopamine levels in the mesolimbic system, achieved through their effects on D2 and 5-HT2 receptors.

Escitalopram[7]

Utilizing escitalopram has displayed encouraging outcomes in the treatment of gratification disorders, particularly in individuals with autistic disorder who exhibit excessive masturbation behavior. The ability of escitalopram to potentially address the compulsive and repetitive behaviors linked to gratification disorders positions; it is a viable therapeutic choice for healthcare professionals managing these conditions. Nevertheless, additional research and controlled studies are required to gain a more comprehensive understanding of the long-term effectiveness and safety of escitalopram within this specific context.

Dose: Starting dose of 5 mg/day and titrated to 10 mg/day during the second week.

Aripiprazole[8]

Studies have shown that aripiprazole may help in managing impulsivity and associated behavioral issues. In some cases, children with obsessive compulsive disorder (OCD) may engage in compulsive behaviors, and gratification could be one of those repetitive behaviors.

One of the distinguishing features of aripiprazole is its ability to act as both an agonist and an antagonist at the D_2 dopamine receptors, depending on the dopamine levels in the brain. When dopamine levels are high, aripiprazole acts as a D_2 receptor antagonist, helping to reduce the excessive dopamine activity and alleviate symptoms of psychosis, such as hallucinations and delusions.

Conversely, in situations where dopamine levels are low, aripiprazole acts as a D_2 receptor agonist, stimulating the receptors to increase dopamine activity and help maintain a balanced dopaminergic system. The partial agonistic effect on dopamine receptors and serotonin 1A receptors likely plays a role in modulating impulsive behaviors by affecting neurotransmitter activity in the brain.

- *Dose:* Initial dose—2 mg orally once a day
- *Dose titration:* Increase dose to 5 mg orally once a day, with subsequent increases to 10 mg or 15 mg orally once a day if needed

SUMMARY AND CONCLUSION

Gratification disorder can be found in children and it is not pathological. Sometimes, clinician may misdiagnose it as seizure disorder leading to unnecessary diagnostic tests and initiation of anticonvulsant medicine. A careful history along with videography of the event can diagnose this behavioral disorder. Reassuring the parents and following regular behavior techniques by parents are the mainstay of the management.

REFERENCES

1. Nemati H, Ahmadabadi F, Shahisavandi M, Farjoud Kouhanjani M, Rostamihosseinkhani M. Treatment of child gratification disorder. Iran J Child Neurol. 2022;16(2):9-16.
2. Nechay A, Ross LM, Stephenson JB, O'Regan M. Gratification disorder ("infantile masturbation"): A review. Arch Dis Child. 2004;89:225-6.
3. Kellogg ND. Clinical report: The evaluation of sexual behaviours in children. Paediatrics. 2009;124:992-8.
4. Rai R, Elon N, Inamdar P, Chowdary S, Kaniti B. Gratification disorder in a toddler: perils of excess screen time. Int J Contemp Pediatr. 2022;9(3):289-91.
5. Yang ML, Fullwood E, Goldstein J, Mink JW. Masturbation in infancy and early childhood presenting as a movement disorder: 12 cases and a review of the literature. Pediatrics. 2005;116;1427-32.
6. Moktan S, Karki U, Bista I, Devkota N. Gratification disorder associated with perineal irritation in young children: management and short-term outcome. J Psychosexual Health. 2021;3(3):265-9.
7. Jan MM, Al Banji MH, Fallatah BA. Long-term outcome of infantile gratification phenomena. Can J Neurol Sci. 2013;40(3):416-9.
8. Kul M, Baykan H. A case of excessive masturbation treated with aripiprazole. Bull of Clin Psychopharmacol. 2014;24(1):93-6.

Chapter 24: Mobile Phone Addiction in Children

Srikant Sharma

INTRODUCTION

"The difference between technology and slavery is that slaves are fully aware that they are not free".
—**Nassim Nicholas Taleb**

In today's digital age, mobile phone addiction among children has emerged as a pressing concern. The widespread use of smartphones among young individuals has raised concerns about its impact on their physical and psychological wellbeing. Problematic smartphone use is defined as behavior characterized by compulsive device usage, which can lead to physical, psychological, or social harm.[1] A study conducted by the American Academy of Pediatrics found that children aged 3-5 years who had their own devices had an average daily usage of 115.3 min/day.[2] Another study by Childwise found that, on average, children spend about 3 hours and 20 minutes each day messaging, playing games, and being online.[3] According to a survey conducted by the Pew Research Center, 60% of children were exposed to smartphones before the age of 5 years. In that group, 31% had been introduced to phones before the age of 2.[4]

While several advantages are observed related to smartphone use, such as improving academic skills, reading recognition, and enriching vocabulary and expressive language, there is also a growing concern over the potential for excessive smartphone use to become problematic. Due to this concern, great efforts have been made through research to evaluate, label, and identify problematic smartphone use, mostly through the development and administration of scales assessing the behavior.[5] Currently, there is no consensus on the definition of smartphone "addiction." As a result, the term "problematic smartphone use" is widely used to characterize a pattern of inability to restrain a compulsive activity that causes functional impairment or suffering and so satisfies the requirements for behavioral addiction.[6]

EPIDEMIOLOGY

A study conducted in 31 countries found that the global prevalence of internet use disorder among 12-41-year-old was estimated at 6.0%, with the Middle East having the highest plurality.[7] Another three-decade meta-analysis found a global Internet Gaming Disorder (IGD) prevalence of 4.6% among adolescents aged 10-19 years.[8] The prevalence of cell phone addiction has varied widely across countries, as have the scales for that addiction. The prevalence of cell phone addiction in adolescents ranged from 2% in Barcelona to 89% in Turkey. In India, the prevalence of mobile phone addiction ranged from 6 to 49%.[9] Among a group of adolescents in Mumbai, a study revealed that as many as 31% of eighth, ninth, and tenth-grade students exhibited signs of cell phone dependence.

Various studies conducted worldwide have consistently indicated that adolescent females exhibit a higher level of smartphone dependence compared to their male counterparts. Moreover, these studies have also revealed that adolescent females face a greater risk of depression.[10,11] It was shown that while males spend more time playing video games, females spend more time online browsing, social networking, and online conversation.[12]

Insecure feelings, staying up late, strained parent-child interactions, strained school relationships, compulsive shopping, pathological gambling, low mood, tension and anxiety, boredom in leisure time, hyperactivity, conduct issues, and emotional symptoms are all linked to problematic phone use.

ETIOPATHOGENESIS

Risk Factors

Mobile addiction in children can result from various risk factors that encompass environmental, psychological, and social aspects. Understanding these risk factors is essential

TABLE 1: Risk factors for mobile addiction in children.		
Risk factors	**Subcategories**	**Definitions**
1. Environmental factors[13-17]	a. Parental addiction	Parents' addiction to smartphones was significantly associated with smartphone addiction in adolescents
	b. Parental neglect	Less authoritative parenting may make kids and teenagers less capable of self-control and impulse management, making them more susceptible to problematic smartphone use
	c. Domestic violence and abuse	Children who experience domestic abuse and violence are more likely to exhibit antisocial behaviors, post-traumatic stress disorder, anxiety disorders, and substance use disorders
2. Psychological factors[18-25]	a. Attachment style	Different attachment styles lead to distinct views of one self and others. Insecure attachment can serve as a predictor of possible problematic smartphone use
	b. Self-regulation	Self-regulation is linked to a person's emotional and impulse control patterns; low self-regulation may contribute to problematic behavior or substance use in adolescents
	c. Self-esteem	Self-esteem is a good indicator of people's adjustment skills and relationship satisfaction levels. Adolescents with low self-esteem have higher chances of depending on a smartphone to interact with others
	d. Checking behavior	The proclivity to check the smartphone often, even when there are no notifications, may contribute to problematic smartphone use
	e. Personality and premorbidities	Addiction is more likely in people who have high neuroticism and low or high extraversion. Premorbid disorders in social communication, such as social anxiety disorder, loneliness, or other psychosocial issues, can make a person vulnerable to excessive smartphone use
3. Social factors[4,26-28]	a. School	In the classroom, adolescents use smartphones to connect and arrange activities. In India, elementary and secondary school pupils spent an average of 2.11 hours per day on digital gadgets, with a 28.1% incidence rate of digital addiction
	b. Peer groups	Increased smartphone usage can also be attributed to a lack of peer support and a need to belong. Their compromised privacy may expose them to cyber attacks and cyber victimization

for developing effective intervention strategies. **Table 1** depicts a list of the main risk factors.

CLINICAL FEATURES AND DIAGNOSIS

Consequences of Excessive Smartphone Use

Cognitive Problems

Excessive smartphone use can result in neurological alterations, such as significantly greater levels of gamma-aminobutyric acid (GABA) in the affected individual's brain, which leads in worse attention and control as well as being more easily distracted.[29] Adolescents may become more reliant on rapid benefits connected with smartphones due to neurological immaturity, as opposed to natural and/or delayed rewards associated with interactions with friends and family members or hobbies.[30] It has been scientifically shown that smart phones influence brain development in toddlers by decreasing growth and interfering with other stimulations that the brain needed to develop, resulting in cognitive deficiencies.

Sleep Disturbances

Blue light exposure at night promotes attentiveness, which affects sleep duration and quality. Blue light inhibits the brain's release of melatonin, causing disruptions in the body's circadian rhythm and disrupted sleep patterns.[31,32] In a 2-year longitudinal research, teenagers who owned a smartphone reported lower sleep duration on weekdays and more sleep disorders than those who did not possess a smartphone.[33] Sleep disruption is a risk factor for attention and concentration issues, mental disorders, and cardiovascular disease.

Psychological

Mobile addiction, like any other type of reliance, serves as an escape route for a youngster from personal and professional difficulties. It may provide temporary relief, but it ultimately opens the door to greater loneliness, worry, and sadness. Depression has been examined as both an outcome and a risk factor or predictor variable for mobile phone addiction. A longitudinal research of 126 US adolescents found that those who used their phones more had higher depressive scores even after a year of follow-up, even when baseline depression was controlled for.[34] Excessive smartphone use may be a maladaptive coping mechanism (avoidant or emotion-based) rather than a problem-solving strategy. If a toddler is kept away from mobile devices, withdrawal symptoms such as temper tantrums and food exclusion can be quite distressing for parents. A toddler who spends too much time on his or her phone or tablet will also experience a delay in the development of social skills.

Physical Disturbances

Elevated blood pressure, obesity, low HDL (high-density lipoprotein) cholesterol, poor stress management (i.e., excessive sympathetic arousal and cortisol dysregulation), and insulin resistance were discovered to be higher in children with mobile addiction. Other physical health effects included impaired vision and decreased bone density, tendon injuries, carpal tunnel syndrome, text neck (cramping, stabbing pain caused by looking at a phone for an extended period of time with poor posture), radiation-related issues, inattention blindness, and computer vision syndrome.[35,36]

Accidents and Mishaps

Unintentional injuries, such as car accidents, pedestrian collisions, and falls, have increased as the number of smartphone users who talk, text, or listen to music while driving has increased.[37-39]

Comorbidity

Excessive smartphone use is also associated with other mental diseases such as social anxiety, depression, conduct disorder, impulsivity, loneliness, and attention deficit problems.[40] For a better outcome, a thorough evaluation of a child with smartphone addiction must entail addressing these comorbidities.

Diagnosis

As researchers and clinicians, it is crucial to employ reliable scales to accurately assess and diagnose smartphone addiction in children. **Table 2** presents a comprehensive review of five commonly used scales to measure smartphone addiction in children, along with their main constructs **(Annexures 1 and 2)**.

TABLE 2: Scales for measuring smartphone addiction in children.

Scale	Description
Smartphone Addiction Scale-Short Version (SAS-SV)[41]	It comprises a set of items that measure the extent of dependency and the negative consequences associated with smartphone use
Smart Phone Addiction Proneness Scale (SPAPS)[42]	Designed to gauge proneness to smartphone addiction, the SPAPS focuses on subjective health complaints, depression, and suicidal ideation related to smartphone use
Mobile Phone Problem Use Scale (MPPUS)[43]	MPPUS targets problematic mobile phone use, capturing behaviors that indicate excessive dependence and interference with daily life
Problematic Mobile Phone Use Scale (PMPUS)[44]	PMPUS delves into impulsive behaviors and problematic usage of mobile phones, allowing for an assessment of addictive tendencies among young users
Nomophobia Questionnaire[45]	Focusing on the fear of being without a mobile phone, it assesses the emotional dependence and anxiety associated with smartphone use

Smartphone addiction is characterized by a behavioral pattern similar to internet addiction or substance addiction; however, the symptomatology of problematic smartphone use may not be immediately observed or may differ depending on context due to the smartphone's multitude of functions. As a result, the proposed symptoms or indicators acquired from self-report questionnaires may be ineffective for detecting problematic smartphone use.[6] Because growing smartphone usage may be normal for certain groups of people, motivation and reward must be considered when identifying problematic smartphone use.[46]

Although excessive smartphone use is not currently recognized as a formal clinical disorder in the Diagnostic and Statistical Manual of Mental Disorders, Fifth Edition (DSM-5) or the International Classification of Diseases, Tenth Revision (ICD-10), many aspects of the behavior appear to resemble other recognized behavioral addictions.[47] So far, gambling disorder is the only

TABLE 3: Symptomatology of smartphone addiction.	
Characteristic	Problematic mobile use
Increased tolerance	Requires prolonged duration and increased frequency to attain satisfaction or alleviate-associated negative emotions
Preoccupied or obsessive thoughts	Experiences an intense urge to frequently check the smartphone
Persistence despite negative impact	Exhibits insomnia or sleep disturbances due to frequent smartphone checking
Difficulty in behavioral control	Demonstrates repeated, unsuccessful attempts to regulate, decrease, or cease compulsive smartphone use
Impairment in occupational, social, and daily life	Engages in withdrawal from familial or communal gatherings due to smartphone usage. Displays detrimental effects on academic, familial, social, or emotional functioning
Withdrawal symptoms	Experiencing sensations of unease, intense craving, abstinence, dependency, and irritability upon inability to access the phone. Furthermore, this condition may lead to heightened anxiety and irritability when the smartphone is not readily available

behavioral addiction recognized by the DSM-5, whereas other addictive behaviors such as "Internet gaming," "sex addiction," "exercise addiction," or "shopping addiction" are classed as impulsive disorders[48] based on DSM-5 criteria for gambling disorder and substance abuse. **Table 3** depicts the suggested symptomatology of smartphone addiction (APA, 2013).

TREATMENT

In the context of problematic smartphone use, which exhibits considerable resemblance to internet addiction, adopting treatment strategies used for internet addiction could serve as a potential approach to mitigate and address the issues associated with problematic smartphone use.[49]

Effective interventions for problematic smartphone use typically encompass five key components:[50]
1. Involuntary restriction
2. Self-awareness and self-control (which is not only the most effective strategy but also serves as a protective factor)
3. School factors
4. Peer support
5. Professional services

Addressing smartphone addiction among children involves a multifaceted approach that encompasses various interventions. The following section addresses the treatments available to children.

Cognitive Behavioral Therapy

Cognitive behavioral therapies (CBTs) are based on the cognitive behavioral model, which asserts that ideas determine feelings and that changing one's thoughts can aid in behavioral change.[51] CBT is divided into three stages:
1. The first stage is *behavior modification*, which focuses on gradually minimizing people's online time and establishing a healthy internet usage schedule.
2. The second stage involves *cognitive reconstruction and rationalizations* for excessive internet use. This stage aims to discover and counteract the causes of overuse, as well as to correct the cognitive training that motivates the individual to begin using the internet.
3. The third stage focuses on the individuals' functional issues connected to their internet use, both individually as well as professionally, in order to aid in recognizing and managing coexisting issues that may have led to the development of problematic internet use, with the goals of maintaining recovery and preventing relapse.[52]

Mindfulness

Mindfulness is a type of meditation that entails paying complete, concentrated, and active attention to an internal experience.[53] For various reasons, the mindfulness technique may be suitable for individuals with behavioral addictions:[54]
- Meditation can be used to replace addictive behaviors and lessen relapse and withdrawal symptoms.
- Compassion cultivation aids in the management of negative emotions associated with addiction.
- Changing the primary focus from the immediate reward of addictive activities to the intrinsic worth of life.
- Reduces salience
- Improves patience

Journaling Smartphone Use

In a South Korean study, participants who kept a daily log of their smartphone use at home (home-based daily journaling) had much lower levels of smartphone addiction. Concurrently, there was a significant increase in ratings expressing parents' concerns about their adolescents' smartphone activities.[55]

Parental Interventions

Promising results have emerged from studies on the use of *authoritative parenting styles*. Authoritative parents can perceive the severity of the threat (problematic smartphone use) and thus be more readily engaged in a parental mediation role.[56] The parents emphasize involuntary restrictions, i.e., boundaries, and have sensible expectations, such as setting rules to limit the amount of time spent and the type of content viewed.[57] Four core strategies are proposed for parents to use in managing children's and adolescents' problematic smartphone use: *instructive strategies, rule setting, usage checking, and content filtering*.[58] Parents should behave as role models by depicting a reduced use of mobile devices and spending more time with adolescents with healthy activities to direct them away from using smartphones excessively.[59,60]

Family Therapy

Family therapy can play a crucial role in the treatment of smartphone addiction in children, as it addresses not only the individual's addictive behaviors, but also the family dynamics that may contribute to or perpetuate the addiction. Through family therapy, parents and caregivers can gain a deeper understanding of their child's smartphone usage patterns and their impact on their wellbeing. Family therapy interventions can foster open communication, set healthy boundaries, and promote collective efforts to establish healthier screen time habits for the child.[61]

School Policy

Educational institutions also play an essential role in monitoring or prohibiting the usage of cellphones in the classroom. School officials and teachers should create awareness among students about the negative implications of problematic smartphone use and educate them on healthy activities and how to be regulated regarding smartphone use. The emphasis should not be on the negative repercussions, but rather on guiding pupils to be clever users who optimize its functionality, bringing positive learning outcomes into everyday life.[62]

Exercise Rehabilitation

Rehabilitation helps individuals recover from musculoskeletal conditions such as carpal tunnel syndrome, stick neck, backache, poor posture, chronic pain, fatigue, and neurological or metabolic conditions. Exercise rehabilitation has also been proven to enhance mental resilience by increasing confidence and happiness, which aids in the recovery of anxiety and depression.

Intervention Applications

Intervention applications (apps) can be valuable tools in reducing smartphone use and addressing problematic behaviors. These apps are designed to promote awareness and self-regulation by providing real-time feedback, setting usage limits, and offering behavioral interventions. They often include features such as screen time tracking, app usage monitoring, and personalized goal setting to help individuals manage their smartphone usage more effectively. Various smartphone overuse intervention apps like AppDetox and NUGU (No Use is Good Use) have been researched and found to be useful.[63]

Psychopharmacological Treatment

Psychopharmacological treatment typically involves medications that target neurotransmitter systems in the brain to address various psychological and behavioral issues. This approach is meant to address comorbidities such as depression, anxiety disorders, attention-deficit hyperactivity disorder (ADHD), substance abuse, and sleep disorders.

PREVENTION

In the digital age, where smartphones have become an integral part of daily life, it is essential to proactively implement preventive measures to curb the risk of smartphone addiction among children. Early intervention and awareness can significantly reduce the likelihood of developing problematic usage habits.

Self-regulation

Self-regulation refers to the ability to govern one's own desires or actions and to adapt to one's surroundings in order to achieve one's personal goals.[64] People who are more capable of controlling their thoughts, emotions, and impulses may be far more unlikely to develop smartphone addiction.[65]

Role of Parents

A more positive parenting style has been linked to better self-regulation.[14] Young people who have had more authoritative parenting styles, e.g., have more solid bonds and develop higher trust and a sense of authority in their relationships with others.

Regarding managing a toddler's mobile dependence, the treating pediatrician should advise parents to:
- Spend more time with their child
- Increase outdoor activities
- Keep phone and gadgets out of reach
- Play audio of rhymes than video
- Being a role model by decreasing their own screen time

Good Peer Relationships and Social Support

According to research, there is an inverse link between friend relationships and social avoidance.[66] Adolescents who are more engaged with their friends and at school are more likely to face fewer prejudices and greater acceptance, which encourages positive thoughts and emotions, which may help buffer psychological issues such as anxiety and depression, as well as higher self-esteem, that promotes healthy identity development.[67]

Comorbidities

Addressing comorbidities such as ADHD, depression, conduct disorder, and anxiety disorders with the help and guidance of mental health experts could play a major role in preventing mobile addiction in childhood.[8]

CONCLUSION

Adolescents commonly exhibit a propensity for risk-taking, novelty-seeking, and social interaction to foster independence during maturation.[68] These behaviors may intensify in response to life stressors or brain structural changes.[69] Given the mobile phone's capacity to provide diverse and intense stimulation, adolescents may be particularly vulnerable to problematic smartphone use. However, excessive reliance on mobile phones can diminish resilience and give rise to challenges across various life domains, warranting the inclusion of mobile addiction in the international classification system. The development of culturally appropriate screening tools can benefit from such inclusion. Effective interventions addressing physical, psychological, legal, and ethical concerns imperative, with parental influence, peer relationships, and the school environment serve as both risk factors and potential treatment modalities. A comprehensive approach encompassing biological, psychological, and social aspects of adolescents' lives is advocated for optimal management, involving collaboration between pediatricians and psychiatrists.

REFERENCES

1. Horwood S, Anglim J. Personality and problematic smartphone use: A facet-level analysis using the Five Factor Model and HEXACO frameworks. Comput Human Behav. 2018;85:349-59.
2. Radesky JS, Weeks HM, Ball R, Schaller A, Yeo S, Durnez J, et al. Young Children's use of smartphones and tablets. Pediatrics. 2020;146(1):1-8.
3. ChildWise. (2020) Childhood 2020: new independent report. [online] Available from www.childwise.co.uk. [Last accessed October, 2023].
4. Auxier BYB, Anderson M, Perrin A, Turner E. Parenting children in the age of screens. Pew Res Cent [Internet]. 2020;1-28.
5. Bottaro BA. (2022). Phone addiction : What you need to know [Internet]. [online] Available from: https://www.verywellhealth.com/phone-addiction-5218743. [Last accessed October, 2023].
6. Kardefelt-Winther D, Heeren A, Schimmenti A, Van Rooij A, Maurage P, Carras M, et al. How can we conceptualize behavioural addiction without pathologizing common behaviours? Addiction. 2017;112(10):1709-15.
7. Lindenberg K, Halasy K, Szász-Janocha C, Wartberg L. A phenotype classification of internet use disorder in a large-scale high-school study. Int J Environ Res Public Health [Internet]. 2018;15(4).
8. Ding K, Li H. Digital addiction intervention for children and adolescents: a scoping review. Int J Environ Res Public Health [Internet]. 2023;20(6).
9. Field T. Cell Phone Addiction in adolescents: A narrative review. Open Access J Addict Psychol. 2020;3(4).
10. Sahu M, Gandhi S, Sharma MK. Mobile phone addiction among children and adolescents: A systematic review. J Addict Nurs. 2019;30(4):261-8.
11. Yang S-Y, Lin C-Y, Huang Y-C, Chang J-H. Gender differences in the association of smartphone use with the vitality and mental health of adolescent students. J Am Coll Health. 2018;66(7):693-701.
12. Nishida T, Tamura H, Sakakibara H. The association of smartphone use and depression in Japanese adolescents. Psychiatry Res. 2019;273:523-7.
13. Kim H-J, Min J-Y, Min K-B, Lee T-J, Yoo S. Relationship among family environment, self-control, friendship quality, and adolescents' smartphone addiction in South Korea: Findings from nationwide data. PLoS One [Internet]. 2018;13(2):1-13.
14. Bae SM. The relationships between perceived parenting style, learning motivation, friendship satisfaction, and the addictive use of smartphones with elementary school students of South Korea: Using multivariate latent growth modeling. Sch Psychol Int. 2015;36(5):513-31.

15. Lian L, You X, Huang J, Yang R. Who overuses smartphones? Roles of virtues and parenting style in smartphone addiction among Chinese college students. Comput Human Behav. 2016;65:92-9.
16. Cao Y, Li L, Zhao X, Zhang Y, Guo X, Zhang Y, et al. Effects of exposure to domestic physical violence on children's behavior: A Chinese community-based sample. J Child Adolesc Trauma. 2016;9:127-35.
17. Steinberg L. Youth violence: Do parents and families make a difference?. Natl Inst Justice J. 2000;243:31-8.
18. Ching KH, Tak LM. The structural model in parenting style, attachment style, self-regulation and self-esteem for smartphone addiction. IAFOR J Psychol Behav Sci. 2017;3(1):85-103.
19. Huis EMJ, Vingerhoets AJJM, Denollet J, others. Attachment style and self-esteem: The mediating role of Type D personality. Pers Individ Dif. 2011;50(7):1099-103.
20. Moilanen KL. The adolescent self-regulatory inventory: The development and validation of a questionnaire of short-term and long-term self-regulation. J Youth Adolesc. 2007;36:835-48.
21. Sanders MR, Mazzucchelli TG. The promotion of self-regulation through parenting interventions. Clin Child Fam Psychol Rev. 2013;16:1-17.
22. Li C, Liu D, Dong Y. Self-esteem and problematic smartphone use among adolescents: A moderated mediation model of depression and interpersonal trust. Front Psychol. 2019;10:2872.
23. Gao Q, Fu E, Xiang Y, Jia G, Wu S. Self-esteem and addictive smartphone use: The mediator role of anxiety and the moderator role of self-control. Child Youth Serv Rev. 2021;124:105990.
24. Oulasvirta A, Rattenbury T, Ma L, Raita E. Habits make smartphone use more pervasive. Pers Ubiquitous Comput. 2012;16:105-14.
25. Enez Darcin A, Kose S, Noyan CO, Nurmedov S, Yilmaz O, Dilbaz N. Smartphone addiction and its relationship with social anxiety and loneliness. Behav Inf Technol. 2016;35(7):520-5.
26. Gökçearslan S, Mumcu FK, Hacslaman T, Çevik YD. Modelling smartphone addiction: The role of smartphone usage, self-regulation, general self-efficacy and cyberloafing in university students. Comput Human Behav. 2016;63:639-49.
27. Ouyang M, Cai X, Yin Y, Zeng P, Chen Y, Wang X, et al. Student-student relationship and adolescent problematic smartphone use: the mediating role of materialism and the moderating role of narcissism. Child Youth Serv Rev. 2020;110:104766.
28. Herrero J, Urueña A, Torres A, Hidalgo A. Socially connected but still isolated: Smartphone addiction decreases social support over time. Soc Sci Comput Rev. 2019;37(1):73-88.
29. Seo HS, Jeong E-K, Choi S, Kwon Y, Park H-J, Kim I. Changes of Neurotransmitters in Youth with Internet and Smartphone Addiction: A Comparison with Healthy Controls and Changes after Cognitive Behavioral Therapy. AJNR Am J Neuroradiol. 2020;41(7):1293-301.
30. Chen J, Liang Y, Mai C, Zhong X, Qu C. General deficit in inhibitory control of excessive smartphone users: Evidence from an event-related potential study. Front Psychol. 2016;7:511.
31. Demirci K, Akgönül M, Akpinar A. Relationship of smartphone use severity with sleep quality, depression, and anxiety in university students. J Behav Addict. 2015;4(2):85-92.
32. Randler C, Wolfgang L, Matt K, Demirhan E, Horzum MB, Beşoluk S. Smartphone addiction proneness in relation to sleep and morningness—eveningness in German adolescents. J Behav Addict. 2016;5(3):465-73.
33. Schweizer A, Berchtold A, Barrense-Dias Y, Akre C, Suris J-C. Adolescents with a smartphone sleep less than their peers. Eur J Pediatr. 2017;176:131-6.
34. Sansone RA, Sansone LA. Cell phones: the psychosocial risks. Innov Clin Neurosci. 2013;10(1):33.
35. Berolo S, Wells RP, Amick III BC. Musculoskeletal symptoms among mobile hand-held device users and their relationship to device use: A preliminary study in a Canadian university population. Appl Ergon. 2011;42(2):371-8.
36. Park JS, Choi MJ, Ma JE, Moon JH, Moon HJ. Influence of cellular phone videos and games on dry eye syndrome in university students. J Korean Acad Community Heal Nurs. 2014;25(1):12-23.
37. Kong X, Xiong S, Zhu Z, Zheng S, Long G. Development of a conceptual framework for improving safety for pedestrians using smartphones while walking: Challenges and research needs. Procedia Manuf. 2015;3:3636-43.
38. Shabeer HA, Wahidabanu RSD. Averting mobile phone use while driving and technique to locate the mobile phone used vehicle. Procedia Eng. 2012;30:623-30.
39. Walsh SP, White KM, Hyde MK, Watson B. Dialling and driving: Factors influencing intentions to use a mobile phone while driving. Accid Anal Prev. 2008;40(6):1893-900.
40. Elhai JD, Dvorak RD, Levine JC, Hall BJ. Problematic smartphone use: A conceptual overview and systematic review of relations with anxiety and depression psychopathology. J Affect Disord. 2017;207:251-9.
41. Kwon M, Kim D-J, Cho H, Yang S. The smartphone addiction scale: development and validation of a short version for adolescents. PLoS One. 2013;8(12):e83558.
42. Kim D, Lee Y, Lee J, Nam JK, Chung Y. Development of Korean smartphone addiction proneness scale for youth. PLoS One [Internet]. 2014;9(5):1-8.
43. Bianchi A, Phillips JG. Psychological predictors of problem mobile phone use. Cyberpsychol Behav.. 2005;8(1):39-51.
44. Billieux J, der Linden M, Rochat L. The role of impulsivity in actual and problematic use of the mobile phone. Appl Cogn Psychol. 2008;22(9):1195-210.

45. Yildirim C, Correia A-P. Exploring the dimensions of nomophobia: Development and validation of a self-reported questionnaire. Comput Human Behav. 2015;49:130-7.
46. Panova T, Carbonell X. Is smartphone addiction really an addiction? J Behav Addict. 2018;7(2):252-9.
47. Rennert L, Denis C, Peer K, Lynch KG, Gelernter J, Kranzler HR. DSM-5 gambling disorder: prevalence and characteristics in a substance use disorder sample. Exp Clin Psychopharmacol. 2014;22(1):50.
48. America Psychiatric Association. What is gambling disorder and it effect. 2021;1-5.
49. Liu H, Soh KG, Samsudin S, Rattanakoses W, Qi F. Effects of exercise and psychological interventions on smartphone addiction among university students: A systematic review. Front Psychol [Internet]. 2022;13.
50. Kent S, Masterson C, Ali R, Parsons CE, Bewick BM. Digital intervention for problematic smartphone use. Int J Environ Res Public Health. 2021;18(24).
51. Chun J, Shim H, Kim S. A meta-analysis of treatment interventions for internet addiction among Korean adolescents. Cyberpsychology Behav Soc Netw. 2017;20(4):225-31.
52. Young KS. CBT-IA: The first treatment model for internet addiction. J Cogn Psychother. 2011;25(4):304-12.
53. Shonin E, Van Gordon W, Griffiths MD. Mindfulness as a treatment for behavioural addiction. J Addict Res Ther. 2014;5(1).
54. Van Gordon W, Shonin E, Garcia-Campayo J. Are there adverse effects associated with mindfulness? Aust N Z J Psychiatry. 2017;51(10):977-9.
55. Lee H, Seo MJ, Choi TY. The effect of home-based daily journal writing in Korean adolescents with smartphone addiction. J Korean Med Sci. 2016;31(5):764-9.
56. Hwang Y, Choi I, Yum J-Y, Jeong S-H. Parental mediation regarding children's smartphone use: Role of protection motivation and parenting style. Cyberpsychology Behav Soc Netw. 2017;20(6):362-8.
57. Chun J-W, Choi J, Kim J-Y, Cho H, Ahn K-J, Nam J-H, et al. Altered brain activity and the effect of personality traits in excessive smartphone use during facial emotion processing. Sci Rep. 2017;7(1):12156.
58. Lee EJ, Ogbolu Y. Does parental control work with smartphone addiction?: A cross-sectional study of children in South Korea. J Addict Nurs. 2018;29(2):128-38.
59. Cheever NA, Moreno MA, Rosen LD. When does internet and smartphone use become a problem? Technol Adolesc Ment Heal. 2018;121-31.
60. Terras MM, Ramsay J. Family digital literacy practices and children's mobile phone use. Front Psychol. 2016;7:1957.
61. Kwak JY, Kim JY, Yoon YW. Effect of parental neglect on smartphone addiction in adolescents in South Korea. Child Abus Negl. 2018;77:75-84.
62. Mahapatra S. Smartphone addiction and associated consequences: Role of loneliness and self-regulation. Behav Inf Technol. 2019;38(8):833-44.
63. Löchtefeld M, Böhmer M, Ganev L. AppDetox: helping users with mobile app addiction. In: Proceedings of the 12th international conference on mobile and ubiquitous multimedia; 2013. pp. 1-2.
64. Forgas JP, Baumeister RF, Tice DM. The psychology of self-regulation: An introductory review. Psychol self-regulation Cogn Affect Motiv Process. 2009;11:1-17.
65. De Ridder DTD, Lensvelt-Mulders G, Finkenauer C, Stok FM, Baumeister RF. Taking stock of self-control: A meta-analysis of how trait self-control relates to a wide range of behaviors. Personal Soc Psychol Rev. 2012;16(1):76-99.
66. Chen C, Shen Y, Lv S, Wang B, Zhu Y. The relationship between self-esteem and mobile phone addiction among college students: The chain mediating effects of social avoidance and peer relationships. Front Psychol. 2023;14:1137220.
67. Xiang Z, Tan S, Kang Q, Zhang B, Zhu L. Longitudinal effects of examination stress on psychological well-being and a possible mediating role of self-esteem in Chinese high school students. J Happiness Stud. 2019;20:283-305.
68. Kelley A, Schochet T, Landry C. Risk Taking and Novelty Seeking in Adolescence: Introduction to Part I. Ann N Y Acad Sci. 2004;1021:27-32.
69. Crews F, He J, Hodge C. Adolescent cortical development: a critical period of vulnerability for addiction. Pharmacol Biochem Behav. 2007;86(2):189-99.

Annexure 1
Nomophobia Questionnaire (NMP-Q)

Please indicate how much you agree or disagree with each statement in relation to your smartphone?

Strongly disagree   *Strongly agree*

1   2   3   4   5   6   7

1. I would feel uncomfortable without constant access to information through my smartphone.
2. I would be annoyed if I could not look information up on my smartphone when I wanted to do so.
3. Being unable to get the news (e.g., happenings, weather) on my smartphone would make me nervous.
4. I would be annoyed if I could not use my smartphone and/or its capabilities when I wanted to do so.
5. Running out of battery in my smartphone would scare me.
6. If I were to run out of credits or hit my monthly data limit, I would panic.
7. If I did not have a data signal or could not connect to Wi-Fi, then I would constantly check to see if I had a signal or could find a Wi-Fi network.
8. If I could not use my smartphone, I would be afraid of getting stranded somewhere.
9. If I could not check my smartphone for a while, I would feel a desire to check it.
10. If I did not have my smartphone with me, I would feel anxious because I could not instantly communicate with my family and/or friends.
11. If I did not have my smartphone with me, I would be worried because my family and/or friends could not reach me.
12. If I did not have my smartphone with me, I would feel nervous because I would not be able to receive text messages and calls.
13. If I did not have my smartphone with me, I would be anxious because I could not keep in touch with my family and/or friends.
14. If I did not have my smartphone with me, I would be nervous because I could not know if someone had tried to get a hold of me.
15. If I did not have my smartphone with me, I would feel anxious because my constant connection to my family and friends would be broken.
16. If I did not have my smartphone with me, I would be nervous because I would be disconnected from my online identity.
17. If I did not have my smartphone with me, I would be uncomfortable because I could not stay up-to-date with social media and online networks.
18. If I did not have my smartphone with me, I would feel awkward because I could not check my notifications for updates from my connections and online networks.
19. If I did not have my smartphone with me, I would feel anxious because I could not check my email messages.
20. If I did not have my smartphone with me, I would feel weird because I would not know what to do.

Scoring

Sum up your responses to each item. Higher scores indicate more severe levels of nomophobia. Refer to the following table to determine your nomophobia level.

Score	Nomophobia level
NMP-Q Score = 20	Absent
21 ≤ NMP-Q Score < 60	Mild
60 ≤ NMP-Q Score < 100	Moderate
100 ≤ NMP-Q Score ≤ 140	Severe

Citation

Yildirim C, Correia AP. Exploring the dimensions of nomophobia: Development and validation of a self-reported questionnaire. Computers in Hum Behav. 2015;49:130-7.

Annexure 2
English Version of Smartphone Addiction Scale-Short Version (SAS-SV)

Items		Strongly disagree	Disagree	Weakly disagree	Weakly agree	Agree	Strongly agree
1.	Missing planned work due to smartphone use	1	2	3	4	5	6
2.	Having a hard time concentrating in class, while doing assignments, or while working due to smartphone use	1	2	3	4	5	6
3.	Feeling pain in the wrists or at the back of the neck while using a smartphone	1	2	3	4	5	6
4.	Won't be able to stand not having a smartphone	1	2	3	4	5	6
5.	Feeling impatient and fretful when I am not holding my smartphone	1	2	3	4	5	6
6.	Having my smartphone in my mind even when I am not using it	1	2	3	4	5	6
7.	I will never give up using my smartphone even when my daily life is already greatly affected by it	1	2	3	4	5	6
8.	Constantly checking my smartphone so as not to miss conversations between other people on Twitter or Facebook	1	2	3	4	5	6
9.	Using my smartphone longer than I had intended	1	2	3	4	5	6
10.	The people around me tell me that I use my smartphone too much	1	2	3	4	5	6

Chapter 25

Teenage and Adolescent Behavioral Issues

Piyali Bhattacharya

INTRODUCTION

Adolescence is a time for developing independence and is characterized by intense emotional and behavioral turbulence. Typically, adolescents exercise their independence by questioning or challenging, and sometimes breaking rules. Young people tend to get involved in offending, substance abuse, and truancy and are at risk of developing a constant pattern of problem behavior. Parents and doctors need to distinguish behaviors expected at this age from a pattern of misbehavior that requires further intervention; e.g., regular drinking, frequent episodes of fighting, absenteeism from school/truancy, and theft are much more significant than isolated episodes of the same activities.

DEFINITION

Problem behavior is socially defined as a problem which is undesirable by the social and/or legal norms of accustomed society and its institutions of authority. According to O'Brien, *problem behavior is an act of a person who either forms significant risk to the health and/or safety to oneself or others* or who *exerts momentous negative impact on his/her own quality of life or the quality of life of others.*

Adolescent problem behavior as a clinically relevant phenomenon is described along two dimensions:
1. Externalizing behavioral problems such as aggression and delinquency
2. Internalizing behavioral problems such as anxiety, depression, psychosomatic complaints, and substance abuse.

Children with externalizing behavior problems of conduct disorder (CD) are very likely to become delinquents during adolescence and, criminals and violent individuals during adulthood. Similarly, children with internalizing behavior problems are expected to grow up becoming anxious and depressed individuals.

Some of the commonly observed behavior problems in children are as follows:
- *Classroom disturbance/bullying:* The extent to which the child teases and torments classmates, interferes with others' work, or is quickly drawn into noise making.
- *Impatience:* The extent to which the child starts work too quickly, is sloppy in work, is unwilling to review work, and rushes through work. Physically, the child is more active and restless.
- *Disrespect-defiance:* The extent to which the child speaks disrespectfully to elders, resists doing what is asked of, belittles the work being done, and breaks classroom rules.
- *Achievement anxiety:* The extent to which the child gets upset about tests and scores and is sensitive to criticism or correction.
- *External reliance:* The extent to which the child looks to others for direction, requires precise direction, and has difficulty making his/her own decisions.
- *Inattentive-withdrawn:* The extent to which the child loses attention, seems to be oblivious to what transpires around him and seems difficult to reach, or is preoccupied.
- *Irrelevant-responsiveness:* The extent to which the child tells exaggerated stories, gives irrelevant answers, interrupts when another person is speaking, and makes irrelevant comments during a discussion.
- *Anxiety-depression:* The child seems to be tense with face drawn and rigid, cries easily at the smallest pretext, does not talk to anyone, and does not take interest in things. The child gets upset about test and test scores and is sensitive to criticism or correction.
- *Quiet and withdrawn:* The child is withdrawn and quiet, does not have friends, and is mostly isolated. He/she tends to be very self-centered, preoccupied with own thoughts and problems, and disinterested in or unenthusiastic about anything else.

- *Aggression and violence:* A hostile or angry behavior directed to harm or injure a person or property.
- *Attention deficit:* The child has difficulty in attending to tasks and instructions for any length of time. He/she gets easily distracted, fidgets excessively, or has difficulty in sitting still.
- *Truancy:* It is absenteeism without permission, skipping classes, or other mandatory school activities. The child who is frequently absent in school for vague reasons or minor ailments.
- *Physical injury:* Recurrent and multiple injuries are observed for which no adequate reason is given, delay medication, spots such as strap marks, bites, and burns.

DIFFERENCES BETWEEN BEHAVIORAL PROBLEMS AND PSYCHIATRIC DISORDERS

The primary difference between a behavior disorder and a psychiatric disorder is the presence of choice. Psychiatric conditions are considered to be involuntary while in behavior disorders, choices are essential. While mental disorders can have behavioral disorders, not all behavioral issues are mental illnesses. Behavioral health is the blanket term that includes mental health. For mental disorders or illnesses, internal psychological or physiological factors dominate.

Examples of mental illnesses that affect children: Anxiety, attention-deficit/hyperactivity disorder (ADHD), depression, obsessive-compulsive disorder (OCD), post-traumatic stress disorder.

Examples of behavior disorders that affect children: Oppositional defiant disorder (ODD) and CD.

EPIDEMIOLOGY

According to the World Health Organization (WHO) estimates, up to 20% of adolescents have one or more mental or behavioral issues.[1] It is important to note, however, that while mental disorders are behavioral problems, not all behavioral issues are mental illnesses. According to studies conducted in various regions of the world, the prevalence of behavioral and emotional issues in teenagers ranges from 16.5[2] to 40.8%, with India having a frequency from 13.7[3] to 50%.[4,5]

Robert et al. in a meta-analysis of 52 studies done in 20 countries of the world found that the prevalence of psychopathology among adolescents (12-18 years) varies from 6 to 41%.[2] In a National Family Health Survey (NFHS) reported study on school-going adolescents of Delhi, 50% of the students were found to have problems of emotional maladjustment. A similar study done in adolescents of Bengaluru reported that 20% of the children had psychiatric problems.[6]

In a more recent study,[7] the Youth Self-Report TM (YSR) was used to measure behavioral and emotional difficulties in 1,123 (12-18 year old) Chandigarh school-aged adolescents. According to the study, the total prevalence of behavioral and emotional issues was 30.4% across all age and gender groups. The prevalence increased significantly from the start of adolescence until 17 years of age, when it began to fall.

Adolescent girls had a higher prevalence of behavioral/emotional issues (33.7%) than boys (27.5%). In addition, whereas boys have a peak around 14-15 years of age, followed by a steady fall to 26.3% by 18-19 years of age, girls have a continual rise in psychiatric disorders with age, with 43% having problems by 18-19 years.

Internalizing syndrome was the most common condition among them (28.6%), followed by neither internalizing nor externalizing (19.5%). The majority (22.08%) of pupils in the internalizing group felt anxious/depressed. Social problems were found to be the most common (9.3%) among neither the internalizing nor the externalizing group. Females were more likely than males to experience internalizing difficulties, including anxiety and despair. In comparison to 19.7% of males, 24.8% of females were nervous or depressed.

Aggressive behavior was the most common (11.8%) among the externalizing group. More boys (18.4%) than girls (12%) were found to suffer from externalizing disorders. 13.3% males had an aggressive behavioral problem as compared to 9.7% females. The problem of rule-breaking or delinquency was twice more in boys as compared to girls and more so (41%) among physically abused adolescents. Children with externalizing behavior problems are at higher risks for delinquency and criminal behavior in adulthood. A lack of data on the subject, which is required for proper health care planning, prevents an assessment of the scope of the problem in India.

ETIOPATHOGENESIS

The adolescent struggles to develop his individuality while still conforming to societal norms. Rapid urbanization and modernization, breakdown in family structure, or excessive or minimal control confuses the adolescent and makes him/her especially vulnerable to maladaptive patterns of thinking and behavior. Healthy adulthood depends upon successful resolution of these emotional and behavioral problems.

Though on a tightrope, most adolescents go through to adulthood normally. However, some adolescents may develop maladaptive patterns in emotional and behavioral spheres resulting in depression, delinquency, and suicides among other problems.

In the etiology of delinquency as well as aggression, the environmental and psychological factors have been strongly implicated. Regulation or control of emotion has been found to be closely associated with externalizing behaviors. Children who were found to be low in negative emotionality were also low in externalizing behaviors, whereas children high in negative emotionality displayed higher levels of problem behavior. Exposure to physical and sexual abuse is a significant factor to influence delinquency and aggression. Children who were rated higher on this scale were also found to have disrupted parent relations, had poor school achievement and peer relations, and were also considered as high risk for future delinquency.

When the association of various socioenvironmental factors and emotional and behavioral problems among adolescents was assessed, it was discovered that children of parents with alcoholism or illicit drug addiction developed up to three times as many behavioral and emotional problems as children of parents without addiction.[7]

Along with the presence of externalizing behavior problems, a wide range of other associated negative consequences such as impaired social cognitive development, academic problems, and irregularities in emotions have simultaneously been found to be present in such children. While examining the natural histories of antisocial and delinquent behavior in children, the pathway research has shown that there exists a series of trajectory of escalating behavior which lead from less serious to more serious.

CLINICAL FEATURES

Aggression

Aggressive behavior, such as fighting or hitting out, also includes various aspects of aggressive personality such as hot temper, arguing, and bragging. Aggression is one component of CD which consists of physical or verbal behavior that harms or threatens others. Whereas boys tend to frequently engage in physical aggression, girls are more likely to exhibit "relational aggression" in various forms such as exclusion of others from their social group and slander.

In all likelihood, both environmental and generic/biological factors contribute toward aggressive behavior. Research on the causes of aggression encompasses work on school aggression, social learning, family violence, imitation, malnutrition, child abuse, neglect, TV, violence, functional and structural brain abnormalities, hormones (e.g., testosterone), and neurotransmitters.

Delinquency

The delinquent behavior syndrome reflects varied antisocial acts such as theft, vandalism, drug use, burglary, violence, and robbery. It seems that there exists continuity in criminal behavior in juvenile offenders who are more likely to become adult offenders. The Child Behavior Checklist (CBCL Achenbach, 1991)[7] has vividly described delinquency with antisocial behavior such as stealing, lying, cheating, and committing antisocial acts with bad companions.

Anxiety

Anxiety disorders in children fall into Diagnostic and Statistical Manual of Mental Disorders, Fifth Edition (DSM-5) diagnostic categories of generalized anxiety disorder, social anxiety disorder, specific phobia, panic disorder, agoraphobia, separation anxiety disorder, and selective mutism.

Children diagnosed with generalized anxiety disorder often have a consistent pattern of uncontrollable and excessive anxiety/worry, with concerns covering a broad range of events or activities lasting 6 months or more. In addition to worry, symptoms may also include fatigue, irritability, restlessness, sleep disturbances, difficulty in concentrating, and muscle tension. Anxiety disorders are typically treated with medication, psychotherapy, or a combination of both.

Social Anxiety Disorder

Social anxiety disorder is a marked and persistent fear of one or more social or performance situations in which the person is exposed to unfamiliar people or to possible scrutiny by others. The individual fears that he or she will act in a way (or show anxiety symptoms) that will be humiliating or embarrassing. The fear or anxiety is out of proportion to the actual threat posed by the social situation and to the sociocultural context. The fear, anxiety, or avoidance is persistent, typically lasting for 6 months or more. The fear, anxiety, or avoidance is not attributable to the physiological effects of a substance (e.g., a drug of abuse, a medication) or another medical condition.

Cognitive behavioral therapy (CBT) psychotherapy is commonly used to treat social anxiety disorder. CBT teaches a different way of thinking, behaving, and reacting to situations to help one feel less anxious and fearful. It can involve breathing, the 5-4-3-2-1 coping technique, or distracting oneself.

Specific Phobia

Specific phobia is marked fear or anxiety about a specific object or situation (e.g., flying, heights, and animals, receiving an injection, seeing blood). The phobic object or situation is actively avoided or endured with intense fear or anxiety with clinically significant distress or impairment in social, occupational, or other important areas of functioning.

The disturbance is not better explained by the symptoms of another mental disorder, including fear, anxiety, and avoidance of situations associated with panic-like symptoms or other incapacitating symptoms (as in agoraphobia), objects or situations related to obsessions (as in OCD), reminders of traumatic events (as in stress disorder), separation from home or attachment figures (as in separation anxiety disorder), or social situations (as in social anxiety disorder).

The best treatment for specific phobias is a form of therapy called exposure therapy. Typically, one specific phobia is treated at a time. Gradual, repeated exposure to the source of specific phobia, and the related thoughts, feelings and sensations, may help the adolescent to manage anxiety. For example, if the child is afraid of elevators, therapy may progress from simply thinking about getting into an elevator, to looking at pictures of elevators, to going near an elevator, to stepping into an elevator. Next, the child may take a one-floor ride, and then ride several floors, and then ride in a crowded elevator.

Panic Disorder

Panic disorder is an anxiety disorder based primarily on the occurrence of panic attacks, which are recurrent and often unexpected. DSM-5 criteria for panic disorder include the experience of recurrent panic attacks, with one or more attacks followed by at least 1 month of fear of another panic attack or significant maladaptive behavior related to the attacks. A panic attack is an abrupt period of intense fear or discomfort accompanied by 4 or more of the following 13 systemic symptoms:
1. Palpitations, pounding heart, or accelerated heart rate
2. Sweating
3. Trembling or shaking
4. Sensations of shortness of breath or smothering
5. A feeling of choking
6. Chest pain or discomfort
7. Nausea or abdominal distress
8. Feeling dizzy, unsteady, lightheaded, or faint
9. Feelings of unreality (de-realization) or being detached from oneself (de-personalization)
10. Fear of losing control or going crazy
11. Fear of dying
12. Numbness or tingling sensations (paresthesias)
13. Chills or hot flushes.

The main treatment options are psychotherapy (CBT) and medications [selective serotonin reuptake inhibitors (SSRIs)]. One or both types of treatment may be recommended, depending upon history and severity of panic disorder.

Selective Mutism

Selective mutism is a childhood disorder typified by an inability to speak in certain circumstances. Specifically, it is a consistent failure to speak in certain social situations where there is a natural expectation of speaking.

The most research-supported treatment for selective mutism is behavioral and cognitive behavioral therapy. Behavioral therapy approaches including gradual exposures, contingency management, successive approximations/shaping, and stimulus fading, are successful in the treatment of childhood anxiety.

Depression (Mood Disorders)

Depression is a common behavioral problem which generally appears at a very young age. According to DSM-5, mood disorders have been broadly categorized as follows:
- Bipolar disorders
- Depressive disorders.

Bipolar disorders are further categorized as bipolar I, bipolar II, cyclothymic disorder, bipolar and related disorder to another medical condition, substance/medication-induced bipolar and related disorder, other specified bipolar and related disorder, and unspecified bipolar and related disorder. Bipolar I disorder is defined as a syndrome in which a complete set of mania symptoms (elevated mood with three or more of the following symptoms: increased goal-directed activity, grandiosity, a diminished need for sleep, distractibility, racing thoughts, increased/pressured speech, and reckless behaviors) has occurred lasting for at least 1 week or requiring hospitalization. If the mood is irritable instead of elevated, four or more of the aforementioned symptoms are needed to meet the criteria for a manic episode.

Hypomania is defined as a nonpsychotic, milder, or subthreshold manic state of short duration lasting for at least 4 consecutive days and without marked social and occupational impairment. It requires elevated mood with three or more symptoms or irritable mood with four or more of the following symptoms: Increased goal-directed activity, grandiosity, a diminished need for sleep, distractibility, racing thoughts, increased/ pressured speech, and reckless behavior. According to the International Classification of Diseases 11th Revision (ICD-11), cyclothymia and hypomania are considered as a prodrome of bipolar disorders, and as per DSM-5, hypomania is a component of bipolar II disorder. A major depressive disorder is diagnosed by the presence of five out of the nine symptoms of sad mood, insomnia, feelings of guilt, decreased energy levels, decreased concentration, decreased appetite, decrease in pleasurable activities (anhedonia), increased or decreased psychomotor activity, and recurrent suicidal ideation/acts of self-harm/ suicide attempt existing over a period of 2 weeks. Three new depressive disorders have been incorporated under mood disorders in DSM-5:

1. Disruptive mood dysregulation disorder (DMDD) is seen in children and adolescents with frequent anger outbursts and irritability out of proportion to the situation.
2. Persistent depressive disorder (PDD) or dysthymia means a depressed mood not severe enough to meet the criteria for major depression. PDD is defined as the depressed mood for at least 2 years in adults and 1 year in children and adolescents.
3. Premenstrual dysphoric disorder (PMDD) is characterized by irritability, anxiety, depression, and emotional lability occurring in a week before the onset of menses followed by resolution of the symptoms after onset.

Other depressive disorders include depressive disorder due to another medical condition, substance or medication-induced depressive disorder, other specified depressive disorder, and unspecified depressive disorder.

PHARMACOLOGICAL TREATMENT

1. *SSRIs:* These are the first-line treatment option for depressive disorder, as they are tolerated better with lesser side effects (e.g., sertraline, fluvoxamine, fluoxetine, citalopram, escitalopram, and paroxetine).
2. *If a presenting episode is a manic episode with severe symptoms or is a mixed episode:* Start with a mood stabilizer (lithium or valproic acid) and an atypical antipsychotic (risperidone, olanzapine, quetiapine, ziprasidone, aripiprazole).
3. *If the patient presents with a less severe episode:* Monotherapy with lithium, an anticonvulsant, or an atypical antipsychotic is recommended. Alternatives to lithium or valproic acid are carbamazepine or oxcarbazepine.
4. *If a presenting episode is a depressive episode:* Prescribe quetiapine or lurasidone or lamotrigine, or a combination of olanzapine and fluoxetine.

PREVENTION

Multipronged intervention at home, school, and society may be required.

Role of Parents

A sizeable population of our adolescents needs support in coping with emotional and behavioral problems. *Authoritative parenting* is a parenting style in which children participate in establishing family expectations and rules. Adolescents who feel warmth and support from their parents and whose parents convey clear expectations regarding their children's behavior and show consistent limit setting and monitoring are less likely to develop serious problems. Such children are less vulnerable and show resilience in adverse conditions.

Family Psychoeducation

Home is the first school and parents are the role model to their children. Behavior therapy teaches children and their families how to strengthen positive child behaviors and eliminate or reduce unwanted or problem behaviors. Improving communication, reducing punishment, positive reinforcement, and praise go a long way in allying aggression and anxiety.

Media

Violence prevention begins in early childhood with violence-free discipline. Limiting exposure to violence through media and video games may also help because exposure to these violent images has been shown to desensitize children to violence and cause children to accept violence as part of their life.

Life Skills

It is important to impart life skills training, e.g., competence, coping skills, resilience, self-efficacy, decision-making. The approach should include multiple members of the family and focus on learning better communication skills and ways to settle conflicts.

Cognitive-behavior Therapy

It works well for disruptive behavior disorder, depression, anxiety, and post-traumatic stress disorder.

Adolescents with depression may respond well to interpersonal psychotherapy, an approach in which the therapists help the adolescents learn ways to handle relationship problems.

Role of Teachers

Schools/colleges are important institutions where the social development takes place. School-based mental health services with a counselor/psychologist in every school are recommended for proper guidance and counseling in solving the day-to-day problems of the adolescent. The academic achievement and assistance for the same may also be required as it is an important determinant of psychological well-being. School-age children should have access to a safe school environment. Older children and adolescents should not have access to weapons.

CONCLUSION

Substance abuse is a common cause of behavioral issues, and substance-use disorders necessitate specialized care. A community intervention for addiction may be required, and schools can serve as the foundation by implementing innovative initiatives such as student theater clubs, street plays, and so on, hence educating both the family and the school children about addiction. Despite their parents' best efforts, adolescents whose behavior is harmful or otherwise inappropriate may require professional intervention.

Lifestyle remedies

Lifestyle and other strategies help to manage the anxiety caused by specific phobias.
- Mindfulness strategies may help to manage anxiety and reduce avoidance behaviors.
- Relaxation techniques, such as deep breathing, progressive muscle relaxation or yoga, may help cope with physical symptoms of anxiety and stress.
- Physical activity and exercise may help manage anxiety related to specific phobias.

Behavioral problems also may be symptoms of learning disabilities, depression, or other mental health disorders. Such disorders typically require counseling, and adolescents who have mental health disorders may benefit from treatment with drugs.

REFERENCES

1. The World Health Report. (2001). Mental Health: New Understanding, New Hope. Geneva: World Health Organization; 2001. pp. 39-44.
2. Roberts RE, Attkisson CC, Rosenblatt A. Prevalence of psychopathology among children and adolescents. Am J Psychiatry. 1998;155(6):715-25.
3. Mishra A, Sharma AK. A clinico-social study of psychiatric disorders in 12–18 years school going girls in urban Delhi. Indian J Community Med. 2001;26(2):71-5.
4. Belfer ML, Sharma AK. Child and adolescent mental health around the world: Challenges for progress. J Indian Assoc Child Adolesc Ment Health. 2005;1:31-6.
5. Jenson PS, Watanabe HK, Richters JE, Cortes R, Roper M, Liu S. Prevalence of mental disorder in military children and adolescents: finding from a two stage community survey. J Am Acad Child Adolesc Psychiatry. 1995;34:1514-24.
6. Srinath S, Girimaji SC, Gururaj G, Seshadri S, Subbakrishna DK, Bhola P, et al. Epidemiological study of child & adolescent psychiatric disorders in urban & rural areas of Bangalore, India. Indian J Med Res. 2005;122: 67-79.
7. Pathak R, Sharma RC, Parvan UC, Gupta BP, Ojha RK, Goel N. Behavioural and emotional problems in school going adolescents. Australas Med J. 2011;4(1):15-21.

FURTHER READING

1. Achenbach System of Emperically Based Assessment (ASEBA). Available from: URL: https://aseba.org/aseba-subsequent-developments/
2. Barman N, Khanikor MS. Prevalence of Behavioural Problems among School Children: A Pilot Study. Int J Health Sci Res. 2018;8(12):95-101.
3. Centers for Disease Control and Prevention. (2020). Behavior or conduct problems in children. [online] Available from: https://www.cdc.gov/childrensmentalhealth/behavior html [Last accessed October, 2023].
4. Datta P, Ganguly S, Roy BN. The prevalence of behavioral disorders among children under parental care and out of parental care: A comparative study in India. Int J Pediatr Adolesc Med. 2018;5(4):145-51.
5. Joseph N, Sinha U, D'Souza M. Assessment of determinants of behavioral problems among primary school children in Mangalore city of South India. Current Psychol. 2021;40:6187-98.
6. Ogundele MO. Behavioural and emotional disorders in childhood: A brief overview for paediatricians. World J Clin Pediatr. 2018;7(1):9-26.
7. World Health Organization. (2019). Global Health Estimates, 2020. online] Available from: https://www.who.int/data/global-health-estimates [Last accessed October, 2023].

Counseling of Parents and Children with Behavioral Disorder

Chapter 26

JS Tuteja

INTRODUCTION

Excellent mental health is defined as a state of well-being of a person which is beyond stress, productive, and gives life to family and to the community to which he/she belongs [World Health Organization (WHO), 2022].[1] Behavioral disorders are common in children. These disorders involve a pattern of untoward behaviors that create problems at school and/or home and also in various social situations. Most of the children and adolescents show such behaviors occasionally. Mental health issues encompass a wide spectrum of concerns that differ in their persistence and severity. It refers to the child's or young person's symptoms and sufferings that are deemed to fulfill the clinical threshold for a specific mental disease by a mental health care provider such as a pediatrician or an adolescent physician.[2]

Common mental health disorders seen in children and adolescents include anxiety, depression, oppositional defiance disorders, conduct disorders, obsessive-compulsive disorder (OCD), and attention-deficit hyperactive disorder (ADHD). These disorders can be classified as externalizing or internalizing disorders. Studies have shown that 80% of preschoolers have mild-grade temper tantrums; however, challenging behavior issues are more commonly seen during the first 2 years of life.[3-5]

Emotional issues such as anxiety, sadness, and post-traumatic stress disorder are more common in later childhood. They are frequently difficult for parents to discover at an earlier stage as children are in a psychosocial developing stage, and parents are unable to distinguish between normal and pathological behavior. Even many times, clinicians also face difficulty in differentiating normal from abnormal behavior.[6,7]

ADOLESCENT PERIOD

Adolescents constitute approximately 23% of population of India. Adolescence is the second phase of life. It is considered as a thrilling phase of life, due to many reasons and developmental changes in the body of the growing child. It is characterized by the physical, mental, emotional, social, and spiritual changes in which a growing child experiences a mixture of excitement to deal with in future life. This precious time of child life needs helping hands from the gatekeepers of society to overcome the excitements and thrills in this period.

It is the time in which a child is passing through physical changes of growth, emotional instability, cognitive development, risk-taking behavior, emerging self-identity, social adjustments, facing adversities and trying to overcome, and envision future to set goals for the future life. Though adolescence is a thrilling period, stress, peer pressure, academic pressure, and emotional turbulence are also high. All these facts combine to make the adolescence period a more complex and dynamic phase of life.[8]

NEUROBIOLOGY STUDIES

Neurobiology studies of the brain show reduced gray matter in the regions of frontal cortex, amygdala, temporal lobes, and the anterior insula in patients with behavior disorders. This is the network which is related to empathetic concern when dealing with other people. There is a decreased thickness of cortical regions in the brain in areas of cingulate and prefrontal cortex.[9,10]

Changes have been detected in hypothalamus, inferior superior parietal lobes, right amygdala, and anterior insula also. It has also been reported that there is decreased activation of the temporal cortex in children who are violent and socially not compatible.[11-13] There have been reports of diminished activity of the hypothalamic–pituitary–adrenal axis in individuals with behavior disorders. It is probably due to a high level of prenatal testosterone as there is a high prevalence of behavior disorders in male children. It may also be due to increased susceptibility to a high level of exposure to alcohol and nicotine during the antenatal period.[14,15]

HISTORY OF COUNSELING IN INDIA

Counseling in India dates back to ancient times as people in India seek guidance and support from knowledge from individuals like parents, grandparents, spiritual and religious celebrities, and friends. Counseling has been an integral part of the Indian society for many centuries. It was in the era of the joint family system where counseling was used to be done for children and adolescents as per their issue of growth and development, sexuality and sex education, marriages, mental health issues, and future working in life by the parents, grandparents, and close relatives in families. These counselors would draw upon their wisdom, spiritual knowledge, and life experiences to provide support and help individuals through difficult situations.

In education, it used to be "Guru Shishya Parampara" which emphasized a deep mentor–student relationship where Guru would guide the disciple not only in academic pursuits but also in matter of character development, ethics, and life choices. But still, we have a long story of counseling in India if we go through our epic—Mahabharata. In true sense, Lord Shree Krishna was the first renowned counselor if one goes through the most revered ancient text. As per our Hindu mythology, he was a great counselor. He had remarkable ability to deal with any crisis for his followers through his ability of perfect empathetic communication, compassion, and intelligence dealing with problem with love and affection which is needed in counseling sessions.[16] In the present era in India, counseling was recognized as early as 1938 by Dr Acharya Narendra Dev, who underlined the importance of counseling in education.[17]

With time, counseling in India has evolved to incorporate western psychological theories and practices. In influence of western education, and growth of psychology as a discipline, counseling started incorporating evidence-based approaches and therapeutic techniques.

Today, counseling in India encompasses a wide range of approaches and techniques. It is provided by adolescent pediatricians/pediatricians/psychologist/psychotherapists, counselors, and social workers. Counseling services are available in various settings, including schools and colleges, universities, hospitals, adolescent-friendly clinics, nongovernmental organizations (NGOs), and private clinics run by pediatricians.

The practice of counseling in India is guided by ethical principles and cultural sensitivities. Indian counselors often take into account cultural norms, values, and traditions when working with clients. They recognize the importance of family systems, community support, and spiritual beliefs in lives of individuals and integrate all these factors in the counseling sessions. In recent years, there has been an increased recognition of the importance of mental health counseling in India. All efforts are being made to raise awareness, reduce stigma, and improve counseling services across the country. The government organizations have been working to develop policies, programs, and initiatives to promote mental health counseling in the whole of India.

CHALLENGES AFFECTING THE DEVELOPMENT OF GUIDANCE AND COUNSELING IN INDIA

There are several challenges affecting guidance and counseling in India, some of which are as follows:

Lack of awareness: Many people in India are not aware of the benefits of guidance and counseling. As a result, they may not seek out these services when they need them.

Limited availability: Guidance and counseling services are not widely available in India, particularly in rural areas and even in urban areas. This makes it difficult for people who live in these areas to access the support they need.

Stigma and cultural barriers: There is still a significant stigma attached to seeking help for mental health and emotional issues in India. In addition, some cultural and religious beliefs may discourage people from seeking counseling.[18]

Shortage of trained professionals: There is a shortage of trained guidance and counseling professionals in India. This limits the availability and quality of available services.[19]

Insufficient funding and resources: Guidance and counseling services require funding and resources to operate effectively. In India, resources available to support these services are limited.[20]

Language and cultural barriers: India is a diverse country with many different languages and cultures. This makes it difficult for counselors to communicate effectively with their clients and understand their unique needs.[21]

WHAT IS COUNSELING?

In counseling, children can learn important tools to help them to navigate the ups and downs of this important life stage. Together, counselor, parents, and adolescents work together through tough issues by building self-confidence and improve family communication so that they feel self-prepared to enter in the adult world. Raising children is difficult, and raising difficult children can make life disrupting.[22]

It is not very easy for the counselor to commit about the child who is coming for the therapy session that which stage the child is passing through. Parents may be more concerned when their child is in the stage of psychosocial development for which they are not aware. It is very necessary for the parents to update themselves about the developmental stages of their children.[23]

Precisely, "counseling is a professional relationship that empowers diverse individuals, families, and groups to accomplish mental health, wellness, education, and career goals". Counseling is a skill process, not just a technique that assists clients in changing their behavior and efficiently coping with their situation. Counseling is not immediately telling or giving advice, a passing concern, a confession, or prayer.[24,25]

Counseling evolved from the 1900s. Progressive guidance movement emphasizes on prevention and purposefulness. It attempts to prevent mental health concerns such as anxiety, stress, and depression as well as to assist the client in discovering his or her purpose and realizing their full potential **(Box 1)**.

COUNSELING VERSUS GUIDANCE

Counseling differs from guidance that assists people in making decisions among many possibilities, whereas counseling makes a person aware of their potential and assists them in making positive changes in their lives. Psychotherapy or therapy is a long-term process that takes place between the client and the therapist, and the duties of counsellors and therapists frequently overlap.

GOALS OF COUNSELING

Counseling includes specific purposes such as encouraging people to make their own decisions, teaching stress management, and advising on how to maintain love and pleasant relationships.

COUNSELING VERSUS HEALTH EDUCATION

There is some confusion that prevails regarding counseling and health education. The differences between the two are given in **Table 1**.

COGNITIVE BEHAVIOR THERAPY

Cognitive behavior therapy is a skill that is based on the principle that many emotions are always driven by our thoughts, and how one processes and interprets it followed by one's behavior. Many times, thoughts are unrealistic and may not be very helpful in life. Such thoughts may create expectations from others or may not be accepted by the other peer group or in family. These kinds of beliefs can contribute to unrealistic, prejudiced, or maladaptive thinking, which can lead to negative feelings and ineffective behavior. Cognitive therapy encourages the adolescent to question erroneous thoughts, appraise situations more accurately, and make judgments.[26-29] It is founded on more balanced reasoning. Working with children and teenagers to shift their interpretations of events or sensations might result in very different emotional responses.

Cognitive behavior therapy is to help children break through major barriers in their lives. It is a tool that works well for the counselor and for the client. Cognitive behavior therapy has a value of having another person to

---

BOX 1: Stages of counseling—GATHER approach.[25]

G = Greet client in a friendly, helpful, and respectful manner
A = Ask client about needs and concerns
T = Tell client about different options and methods
H = Help client to make decision about choice of methods she/he prefers
E = Explain to client how to use the method
R = *Return:* Schedule and carry out return visit and follow-up of client

---

TABLE 1: Counseling versus health education.

Counseling	Health education
Confidential	Nonconfidential
One-to-one process/small group	For a group of people
Focused, specific, and directed	Generalized
Facilitate change attitude and motivate behavior change	Information provided to increase the knowledge
Problem oriented	Content oriented
Based on the need of client	Based on public health needs

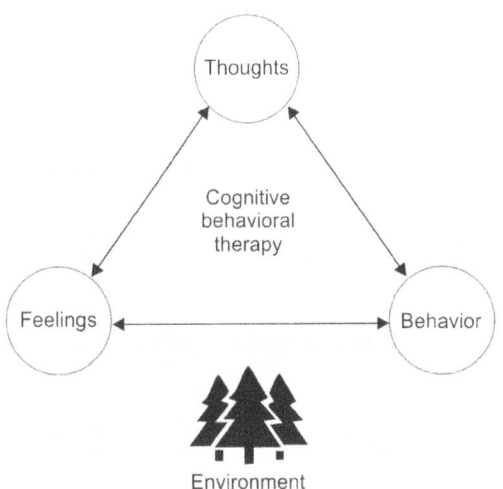

Fig. 1: Cognitive behavioral therapy.

listen to client, to validate his/her perspective, and gently challenge when needed. It is a tool where whatever said is accepted. Cognitive behavior therapy is a tool which provides relief anxiety and depression.[30]

How does Cognitive Therapy Help?

Cognitive therapy helps children and adolescents to (Fig. 1):
- Distinguish between their thoughts, feelings, and actions
- Become aware of the ways in which thoughts can influence feelings and actions that are not helpful
- Learn about thoughts that seem to occur automatically, without the person even realizing how their thoughts may affect their emotions
- Evaluate critically whether these "automatic" thoughts and assumptions are accurate or biased
- Develop the skills to notice, interrupt, and correct these biased thoughts independently.

Types of Cognitive Behavioral Therapy

Cognitive behavioral therapy involves a variety of skills and ways for dealing with ideas, emotions, and behaviors. Some of the specific types of therapeutic approaches that involve cognitive behavioral therapy include:
- Cognitive therapy centers on identifying and changing inaccurate or distorted thought patterns, emotional responses, and behaviors.[31]
- Dialectical behavior therapy addresses destructive or disturbing thoughts and behaviors while incorporating treatment strategies such as emotional regulation and mindfulness.
- Multimodal therapy suggests that psychological issues must be treated by addressing seven different but interconnected modalities: Behavior, affect, sensation, imagery, cognition, interpersonal factors, and drug/biological considerations.[32]
- Rational emotive behavior therapy involves identifying irrational beliefs, actively challenging these beliefs, and finally learning to recognize and change these thought patterns.

While each style of cognitive behavioral therapy has a unique methodology, they all aim to address the underlying thought patterns that contribute to psychological suffering. Cognitive behavioral therapy is a prominent skill that teaches people to connect their thoughts and behaviors. It also assists clients in making them more aware of factors that hinder their recovery by demonstrating that many of their detrimental behaviors are not logical or rational.[33]

How does Cognitive Behavioral Therapy Work?

A counselor works to identify negative thoughts that can be obstacles in recovery of the client. These often irrational beliefs are based on misconceptions and internalized feelings of self-doubt or fear. Such clients when come in session learn to reframe their disturbed memories from a different perspective to reduce the pain of those memories. Once these thoughts and memories are reframed, the client can then learn new positive behaviors. Cognitive behavioral therapy is successful at treating anxiety, depression, trauma, attention deficit disorder (ADD), ADHD, bipolar disorder, OCD, substance abuse, and schizophrenia. Cognitive behavior therapy entails more than just recognizing thought patterns. It employs a variety of ways to assist people in breaking free from these routines. A few approaches utilized in cognitive behavioral therapy are as follows:[34]

Identifying negative thoughts: It is critical to understand which thoughts, feelings, and conditions contribute to maladaptive behavior. However, this process can be challenging, especially for individuals who struggle with introspection. Taking the time to identify these thoughts, on the other hand, can lead to self-discovery and provide insights that are critical to the therapy process.[35]

Practicing new skills: People are frequently taught new skills that can be applied in real-world circumstances during cognitive behavioral therapy.

Goal-setting: This can be an important step in recovery from mental illness, helping to make changes to improve their health and life. During cognitive behavioral therapy, a therapist can help to build skills. This might involve teaching, helping, and identifying goals or distinguishing between short- and long-term goals.

Problem solving: Learning problem-solving skills during cognitive behavioral therapy can assist in learning how to recognize and handle problems that may arise as a result of both large and little life pressures. It can also assist to mitigate the harmful effects of mental and physical sickness. In cognitive behavior therapy, problem solving frequently requires five steps:[36]
1. Identify the problem.
2. Generate a list of potential solutions.
3. Evaluate the strengths and weaknesses of each potential solution.
4. Choose a solution to implement.
5. Implement the solution.

Self-monitoring

Self-monitoring, sometimes known as daily diary work, is an important cognitive behavioral therapy strategy. It entails keeping note of habits, symptoms, or experiences over time and sharing them with a therapist. Self-monitoring can offer counselors with the data they need to provide the best possible care. Journaling, role acting, relaxation strategies, and the use of mental diversions are examples of further cognitive behavioral therapy practices.[37-39]

Effectiveness of Cognitive Behavioral Therapy

Cognitive behavior therapy arose in the 1960s as a result of the work of psychiatrist Aaron Beck, who observed that certain forms of thinking contributed to emotional issues. Beck coined the term "automatic negative thoughts" and pioneered cognitive therapy. Previous behavior therapies focused almost entirely on associations, reinforcements, and punishments to improve behavior, whereas the cognitive approach examines how thoughts and feelings influence behavior. Cognitive behavioral therapy is now one of the most thoroughly researched modalities of treatment. It has been proven to be useful in the treatment of anxiety, depression, eating disorders, insomnia, OCD, panic disorder, post-traumatic stress disorder, and drug-use disorder.[40]

Cognitive behavioral therapy has been demonstrated to be effective in treating insomnia. It is useful for people who have a medical condition that prevents them from sleeping, such as pain. Mental illnesses, such as depression, is another option. It has been clinically demonstrated to be useful in treating depressive and anxiety symptoms in children.[41] A 2018 meta-analysis of 41 researches indicated that cognitive behavior therapy helped persons with anxiety and anxiety-related disorders, such as OCD and post-traumatic stress disorder, improve their symptoms.[42,43] It has strong empirical evidence for the treatment of substance-use disorders, assisting people with these disorders in improving self-control, avoiding triggers, and developing coping mechanisms for daily stressors. CBT is one of the most researched types of therapy, in part because treatment is focused on very defined goals and results are relatively easy to quantify.

What Happens during a Cognitive Behavior Session?

In the first session, the counselor learns about the problem and the client hopes to achieve through cognitive behavior therapy. The counselor will then devise a strategy to achieve certain goals. Goals should be specific, quantifiable, attainable, reasonable, and time-bound. Sessions are typically an hour long and held once a week, though this might vary depending on individual needs and availability. Homework is often required as part of the process, so clients may be requested to complete worksheets or execute specific chores in between sessions. Communication with the counselor should be open and comfortable. If the client does not feel entirely at ease with the counselor, attempt to find another counselor with whom the client can connect and open up.[44] Always look for a counselor who is trained in cognitive behavior therapy and has experience in treating a client-specific problem. One can enquire from a health care provider. Practitioners may include pediatricians, adolescent pediatricians, psychiatrists, and psychologists.

Are There Any Risks?

Cognitive behavior therapy is generally not considered a risky therapy, though there are a few things to keep in mind:
- It is a very personal process, but in the beginning, some people may find it stressful or uncomfortable to confront their problems.
- Some types of cognitive behavior therapy, like exposure therapy, can increase stress and anxiety.

- It does not take effect overnight. Working on new strategies between sessions and after therapy requires dedication and willingness.
- It can sometimes be difficult to find a good cognitive behavior therapy counselor.
- It has become fashionable for counselor/pediatricians/family physicians to describe themselves as offering cognitive behavior therapy, even when they do something quite different; it is perfectly appropriate to ask what kind of training potential a counselor has received.
- It may be difficult to find a well-trained cognitive behavior therapy counselor in some communities. In such cases, medications may represent the best available option.
- Cognitive behavior therapy will not work for everyone, and if it does not work for your child within a reasonable period of time, then it might be wise to consider adding or switching to medications.
- It also may help to add medications if cognitive behavior therapy produces some relief but does not fully resolve the problems that brought the child into treatment.
- Some parents, or even the children or adolescents themselves, may prefer medications to cognitive behavior therapy, since medications typically work a little faster and may involve less time and effort. That is perfectly all right; it is good to live in an age in which there multiple efficacious treatment options are available. But it is always important to remember that adding medications can sometimes help when cognitive behavior therapy alone is not enough; similarly, adding cognitive behavior therapy to medications can also help when drugs alone are not enough.

FAMILY THERAPY

When parents, siblings, and other family members attend therapy sessions alongside their children, they often benefit. Family counseling can help to enhance relationships and communication while decreasing conflict. Family therapy is a type of treatment in which psychological issues and their treatment are viewed through the interactions of family members. Families are viewed as an integrated, interconnected unit in which each family member influences psychological functioning both individually and collectively as a complete system.[45]

There is no formal designated patient in family therapy; instead, the emphasis is on interpersonal patterns and communication among family members. When a child has a behavior problem, for example, a family counselor is more likely to see the child's difficulties within the greater framework of the family system than his/her particular limitations. The counsellor avoids criticizing any particular family member for the problem during family therapy. Anorexia nervosa, bulimia nervosa, drug and alcohol misuse, obesity and overweight, parenting, communication challenges, relationship issues, and mental health issues can all benefit from family therapy.[46]

What are Some Forms of Family Therapy?

Family-based Behavioral Treatment

In family-based behavioral treatment, parents set a good example by improving their own behavior in order to help their children modify theirs in the long run. Training parents in child management and problem-solving abilities is an important component of this sort of therapy. This therapy has been shown in studies to be beneficial in treating obesity or overweight disorders in children, as well as anorexia in adolescents.[47]

Parent-only Family-based Treatment

This treatment has been shown as highly beneficial when used with a lifestyle or dietary regimen for children who are obese or overweight. Currently, parent-only family-based behavioral treatment has been shown to be effective for children but not adolescents.[48]

Functional Family Therapy

Functional family therapy is a family-based therapy that was established to assist youngsters with behavioral challenges and has been shown to be successful in the treatment of adolescent substance-use disorders. Functional family therapy's goals are to drive adolescents and their families to reduce negativity in the home and to develop abilities in each family member to reduce harmful behaviors through communication, effective parenting, and conflict resolution.[49]

Multidimensional Family Therapy

Multidimensional family therapy is a family-centered treatment that focuses on the individual, familial, and environmental factors that influence a wide range of behavioral difficulties in children. This treatment is founded on the premise that behavioral issues in adolescents are caused by a variety of circumstances and that treatment should be delivered with dignity and compassion. Youth gain coping, problem-solving, and decision-making abilities are included in this therapy, while the family learns how to improve family functioning. It has been shown in studies to be beneficial in the treatment of substance-use disorders in adolescents.[50]

Multisystemic Therapy

Multisystemic treatment is a family-centered, evidence-based intervention for adolescents who exhibit substantial antisocial behavior, delinquency, and substance abuse issues. It evaluates these behaviors in the context of numerous systems of influence, including individual, family, peer, school, and community impacts. Its interventions minimize problem behaviors and improve youth and family functioning in a cost-effective framework.[51]

ART THERAPY

Art making has been shown to be one of the most powerful ways humans have discovered to express themselves. Art therapy programs are a form of meditative and expressive therapy that has been around for decades. It continues to grow in popularity as it assists individuals in expressing their thoughts and feelings. Expression through art helps people explore, understand, and resolve issues that they may not be able to address using words alone. Art is often a nonverbal process and sometimes the only way an individual can convey ideas or emotions. Art therapy programs provide people with the opportunity to explore their inner thoughts without feeling confined to using words—a valuable service for any person with issues that are too painful to discuss. There are many different art therapy programs that a counselor can use at any stage throughout the healing process—from children up through adulthood.[33]

ADVENTURE THERAPY

Adventure therapy is a unique approach to recovery that uses adventure-based activities to promote healing and growth. Unlike traditional therapy, which often takes place in an office setting, adventure therapy takes advantage of the natural world to provide a more mindful experience. This type of therapy is particularly effective for those struggling with anxiety, depression, trauma, and substance abuse.

By working with a trained counselor, clients can learn to overcome obstacles, develop new skills for managing difficult situations, and build more meaningful relationships with their peers as they connect through these activities. Staying active and getting exercise play a significant role in holistic recovery, so clients also have access to a fully equipped, top-of-the-line gym during designated fitness and free times.

The use of adventure therapies is an engaging way to encourage transformation. These activities are often conducted in groups, using the opportunity to overcome personal challenges. Overall, the process helps people internalize whatever has happened during each activity, allowing counselors to facilitate discussion regarding how those experience apply to their therapeutic goals. Benefits of adventure therapy are pride, mindfulness, movement, courage, respect, cooperation, strength, trust, and physicality.

ROLE OF PARENTING STYLES

There is no doubt that adolescence is one of the most complicated stages of a child's life. Parents have to go through a tough time when they have to take care, teach, and discipline a teen. Indian teens today are forced to live on the extreme environment of completion in life. There is no or little acceptance from the parents, which adds to the peer pressure and the need to get embraced by the society. The path of children growing to adolescent and young adults is lot complicated without guidance at this stage of life. The role of media is not going too well on the preaching side either. The electronic media depicts everything as fair in teenage, whether it is premarital sex, bullying, breaking rules, and violent behavior. With so much happening out there, they are bound to become defiant, rebellious, and out of control. So, here comes the role of parents to save their children for better life by superb parenting styles.[45]

Parenting Styles

Parenting approaches are rarely to blame for behavioral issues in children. Nonetheless, parents play an important role in the treatment of early childhood behavioral disorders. There are four major types of parenting styles, one of which is most helpful in raising well-adjusted and well-behaved children:

1. *Authoritarian parenting:* Strict standards with no wiggle room and no child input.

2. *Authoritative parenting:* Parents are willing to listen and collaborate with their children despite the strict rules. Parenting that is more democratic than dictatorial.
3. *Permissive parenting:* There are few regulations and minimal expectations placed on youngsters. In this home, there is little to no punishment, and parents often play the role of friend.
4. *Uninvolved parenting:* There are no regulations and virtually little engagement. These parents are emotionally distant and may reject or ignore their children.

Authoritative parenting is more likely to result in well-adjusted, happy children. Children raised by uninvolved parents are more prone to lacking self-esteem, self-control, and general competency. These parenting styles teach us that children not only want clear rules and penalties, but also require a parent who is willing to listen and guide.[23]

PREVENTION

Mental health necessitates the development of cognitive, emotional, and social abilities, which educational institutions provide in spades. Educational settings improve mental health by giving children and adolescents a feeling of identity, self-esteem, direction, and meaning in life, mastery, belonging, safety, social support, and involvement in good activities. Better educational and behavioral outcomes are related to good mental health. There are a variety of effective interventions available to promote mental health as well as prevent and reduce mental disease. However, in the school setting, very few children and adolescents receive such interventions. Life skills education should be applied in all educational institutions around the country so that youngsters suffer less and live their lives with a positive attitude.

Patience, empathy, and encouragement are important for helping to boost self-esteem. An authoritative parenting style, which involves listening to children whilst also setting reasonable rules and boundaries, is also helpful. It is important to note that boot camp-style programs and "tough love" are not effective for behavioral disorders. In fact, they can be very damaging. Identification and management of mental health problems in primary care settings such as routine pediatric clinics or family medicine/general practitioner/adolescent friendly clinics are cost-effective due to a number of desirable characteristics that make it acceptable to children and adolescents (e.g., no stigma, in a familiar setting, and familiar providers). Recently, several models for improving mental health service delivery in pediatric/primary care settings/adolescent-friendly clinics have been recommended and evaluated, including coordination with external specialists, joint consultations, improved mental health training, and more integrated on-site intervention with specialist collaboration.[52-54]

CONCLUSION

School guidance is developing very rapidly in many countries around the world. At the secondary level, there is tough competition among students to secure good marks in the exam and to secure a promising career which leads to frustration among students, and this is one of the important causes of anxiety, depression, and suicidal tendency. In such circumstances, the role of a school guidance program is very much important to help the students. Therefore, it is recommended that every school should have a proper guidance unit with several school guidance personnel like pediatricians/adolescent pediatricians/psychiatrist/social workers/active parent–teacher meetings/teens clubs who help the students with their varied problems.

This will in turn help in enhancing the overall quality of education. Career guidance and counseling need to be introduced as an integrated component of the curriculum at all stages of the school curriculum with diverse objectives depending upon the needs of the students in each stage of education and to prevent them from anxiety and depression. There is a need to create a stable, supportive, playful environment in families, to build trust in relationship with children so that they do not hide anything from parents, children taking care of themselves, support from parents during tough times, enforcement of clear boundaries and discipline, and creating balance in families.[24]

In India, we still have a long way to go, but counseling is a well-established system in Western countries. Counseling deals with promoting wellness, concern for social justice and advocacy, leadership, personal growth, etc. This would ensure a strong foundation to make school students responsible and dedicated citizens who are the future wealth of India.[16,55]

REFERENCES

1. World Health Organization. (2022). Mental health. [online] Available from: https://www.who.int/news-room/fact-sheets/detail/mental-health-strengthening-our-response/ [Last accessed October, 2023].

2. Study.com. (2022). Behavioural disorders in children: overview and types. [online] Available from: https://study.com/academy/lesson/behavioral-disorders-in-children-definition-symptoms-quiz.html [Last accessed October, 2023].
3. Parry TS. Assessment of developmental learning and behavioural problems in children and young people. Med J Aust. 2005;183:43-8.
4. Hong JS, Tillman R, Luby JL. Disruptive behavior in preschool children: distinguishing normal misbehavior from markers of current and later childhood conduct disorder. J Pediatr. 2015;166:723-30.e1.
5. Wakschlag LS, Choi SW, Carter AS, Hullsiek H, Burns J, McCarthy K, et al. Defining the developmental parameters of temper loss in early childhood: implications for developmental psychopathology. J Child Psychol Psychiatry. 2012;53:1099-108.
6. El-Radhi AS. Management of common behaviour and mental health problems. Br J Nurs. 2015;24:586-90.
7. Gardner F, Shaw DS. Behavioral problems of infancy and preschool children (0-5). In: Rutter M, Bishop DVM, Pine DS, Scott S, Stevenson J, Taylor E, Thapar A. Rutter's Child and Adolescent Psychiatry, 5th edition. New York: Wiley; 2008.
8. Bagner DM, Rodríguez GM, Blake CA, Linares D, Carter AS. Assessment of behavioral and emotional problems in infancy: a systematic review. Clin Child Fam Psychol Rev. 2012;15:113-28.
9. Michalska KJ, Decety J, Zeffiro TA, Lahey BB. Association of regional gray matter volumes in the brain with disruptive behavior disorders in male and female children. Neuroimage Clin. 2014;7:252-7.
10. Fahim C, He Y, Yoon U, Chen J, Evans A, Pérusse D. Neuroanatomy of childhood disruptive behavior disorders. Aggress Behav. 2011;37:326-37.
11. Sebastian CL, McCrory EJ, Cecil CA, Lockwood PL, De Brito SA, Fontaine NM, Viding E. Neural responses to affective and cognitive theory of mind in children with conduct problems and varying levels of callous-unemotional traits. Arch Gen Psychiatry. 2012;69:814-22.
12. Raine A, Yang Y, Narr KL, Toga AW. Sex differences in orbitofrontal gray as a partial explanation for sex differences in antisocial personality. Mol Psychiatry. 2011;16:227-36.
13. Kiehl KA, Smith AM, Mendrek A, Forster BB, Hare RD, Liddle PF. Temporal lobe abnormalities in semantic processing by criminal psychopaths as revealed by functional magnetic resonance imaging. Psychiatry Res. 2004;130:27-42.
14. Kohrt BA, Hruschka DJ, Kohrt HE, Carrion VG, Waldman ID, Worthman CM. Child abuse, disruptive behavior disorders, depression, and salivary cortisol levels among institutionalized and community-residing boys in Mongolia. Asia Pac Psychiatry. 2015;7:7-19.
15. Martel MM, Roberts BA. Prenatal testosterone increases sensitivity to prenatal stressors in males with disruptive behavior disorders. Neurotoxicol Teratol. 2014;44:11-7.
16. Hindustan Times. Krishna was world's first counsellor: IMA Chief. [online] Available from: https://www.hindustantimes.com/india-news/mahabharata-offers-answers-on-psychiatric-issues-krishna-counselled-arjuna-ima-chief/story-38PLCVBtWNbVU1bILEssJP.html [Last accessed October, 2023].
17. Counselling in the Indian context. [online] Available from: https://egyankosh.ac.in/bitstream/123456789/23934/1/Unit-4.pdf. [Last accessed October, 2023].
18. Iyejare O. (2022). Traditional guidance and counseling (definition, advantages and limitations). [online] Available from: https://theselfdiscoveryblog.com/traditional-guidance-and-counseling-definition-advantages-and-limitations/#google_vignette [Last accessed October, 2023].
19. Iyejare O. 9 ways of Improving Counsellor Training Programs in Nigeria. [online] Available from: https://theselfdiscoveryblog.com/9-ways-of-improving-counsellor-training-programs-in-nigeria/ [Last accessed October, 2023].
20. Iyejare O. 7 ways to advocate for guidance and counseling. [online] Available from: https://theselfdiscoveryblog.com/7-ways-to-advocate-for-guidance-and-counseling/ [Last accessed October, 2023].
21. Iyejare O. Full history of guidance and counseling in South Africa (1961 to date). [online] Available from: https://theselfdiscoveryblog.com/history-of-guidance-and-counseling-in-south-africa-1961-to-date/ [Last accessed October, 2023].
22. Townsend family therapy. Adolescent and family therapy. [online] Available from: https://www.townsendfamilytherapy.com/adolescent-family-therapy [Last accessed October, 2023].
23. Healthline. (2015). The most common behavior disorders in children. [online] Available from: https://www.healthline.com/health/parenting/behavioral-disorders-in-children. [Last accessed October, 2023].
24. Tutorialspoint. History of counselling psychology. [online] Available from: https://www.tutorialspoint.com/history-of-counselling-psychology. [Last accessed October, 2023].
25. Stages of counselling-Gather. [online] Available from: http://www.ocw.upj.ac.id/files/Slide-PSY308-PSY308-Slide-13.pdf- [Last accessed October, 2023].
26. Beck JS Cognitive Behavior Therapy: Basics and Beyond, 2nd edition. New York: Guilford Press; 2011.
27. Kendall PC (Ed). Guiding theory for therapy with children and adolescents. In: Child and Adolescent Therapy: Cognitive-Behavioral Procedures, 4th edition. New York: Guilford Press; 2012.
28. Weisz JR, Kazdin AE. Evidence-based Psychotherapies for Children and adolescents, 3rd edition. New York: Guilford Press; 2017.

29. Cognitive therapy. [online] Available from: https://tppul.ckcfood.com/children-and-medication-therapy/19745687.
30. Cognitive behavioural therapy in 7 weeks. Introduction. Gillihan; 10.
31. Rnic K, Dozois DJ, Martin RA. Cognitive distortions, humor styles, and depression. Eur J Psychol. 2016;12(3):348-62.
32. Lazarus AA, Abramovitz A. A multimodal behavioral approach to performance anxiety. J Clin Psychol. 2004; 60(8):831-40.
33. Silicon Valley Recovery. Art therapy. [online] Available from: https://siliconvalleyrecovery.com/drug-and-alcohol-treatment-therapy- options/art-therapy-programs/ [Last accessed October, 2023].
34. Cherry K. What is cognitive behavioral therapy (CBT)? [online] Available from: https://www.verywellmind.com/what-is-cognitive-behavior-therapy-2795747 [Last accessed October, 2023].
35. Lincoln TM, Riehle M, Pillny M, Helbig-Lang S, Fladung AK, Hartmann-Riemer M, et al. Using functional analysis as a framework to guide individualized treatment for negative symptoms. Front Psychol. 2017;8:2108.
36. Ugueto AM, Santucci LC, Krumholz LS, Weisz JR. Problem-solving skills training. In: Sburlati ES, Lyneham HJ, Schniering CA, Rapee RM. Evidence-Based CBT for Anxiety and Depression in Children and Adolescents: a Competencies-Based Approach. New York: Wiley; 2014.
37. Lindgreen P, Lomborg K, Clausen L. Patient experiences using a self-monitoring app in eating disorder treatment: Qualitative study. JMIR Mhealth Uhealth. 2018;6(6):e10253.
38. Tsitsas GD, Paschali AA. A cognitive-behavior therapy applied to a social anxiety disorder and a specific phobia, case study. Health Psychol Res. 2014;2(3):1603.
39. Trauer JM, Qian MY, Doyle JS, Rajaratnam SMW, Cunnington D. Cognitive behavioral therapy for chronic insomnia: A systematic review and meta-analysis. Ann Intern Med. 2015;163(3):191.
40. Agras WS, Fitzsimmons-craft EE, Wilfley DE. Evolution of cognitive-behavioral therapy for eating disorders. Behav Res Ther. 2017;88:26-36.
41. Oud M, De winter L, Vermeulen-Smit E, Bodden D, Nauta M, Stone L, et al. Effectiveness of CBT for children and adolescents with depression: A systematic review and meta-regression analysis. Eur Psychiatry. 2019;57: 33-45.
42. Carpenter J, Andrews L, Witcraft S, Powers M, Smits J, Hofmann S. Cognitive behavioral therapy for anxiety and related disorders: A meta-analysis of randomized placebo-controlled trials. Depress Anxiety. 2018;35(6):502-14.
43. Carroll KM, Kiluk BD. Cognitive behavioral interventions for alcohol and drug use disorders: Through the stage model and back again. Psychol Addict Behav. 2017; 31(8):847-61.
44. Healthline. Cognitive behavioural therapy: What is it and how does it work? [online] Available from: https://www.healthline.com/health/cognitive-behavioral-therapy [Last accessed October, 2023].
45. Cherry K. Types of behavioral disorders in children. [online] Available from: https://www.verywellmind.com/behavioral-disorders-in-children-definition-symptoms-traits-causes-treatment-6889450 [Last accessed October, 2023].
46. Altman M, Wilfley DE. Evidence update on the treatment of overweight and obesity in children and adolescents. J Clin Child Adolesc Psychol. 2014;44(4):521-37.
47. Society of Clinical Child and Adolescent Psychology. (2022). What is family therapy? [online] Available from: https://effectivechildtherapy.org/therapies/what-is-family-therapy/ [Last accessed October, 2023].
48. Janicke DM, Sallinen BJ, Perri MG, Lutes LD, Huerta M, Silverstein JH, et al. Comparison of parent-only vs family-based interventions for overweight children in underserved rural settings: outcomes from project STORY. Arch Pediatr Adolesc Med. 2008;162(12):1119-25.
49. CEBC. Functional family therapy. [online] Available from: https://www.cebc4cw.org/program/functional-family-therapy/ [Last accessed October, 2023].
50. Multidimensional Family Therapy. The proven family-centered treatment for youth. [online] Available from: https://www.mdft.org/what-is-mdft [Last accessed October, 2023].
51. MST Services. Multisystemic therapy. [online] Available from: https://www.mstservices.com/ [Last accessed October, 2023].
52. Jawahar P. Comorbidity of conduct disorders and learning disabilities of upper primary children in relation to academic performance. Thesis, Alagappa University, 2016. [online] Available from: http://hdl.handle.net/10603/201864 [Last accessed October, 2023].
53. Kolko DJ, Perrin E. The integration of behavioral health interventions in children's health care: services, science, and suggestions. J Clin Child Adolesc Psychol. 2014;43:216-28.
54. American Academy of Child and Adolescent Psychiatry (AACAP). A Guide to Building Collaborative Mental Health Care Partnerships. In: Pediatric Primary Care; 2010. pp. 1-27. [online] Available from: https://www.aacap.org/App_Themes/AACAP/docs/clinical_practice_center/guide_to_building_collaborative_mental_health_care_partnerships.pdf [Last accessed October, 2023].
55. XNSPY. Surviving teenage: How tough is it for Indian teenagers nowadays. [online] Available from: https://xnspy.com/blog/surviving-teenage-how-tough-is-it-for-indian-teenagers-nowadays.html#:~:text=Indian%20teens%20today%20are%20forced,path%20of%20becoming%20an%20adult [Last accessed October, 2023].

Chapter 27

Mobile and Behavioral Disorders in Children

Pradeep Jain, BD Gupta

INTRODUCTION

As we continue to explore the intersection of technology and child development, it is important to delve into the relationship between mobile device usage and behavioral disorders in children. With the ever-increasing trends of mobile device usage, availability of multiple mobile devices to the majority at affordable prices, from smartphones to tablets, our understanding of their impacts on childhood behavior is of paramount importance. The American Academy of Pediatrics (2016) agreed and recommended children using technology alone should be avoided.[1] This chapter will give view in depth of this complex and rapidly evolving field, examining the current research and discussing the various behavioral disorders that can occur by excessive mobile device usage, and also, offering guidance for parents, educators, and healthcare professionals.

DEFINITION

Excessive Mobile Use

There is no one-size-fits-all definition of excessive mobile use by children, as the amount of time that is excessive will vary depending on the child's age, stage of mental development, and individual needs.[2] Mobile phone use is considered excessive if it fulfils the following criteria:

- Using mobile phone for >2 h/day
- Having difficulty staying off their mobile phone, even when it is not needed
- Becoming irritable or anxious not allowed to use their mobile phone
- Choosing to use their mobile phone over other activities, such as spending time with family and friends or playing outside
- Experiencing problems at school or in other areas of their life due to their mobile phone use.

EXTENT OF USE AND MAGNITUDE OF PROBLEM

The use of mobile devices by children in India has been significantly increasing in recent years driven by factors such as increased affordability, accessibility, and advancements in technology.[3] While specific statistics on the magnitude of the problem in India may vary, several key points highlight the concerns associated with mobile device use among children:

- *Increasing smartphone penetration:* India has witnessed a substantial increase in smartphone penetration, with a significant number of households owning at least one smartphone. This widespread availability of mobile devices has contributed to children having greater access to smartphones and tablets.
- *Age of initiation:* Children in India are starting to use mobile devices at increasingly younger ages. This early exposure to digital technology raises concerns about the potential impact on their development, social interactions, and overall well-being.
- *Internet accessibility:* With the increasing availability of affordable mobile internet plans and the expansion of network coverage, children in India have easier access to online content. While the internet provides valuable educational resources, it also exposes children to potential risks, including inappropriate content, cyberbullying, online predators, and scams.

FACTORS RESPONSIBLE FOR EXCESSIVE MOBILE USE BY CHILDREN

Several factors contribute to the increased mobile device use by children.[4] These factors can vary based on individual, societal, and technological influences. Some key factors are as follows:

- *Technological advancements:* The rapid advancement of mobile technology, including the availability of

affordable smartphones and tablets, has made mobile devices more accessible to children.
- The increasing capabilities, features, and interactive nature of these devices make them attractive and engaging for children.
- *Peer influence:* Children are influenced by their peers, and if their friends or classmates are using mobile devices, they may feel pressure to do the same.
- Social norms and the desire to fit in can drive children to adopt mobile device use at younger ages or spend more time on them.
- *Parental influence and digital parenting:* The attitudes and behaviors of parents play a significant role in shaping a child's mobile device use. Mostly, parents themselves handover their device to children to play while they do their household tasks. If parents themselves are heavy mobile device users or have lax rules and monitoring, children may adopt similar habits. Conversely, if parents set limits and provide guidance, it can help regulate a child's mobile device use.
- *Rise of social media:* Social media platforms such as Facebook, Twitter, and Instagram have become increasingly popular among children, and they provide a way for children to connect with friends and family, as well as to share their thoughts and experiences with the world.
- *Entertainment and media consumption:* Mobile devices provide a wide range of entertainment options, including games, videos, social media, and streaming platforms. Children are drawn to the interactive and engaging nature of these activities, which can lead to increased mobile device use for entertainment and media consumption purposes.
- *Educational opportunities:* Mobile devices offer access to educational apps, e-learning platforms, and online resources that can enhance learning experiences. Parents and educators may encourage mobile device use for educational purposes, leading to increased usage time.
- *Digital connectivity and communication:* Mobile devices facilitate instant communication and connectivity, allowing children to stay in touch with friends and family through messaging apps, social media, or video calls.
- *Desire to maintain social connections* and stay updated can contribute to increased mobile device use.
- *Digital dependency and addiction:* Children, like adults, can develop a dependency on mobile devices. The addictive nature of certain apps, games, and platforms, combined with the constant availability of digital content, can lead to excessive use and difficulty in self-regulation.

UNDERSTANDING THE IMPACT OF MOBILE DEVICES ON CHILDREN

Mobile technology has profoundly changed the way children interact with the world. They can access a wealth of information, communicate with others, and engage in interactive activities.

ADVANTAGES OF MOBILE

- *Increased social interaction:*[5] Mobile phones can help children *stay connected* with their friends and family, even when they are not physically together. This can be especially beneficial for children who live in rural areas or who have difficulty making friends.
- *Access to information:* Mobile phones can provide children with access to a wealth of information, including educational resources, news articles, and entertainment. This can help children learn and grow.
- *Improved safety:* Mobile phones can be used to track children's whereabouts and to contact them in an emergency. This can help to keep children safe.
- *Development of digital skills:* Using mobile phones can help children develop their digital skills, which are increasingly important in today's world.

HARMS ASSOCIATED WITH MOBILE PHONES

While these devices provide numerous benefits, they also pose potential risks to children's mental and emotional health.[1,2,6]

A cross-sectional study was conducted at the OPD in the department of pediatrics at a tertiary care teaching institute. All the children attending the OPD below the age of 15 years were included in the study during the period of January 2017 to March 2017. A total of 450 children were enrolled in the study.[7]

Results: In the study, 277 (61.5%) participants were boys and 173 (38.5%) were girls. 414 (92.1%) parents were using mobile phones and 350 (77.8%) parents had smartphones. Majority (194; 43.1%) of the children were using mobiles for 1–3 hours followed by 130 (28.8%) children who used mobiles for >4 hours. Physical morbidities such as decreased physical activity in 189 (45.8%) children, laziness in 143 (34.7%) children, pain in fingers and wrist in 76 (18.5%) children, and eye symptoms in 148 (35.7%) children were observed. Mental issues faced were throwing tantrums if mobile is not given in 187 (45.3%) children, not obeying parents in 110 (26.6%) children, and reduced grades in school in 89 (21.4%) children.

Conclusions: The study concluded that the use of mobile phones by young generation has increased resulting physical, social, and psychological impact. It is the role of the family to regulate the use and guide the children for proper usage of mobile phones.

The "Always-On" Culture

One significant impact of mobile devices is the creation of an "always-on" culture, where children are constantly connected to their devices. This often results in excessive screen time, which can disrupt normal sleep patterns, lead to sedentary behavior, and reduce the time spent on physical activities and face-to-face social interactions. The constant access to mobile devices can blur the boundaries between school, leisure, and personal life, making it challenging for children to disconnect and engage in other essential activities. This can lead to a decrease in overall well-being and a potential increase in behavioral difficulties.

Impaired Social Skills

Frequent use of mobile devices can hinder the development of essential social skills in children. Excessive screen time may limit face-to-face interactions, affect communication skills, and lead to difficulties in forming and maintaining relationships.

Immersion in Virtual Worlds

Mobile devices allow children to immerse themselves in virtual worlds, often reducing their engagement in real-world activities. Whether it is playing video games, browsing social media, or consuming online content, children may spend significant amounts of time in virtual environments. This can lead to feelings of isolation and loneliness, as well as a disconnection from the physical world and real-life social interactions. Over time, this immersion in virtual worlds can contribute to the development of social anxiety and depression. Moreover, the constant exposure to unrealistic standards portrayed in media can negatively impact body image and self-esteem, particularly among adolescents.

Developmental Considerations

It is important to consider the developmental stage of children when examining the impact of mobile devices. Younger children, for instance, are more vulnerable to the potential negative effects as their brains are still developing. Excessive screen time during crucial developmental periods can interfere with cognitive, social, and emotional development, potentially impacting their ability to regulate emotions, develop empathy, and engage in imaginative play. Additionally, the reliance on mobile devices for entertainment and stimulation may hinder the development of essential life skills such as problem-solving, creativity, and self-regulation in real life.[7]

Sleep Disruptions

The use of mobile devices, especially close to bedtime, can significantly disrupt children's sleep patterns. The blue light emitted by screens can suppress the production of melatonin, the hormone that is responsible for regulating sleep. Consequently, children may experience difficulties falling asleep or maintaining a healthy sleep duration, which can impact their mood, cognitive functioning, and overall behavior.

Impact on Physical Health

Excessive mobile device usage is often associated with sedentary behavior, reducing the time children spend engaging in physical activities. This lack of physical exercise can contribute to an increased risk of obesity, cardiovascular problems, and other physical health issues. Furthermore, prolonged periods of screen time can lead to poor posture.

MOBILE DEVICES AND BEHAVIORAL DISORDERS

Mobile-related behavioral disorders in children refer to the negative behavioral and psychological effects that can arise from excessive or inappropriate use of mobile devices such as smartphones and tablets. Researchers have identified a link between excessive mobile device usage and various behavioral disorders in children. Although the nature of this relationship is complex and multifaceted, it is clear that mobile devices can play a role in the development and exacerbation of these disorders. It can easily be considered as at least a comorbid condition. A few common mobile-related behavioral disorders in children are as given in the following text.

Attention Deficit Hyperactivity Disorder

Negative Impact of Mobile on Attention Deficit Hyperactivity Disorder

- Excessive screen time can lead to problems with attention and concentration, potentially contributing to symptoms of attention deficit hyperactivity disorder (ADHD). Children who spend a lot of time with mobile devices may struggle to focus on tasks that require sustained attention, leading to difficulties in academic and social settings.
  - *Distraction and impulsivity:* Individuals with ADHD often struggle with maintaining focus and regulating impulsivity. Mobile phones, with their constant notifications, social media updates, and access to various apps and games, can exacerbate these difficulties. The instant and frequent distractions provided by mobile devices can make it challenging for individuals with ADHD to stay focused on tasks or activities. The allure of new information and the need for constant stimulation can lead to a cycle of checking and rechecking the phone, hindering productivity, and attention span.
  - *Hyperfocus:* While individuals with ADHD may struggle with maintaining focus in certain situations, they may also experience a state of hyperfocus. Hyperfocus refers to becoming intensely absorbed in a particular task or activity of interest. Mobile phones, with their interactive and engaging features, can capture attention and trigger hyperfocus in individuals with ADHD. This can lead to spending excessive amounts of time on the device, often to the detriment of other responsibilities, such as schoolwork, work tasks, or personal relationships.
- *Time management and productivity:* Managing time and staying organized can be challenging for individuals with ADHD. Mobile phones, with their multitasking capabilities, can make it even more difficult to prioritize tasks, adhere to schedules, and complete assignments or work in a timely manner. The constant availability of entertainment, social media, and online activities can lead to procrastination and difficulty in allocating time effectively.
- *Sleep disturbances:* Sleep difficulties are common in individuals with ADHD, and the use of mobile phones, especially before bedtime, can exacerbate this issue. The blue light emitted by screens can interfere with the body's natural sleep-wake cycle, making it harder to fall asleep and have a restful night. Additionally, the stimulating content and the temptation to engage with the device can keep individuals with ADHD awake for longer periods, further disrupting their sleep patterns.

Positive Impact of Mobile on Attention Deficit Hyperactivity Disorder

Digital organization and reminders: On a positive note, mobile phones can also be a helpful tool for individuals with ADHD in terms of organization and reminders. Various apps and features can assist individuals in keeping track of appointments, tasks, and deadlines. Calendar apps, to-do lists, and reminder notifications can provide structure and assistance in managing daily routines and responsibilities.

Anxiety and Depression

The overuse of mobile devices can also contribute to feelings of anxiety and depression. Children may feel pressured to maintain a constant online presence or may experience cyberbullying. Furthermore, excessive use of social media apps can lead to unhealthy comparisons with others, resulting in low self-esteem and depressive symptoms.

Mobile Phone Use and Autism

The relationship between mobile and autism, a neurodevelopmental disorder, has been a subject of interest and research. Autism is a complex condition, and while we can provide some general information, it is important to note that individuals with autism can have diverse experiences and responses to mobile phone usage.

- *Sensory sensitivities:* Many individuals with autism have sensory sensitivities, which can include sensitivity to auditory, visual, and tactile stimuli. Mobile phones, with their bright screens, notifications, and sounds, may contribute to sensory overload for some individuals with autism. The constant stimulation and unpredictability of mobile devices can be overwhelming and lead to increased anxiety or discomfort.
- *Special interests and routines:* Individuals with autism often have special interests and may adhere to specific routines and patterns. Mobile phones can provide a platform for individuals with autism to engage with their special interests or establish comforting routines.

They might find solace in using specific apps or engaging with particular content on mobile devices.
- *Social communication and interaction:* Mobile phones can have both positive and negative impacts on social communication and interaction skills for individuals with autism. On one hand, mobile devices can provide a means for social connection, particularly through text-based communication or social media platforms. This can offer individuals with autism an opportunity to communicate and connect with others in a way that is comfortable for them. On the other hand, excessive mobile phone use can lead to social isolation or difficulty engaging in face-to-face interactions.
- *Technology-assisted communication:* Mobile phones and related apps can be valuable tools for individuals with autism who use augmentative and alternative communication (AAC) systems. AAC apps on mobile devices can support communication for individuals who have limited verbal speech or face challenges in expressive language. These apps can enhance communication abilities and provide a portable and accessible means of expression.

Parental Concerns and Monitoring

Parents of children with autism may have concerns about their child's mobile phone use. They may worry about potential risks, such as exposure to inappropriate content or excessive screen time. Parental monitoring and setting appropriate boundaries around mobile phone usage can help address these concerns and ensure a safe and balanced use of technology.

It is essential to recognize that every individual with autism is unique, and their experiences and responses to mobile phone usage can vary. It is important for parents, caregivers, and professionals to assess the specific needs of individuals with autism and make informed decisions regarding mobile phone use based on individual strengths, challenges, and developmental goals. Consulting with healthcare professionals or autism specialists can provide more personalized guidance on managing mobile phone usage for individuals with autism.

Behavioral Addiction

Children can develop behavioral addictions to their mobile devices, exhibiting signs of withdrawal when separated from their devices. This can have a significant impact on their emotional well-being and daily functioning, leading to a decline in academic performance and physical health.

Internet Addiction

Excessive use of mobile devices, particularly the internet, can lead to internet addiction. Children may become preoccupied with online activities, experience withdrawal symptoms when not using their devices, and neglect other important areas of their life.

Nomophobia

Nomophobia, short for "no-mobile-phone phobia", is the fear of being without a mobile device. Children may experience anxiety or panic when they do not have access to their smartphones or when the battery is low.

Cyberbullying

Mobile devices provide a platform for cyberbullying, which involves the use of technology to harass, intimidate, or humiliate others. Children who are victims of cyberbullying may display emotional distress, social withdrawal, and declining academic performance.

Some authors have also described the following disorders:
- *Textaphrenia* (thinking that they have heard a message come in or felt the device vibrate when it actually has not)
- *Textiety* (feeling anxious of not receiving any texts or not being able to send any)
- *Post-traumatic text disorder* (physical and mental injuries related to texting)
- *Binge texting* (sending multiple texts to feel good about themselves and to attract responses).[8]

STRATEGIES FOR MANAGING EXCESSIVE MOBILE DEVICE USAGE

Given the potential risks associated with excessive mobile device usage, it is crucial for parents and educators to implement strategies to manage children's screen time.[9] Excessive mobile use by children can have negative impacts on their physical and mental health, as well as their overall development. Some strategies for managing excessive mobile use are as follows:
- *Set clear limits and boundaries*: Establish clear guidelines regarding mobile phone usage, including specific time limits and designated "phone-free" zones

or times, such as during meals or before bedtime. Consistency is key in enforcing these rules.
- *Lead by example:* Children are more likely to follow rules if they see their parents or caregivers adhering to them as well. Model healthy mobile phone habits by reducing your own screen time and being present and engaged when interacting with your child.
- *Encourage alternative activities:* Encourage children to engage in a variety of activities that do not involve mobile phones. This could include physical activities, hobbies, reading, creative play, or spending time with friends and family. Provide them with options and support their interests.
- *Foster open communication:* Create an environment where children feel comfortable discussing their mobile phone usage and any challenges they may face. Encourage open conversations about the benefits and drawbacks of excessive screen time and work together to find solutions.
- *Establish tech-free zones:* Designate certain areas of the house, such as bedrooms or study areas, as tech-free zones. Keep mobile phones and other screens out of these areas to promote healthier habits and minimize distractions.
- *Use parental control apps:* Utilize parental control apps or features available on mobile devices to monitor and limit your child's screen time. These tools can help you set restrictions, block certain apps or websites, and track usage patterns.
- *Encourage outdoor and social activities:* Encourage children to participate in outdoor activities, sports, and social interactions. Plan family outings, involve them in community activities, and encourage face-to-face interactions with peers.
- *Educate about responsible mobile phone use:* Teach children about responsible mobile phone use, including the importance of privacy, online safety, and the potential consequences of excessive screen time. Help them understand the value of balance and self-regulation.
- *Provide alternative entertainment:* Ensure that your child has access to other forms of entertainment, such as books, puzzles, board games, or art supplies. Provide a variety of stimulating activities that can capture their interest and attention.
- *Monitor and track usage:* Keep an eye on your child's mobile phone usage and monitor the apps they use and the content they access. Regularly reviewing their activity can help you identify excessive use and address it promptly.

Remember that it is important to approach the management of excessive mobile use with empathy and understanding. Be supportive of your child's challenges and help them develop healthy habits that will benefit them in the long run.

TREATMENT OF MOBILE ADDICTION

Mobile addiction, also known as smartphone addiction or problematic mobile device use, is a condition where individuals develop a compulsive and excessive reliance on their mobile devices, leading to negative consequences in various areas of their lives. Some strategies for treating mobile addiction are as follows:[10]

- *Recognize the problem:* The first step in addressing mobile addiction is acknowledging the issue and understanding its impact on your life. Reflect on the negative consequences it has caused in your relationships, work or school performance, physical health, and overall well-being.
- *Set goals:* Establish clear goals related to reducing mobile device use and regaining control over your time and attention. Define specific objectives, such as limiting screen time, restricting usage in certain situations, or focusing on alternative activities.
- *Create a schedule:* Develop a structured schedule that includes designated times for using mobile device and times of off-limits. Stick to the schedule and gradually reduce the amount of time spent on your device.
- *Practice digital detox:* Consider taking regular breaks or engaging in digital detox periods where you completely abstain from using your mobile device. This allows you to reset your habits and develop healthier relationships with technology.
- *Use productivity apps:* Utilize productivity apps or features on your mobile device that help you manage and limit your usage. These can include apps that track your screen time, set reminders for breaks, or block access to certain apps or websites.
- *Establish device-free zones:* Designate certain areas or times in your home or workplace where mobile devices are not allowed. This helps create boundaries and encourages you to focus on other activities or interactions.

CONCLUSION

It is important to approach the management of excessive mobile use with empathy and understanding. Be supportive of your child's challenges and help them develop healthy habits that will benefit them in the long run. Parents are role model for their children and kids follow the pattern their parents are creating; hence, parents have to themselves restrict use of mobile phones, especially in front of their children to prevent over-relying on mobile to tackle boredom at its earliest. Parents can get involved into creative activities with their children which improve family bonding as well as negate the craving for attention in the child.

REFERENCES

1. American Academy of Pediatrics. Media and young minds. Pediatrics. 2016;138(5):1-6.
2. Gangadharan N, Borle AL, Basu S. Mobile phone addiction as an emerging behavioral form of addiction among adolescents in India. Cureus. 2022;14(4):e23798.
3. Sun S. Statista. Smartphone penetration rate in India from 2009 to 2023, with estimates until 2040. Statista. [online] Available from: https://www.statista.com/statistics/1229799/india-smartphone-penetration-rate/ [Last accessed October, 2023].
4. Olasina G, Kheswa S. Exploring the factors of excessive smartphone use by undergraduate students. Knowledge Management ELearning. 2021;13(1):118-41.
5. Krista W. (2020). The Effects of Technology in Early Childhood. Master's Theses & Capstone Projects. [online] Available from: https://nwcommons.nwciowa.edu/education_masters/246 [Last accessed October, 2023].
6. Wacks Y, Weinstein AM. Addictive disorders. Front Psychiatry. 2021;12. [online] Available from: https://doi.org/10.3389/fpsyt.2021.669042 [Last accessed October, 2023].
7. Miyashita C, Yamazaki K, Tamura N, Ikeda-Araki A, Suyama S, Hikage T, et al. Cross-sectional associations between early mobile device usage and problematic behaviors among school-aged children in the Hokkaido Study on Environment and Children's Health. Environ Health Prev Med. 2023;28:22.
8. Nehra R, Kate N, Grover S, Khehra N, Basu D. Does the Excessive use of Mobile Phones in Young Adults Reflect an Emerging Behavioral Addiction? J Postgrad Med Edu Res. 2012;46(4):177-82.
9. Terras MM, Judith R. Family digital literacy practices and children's mobile le Phone use. Front Psychol. 2016;7. [online] Available from: https://doi.org/10.3389/fpsyg.2016.01957 [Last accessed October, 2023].
10. Young KS, De Abreu CN. Internet Addiction in Children and Adolescents: Risk Factors, Assessment. [ebook]. Springer; 2017.

Chapter 28: Pharmacology of Behavioral Disorders

Archana Vyas

INTRODUCTION

Mental health disorders in children are very common and include emotional and behavioral disorders [anxiety, depression, impulsive control, conduct disorders, obsessive compulsive disorder, attention deficit hyperactivity disorder (ADHD), etc.], developmental disorders (Speech and Language Delays, Intellectual Disability, etc.) and pervasive disorders (autistic spectrum disorders). During the first 2 years of life, challenging behaviors and emotional problems are most likely to be considered problems rather than disorders. These problems may include self-harm, physical or verbal violence, nondiscipline, disturbance of the environment, poor vocalization, and stereotypes. When children are unable to adapt to the complex world around them, they may exhibit strange behaviors and this can lead to the development of behavioral disorders or behavioral problems.[1]

While the DSM-V (Diagnostic and Statistical Manual of Mental Disorders, Fifth Edition) and the ICD 11 (International Classification of Diseases, 11th Revision) are generally accepted as the most common criteria for diagnosing mental and behavioral disorders in children and adults but for the sake of clarity and based on the idea of externalizing emotions (emotions and behaviors directed toward the child's environment, causing difficulties for their external world) and internalizing emotions and behaviors (originating from within, causing subjective distress), these disorders can be classified as: Externalizing disorders (ADHD, oppositional defiant disorder, conduct disorder, substance use disorders) and internalizing disorders (depression disorders, anxiety disorders, eating disorders, and post-traumatic stress disorder). Categorizing these disorders into separate groups does not provide a watertight compartment for them and they often have overlapping symptoms such as: A child with ADHD, because of poor school performance may exhibit features of depression and anxiety and likewise, child with substance use disorder may ultimately land up into conduct disorders. These children require holistic management with both pharmacological and nonpharmacological approaches as well as drug polytherapy for concomitant disorders.[2]

PREVALENCE OF BEHAVIORAL AND EMOTIONAL DISORDERS IN CHILDHOOD

The prevalence of various emotional and behavioral disorders in children is difficult to be accurately estimated due to the difficulties of research methodology that relies on subjective assessment and different definitions. As per 2001 World Health Organization (WHO) report, the 6-month prevalence rate of any mental health disorder in children and youth up to 17 years of age was 20.9%, with disruptive behavior disorder being the second most common (10.3%) and anxiety disorders being the most common (13%). Approximately 5% of children in the general population have depression at any time in their lives, and girls are more likely to experience it than boys (54%). A similar survey conducted in the United States in 2005–2011, the National Survey of Children's Health (NSCH), involving 78,042 households, found that 4.2% of children of 3–17 years of age had a past history of disruptive behavior disorder, which was twice as high in boys (6.0% vs. 4.7%), and 3.9% in girls (4.9% vs. 1.1%).[3]

PSYCHOPHARMACOLOGY: HISTORICAL BACKGROUND AND THE PRESENT STATUS

Psychopharmacology is the field of research that focuses on the clinical benefits of psychoactive drugs, their properties that influence how they respond, side effects, toxicity, and interactions between drugs. Psychoactive drugs or psychopharmacologic agents are those that have the greatest impact on psychological processes. In the early and mid-20th century, children with behavioral disorders were classified as "problem children" and, depending on the severity of the disorder, they were treated with psychotherapy and medication in outpatient clinics or in residential institutions. At the time, discoveries of psychotropic drugs for pediatric use were accidental. In 1937, George Bardley, a psychiatrist, conducted a study on 30 children with behavioral disorders at the "Bardley home for Problem Children" in America. He reported a 50% improvement in the children's behavior.

Stimulants started being used in "minimal brain dysfunction" and treatment of enuresis was being carried out by antidepressants. In the 1970s, research methodology developed and in the 1980s, double-blinded studies showed that stimulants were highly effective in treating ADHD in children. This was the start of evidence-based use of drugs for mental health problems. Over the past 50 years, research in psychoactive drugs has made great strides. Psychoactive drug actions are mainly mediated through neurotransmitters in the central nervous system (CNS). The field of psychopharmacological drug research is concerned with the clinical benefits, properties that affect action of psychoactive drugs, adverse reactions, toxicity, and drug–drug interactions. Psychological drugs may be used for emotional and/or behavioral symptoms in the absence of response to evidence-based non-pharmacological therapies, or in the presence of significant distress, functional disability or risk of injury. The selection of drugs is dependent on the predominant behavior and/or the underlying cause of the symptoms. Best practice principles must be followed to ensure that drugs are used safely and appropriately, including planning treatment and monitoring for adverse effects, obtaining consent or asset, implementation of treatment and monitoring of patients for adverse effects.[4]

MANAGEMENT STRATEGIES AND ROLE OF PHARMACOTHERAPY IN TREATMENT OF BEHAVIORAL DISORDERS IN CHILDREN

The success of treatment strategies is dependent on a thorough evaluation of symptoms, socioeconomic factors, the impact of family and caregivers, child's development, and physical health. This requires a multidisciplinary approach that includes experts in psychology, psychiatry, behavior analysis, nursing, social care, speech and language, education, occupational therapy, physical therapy, pediatrician, and pharmacist. Generally, pharmacotherapy is used in conjunction with psychological and other treatments.

Holistic management involves combining a variety of interventions, such as cognitive behavioral therapy (CBT), behavioral modification, and social communication techniques, as well as parenting skill training, psychopharmacology, and psychosocial treatment. Several studies have shown that combining psychosocial and pharmacological therapies can be effective in treating children with emotional and behavioral disorders. A meta-analysis of 16 randomized trials and one randomized controlled trial involving 2,668 children with ADHD showed that the combination of pharmacotherapy and psychotherapy led to clinically significant reductions in core symptoms. The psychosocial treatment itself, which combined behavioral, cognitive behavioral, and skill training techniques, showed small-to-medium-sized improvements in parent-rated ADHD symptoms and in interpersonal functioning.[3,5]

PSYCHOPHARMACOLOGY OF BEHAVIORAL DISORDERS

Drugs are prescribed as part of a comprehensive treatment plan for childhood behavioral disorders in addition to other therapies. The most extensive evidence of pharmacotherapy is for the use of drugs for the treatment of ADHD in children and adolescents. The evidence of pharmacotherapy for the treatment of other behavioral disorders is less extensive, but there is a renewed interest in this area. The main classes of drugs used for various behavioral disorders are presented in **Table 1**.[3]

DRUGS FOR ATTENTION DEFICIT HYPERACTIVITY DISORDER

The following section will provide information on the drugs used in ADHD, their mechanisms of action, clinical effectiveness, pharmacokinetics, side effects, and guidelines. As consistent evidence from studies shows that pharmacological therapy is beneficial and effective in treating ADHD. Psychopharmacological treatments for ADHD include psychostimulants such as methylphenidate (mpH), dexamphetamines and amphetamine (AMP) derivatives, as well as nonpsychoactive medications such as atomoxetine and guanfacine.

TABLE 1: Classes of drugs commonly used in childhood behavioral disorders.

Group	Common examples	Indications for use	Common side effects	Follow-up monitoring
Traditional antipsychotics	Haloperidol, chlorpromazine, trifluoperazine, pimozide	Schizophrenia, bipolar disorder, schizoaffective disorder, obsessive-compulsive disorder, depression, aggression, mood instability, and irritability in autistic disorders	Tremors, muscle spasms, abnormal movements, stiffness, blurred vision and constipation	Blood pressure checks, cholesterol testing, heart rate checks, blood sugar testing, electrocardiogram, height, and weight and blood chemistry tests
Atypical antipsychotics	Aripiprazole, clozapine, olanzapine, quetiapine, risperidone, and ziprasidone	Schizophrenia, bipolar disorder, schizoaffective disorder, obsessive-compulsive disorder, depression, aggression, mood instability, and irritability in ASD	Low white blood cell count (agranulocytosis – with clozapine), diabetes, lipid abnormalities, eight gain, other medication-specific side effects	Frequent blood tests (clozapine), blood pressure checks, cholesterol testing, heart rate checks, blood sugar testing, electrocardiogram, height, and weight and blood chemistry tests
Tricyclic antidepressants	Amitriptyline, desipramine, doxepin, and imipramine	Depression, anxiety, seasonal affective, disorder, OCD, post-traumatic stress disorder, social anxiety, bed-wetting, and premenstrual syndrome	Dry mouth, constipation, blurry vision, urinary retention, dizziness, drowsiness	Watch for worsening of depression and thoughts about suicide. Blood tests and blood pressure monitoring may be needed
Selective Serotonin Reuptake Inhibitors	Citalopram, escitalopram, fluoxetine, fluvoxamine, and sertraline	Depression, anxiety, seasonal affective, disorder, OCD, post-traumatic stress disorder, social anxiety, bed-wetting, and premenstrual syndrome	Headache, nervousness, nausea insomnia, weight loss	Watch for unusual bruises, bleeding from the gums when brushing teeth, if taking other medications, blood tests and blood pressure checks may be needed
Stimulants	Methylphenidate immediate release and modified release (e.g., Concerta XL, Equasym XL), dexamfetamines immediate release and modified release (e.g., Lisdexamfetamine)	ADHD	Decreased appetite/weight loss, sleep problems, jitteriness, restless, headaches, dry mouth, dysphoria, feeling sad, anxiety, increased heart rate, and dizziness, abuse liability	Blood pressure and heart rate will be checked before treatment and periodically during treatment. Child's height and weight are monitored
Nonstimulants	Atomoxetine	ADHD	Diarrhea, xerostomia, appetite loss, insomnia, somnolence, depression, mood swings, and palpitation, hepatitis	Blood pressure and heart rate will be checked before treatment and periodically during treatment. Child's height and weight are Monitored. LFT
Alpha-2 agonists	Clonidine, guanfacine	ADHD	Transient increase in BP, rebound hypertension, hepatotoxicity	Do not stop these medications suddenly without slowly reducing (tapering) the dose as directed by the clinician

Contd…

Contd...

Group	Common examples	Indications for use	Common Side effects	Follow-up monitoring
Benzodiazepines	Lorazepam, clonazepam, diazepam, alprazolam, oxazepam	Anxiety, Panic disorder	Drowsiness, dizziness, sleepiness, confusion, memory loss, blurry vision, balance problems, worsening behavior	
Antihistamines	Hydroxyzine HCl, Hydroxyzine, Pamoate, Alimemazine	Anxiety, bruxism, and sleep problems	Drowsiness, dizziness, sleepiness, confusion, memory loss	
Sleep-enhancers	Zolpidem, Zaleplon, Diphenhydramine, Trazodone	Insomnia (short-term)	Headache, dizziness, weakness, nausea, memory loss, daytime sleepiness, hallucinations, dry mouth, confusion, blurred vision, balance problems, heartburn	

(ADHD: attention-deficit hyperactivity disorder; ASD: autistic spectrum disorder; PTSD: post-traumatic stress disorder; OCD: obsessive-compulsive disorder)
Source: Modified from: Ogundele MO. Behavioural and emotional disorders in childhood: A brief overview for paediatricians. World J Clin Pediatr. 2018;7(1):9-26.

Psychostimulants

Dexamphetamine, amphetamine, and MPH are the most effective drugs for ADHD, with a response rate of around 70%, which may rise to 95% when nonresponders are treated with a second drug. Significant problem with amphetamine is that it is listed under controlled substance, which restricts its use for treatment of children.

Molecular Mechanism of Action

Dexamphetamine, amphetamine, and MPH enhance release and function of noradrenaline (NA) and dopamine (DA) in the CNS, they have a rapid onset of action and act by blocking or even reversing reuptake in respective monoamine transporters. It also increases catecholamine release from synaptic vesicles. Thus, there is increased concentration of NA and DA in the synaptic cleft. The therapeutic effects on behavior and attention are presumed to be related to enhanced neurotransmission of this catecholamine, especially in prefrontal cortex.

At therapeutic doses, DA and NA work in tandem to increase catecholaminergic neuron's firing rate, resulting in enhanced signaling, especially in the prefrontal cortex. When performing cognitive tasks, MPH increases cerebral blood flow to the prefrontal cortex and the posterior parietal cortex, while significantly reducing blood flow to other brain regions. This suggests reduced metabolic activation in brain regions that are not relevant to the task.

In recent studies, both drugs have been shown to modify functional connectivity. For example, in children with ADHD, there is a raised motivational threshold, at which task-relevant stimuli become sufficiently relevant to deactivate a default mode network. Treatment with TMZ normalizes this motivational threshold.[6]

Pharmacokinetics

Amphetamine: Absorption is rapid, onset of action is within 1 hour after administration, peak plasma therapeutic doses, plasma levels reach at about 3 hours. It is metabolized in liver by various P450 enzymes. Food can delay its absorption. Amphetamine requires at least twice daily administration. Mixtures of different d-AMP and dl-AMP salt formulations are available.

Lisdexamphetamine (LDX) is a preparation in which L-lysine is attached to dextroamphetamine (DEX). LDX is not pharmacologically active and does not produce high DEX levels upon injection or snort, making it less likely to be abused. After oral administration, the amide linkages between the two molecules are hydrolyzed, resulting in the release of active DEX. This hydrolysis occurs mainly in red blood cells, and both DEX (Dextroamphetamine) and LDX (Lisdexamphetamine) follow linear kinetics, with no drug accumulation.

Dose: The Food and Drug Administration (FDA) approved for adults and children >3 years of age.
- *<3 years:* Not recommended
- *3-5 years:* Start with 2.5 mg daily; increase by 2.5 mg weekly until optimal response. *Maximum dose:* 40 mg once daily
- *>6 years:* 5 mg/day initially, increase by 5 mg weekly until optimal response. *Max dose:* 40 mg/day.

Methylphenidate: Oral MPH is quickly absorbed from the digestive tract, reaching peak plasma levels 1–3 hours postadministration, with a half-life of approximately 3–3.5 hours. Due to this short half-life, steady state of oral MPH cannot be achieved during normal treatment. Various drug formulations offer a combination of immediate and prolonged release of MPH, they differ in the mechanism of delayed release system, and the ratio of immediate to delayed release of MPH, e.g., the effects of Concreta XL or Matoride XL last 10–12 hours, while Equasym XL or Ritalin LA is a mid-release formulation with effects lasting 6–8 hours. Some transdermal patches (Daytrana), when worn for 9 hours, allow about 12-hour effects. The most recent long-term liquid preparation of MPH is quillivant XR (5 mg/mL). Peak plasma levels appear after 5 hours, and effects last approximately 12 hours.

Drug interactions: These drugs have the potential to block the absorption of anticonvulsive drugs, including phenobarbitone and phenytoin, as well as primidone and the tricyclic antidepressant. They may also potentiate the stimulatory effects of other medications on the cardiovascular and CNS, and may increase the pressor response of vasopressor agents.

Dose: The FDA approved for adults and children >6 years of age.

Initial: 0.3 mg/kg/dose orally before breakfast and lunch. May increase by 0.1 mg/kg/dose per week; *Maximum dose:* 60 mg/day. *Maintenance:* 0.3–1 mg/kg orally before breakfast and lunch. Maximum dose: 2 mg/kg/day in two divided doses.[6,11-13]

Nondopaminergic Medications

Currently, two nondopaminergic drugs are approved for treatment of ADHD: the selective nonadrenaline reuptake inhibitor, atomoxetine (ATX), and the alpha-2 agonist, guanfacine, and clonidine. The primary clinical differences between these drugs and dopaminergic medications are their favorable legal status, their long-term (up to 24 hours) clinical efficacy, and their slower onset of action (at least several weeks).

Atomoxetine

Mechanism of action: The mechanism of action of this drug is to inhibit the reuptake of NA neurotransmitters. It has been demonstrated to be highly selective in vitro and has a high affinity for norepinephrine transporters. In vivo, it has been demonstrated to increase the extracellular concentrations of NA in the prefrontal cortex. Despite its low affinity to its neurotransmitter transporters in this region, it has also been demonstrated to result in a significant increase in extraneuronic dopamine concentrations, which remain stable in both the nucleus accumbens and the striatum, thus reducing the likelihood of abuse or activation of Tic-related events by ATX.

Pharmacokinetics: Absorbed orally, hydroxylated by CYP2D6 and excreted in urine, mainly as glucuronide. Majority of population is extensive metabolizer; few are poor metabolizers, due to polymorphism of CYP2D6.

Adverse effects: Dyspepsia, anorexia, growth retardation, sleep disturbances, mood swings, emotional liability, hepatotoxicity and rarely suicidal thoughts.

Drug interactions: Inhibitors of CYP2D6 such as fluoxetine, paroxetine, quinidine increase concentration and toxicity of atomoxetine. It should not be used with monoamine oxidase (MAO) inhibitors and in glaucoma.[6]

Dose: The FDA approved for children >6 years of age.

Initial: 0.5 mg/kg/day orally, increase every third day to a target total daily dose of approximately 1.2 mg/kg/day as a single daily dose or as evenly divided doses every 12 hourly. Maximum: 1.4 mg/kg or 100 mg.[6,11-13]

Guanfacine and Clonidine

Mechanism of action: Guanfacine is a selective α-2 receptor agonist, with 15–20 times higher affinity for α-2a than other receptors. Clonidine is also an α-2 receptor agonist. These drugs modulate the central sympathetic activity.

Pharmacokinetics: Guanfacine—It is well absorbed orally. Peak plasma concentration is achieved in 5 hours; half-life is 16–17 hours. It follows first-order kinetics.

Dose: The FDA approved for children > 6 years of age.

6–18 years: Starting dose 1 mg/day, may be increased by 1 mg/week, up to 4 mg, the recommended maximum dose. A maintenance dose of 0.05–0.08 mg/kg once daily, up to 0.12 mg/kg, may be considered. Therapy should not be stopped abruptly.

Clonidine: Absorbed orally, peak occurs in 2–4 hours, half of the oral dose is excreted unchanged in urine, rest as metabolites. Half-life is 8–12 hours. Effect of single dose lasts for 6–24 hours.

Dose: The FDA approved for children >6 years of age. Initially 0.05 mg/24 hours OD, increase by 0.05 mg once in 5–7 days up to maximum 0.4 mg/kg/day in three to four divided doses.

Adverse effects: Sedation, mental depression, disturbed sleep, dryness of mouth, nose and eyes, constipation, bradycardia, sudden increase in blood pressure, with missed doses for 1–2 days.

Newer Drugs under Trial for ADHD

Modafinil

It is a "wakefulness-promoting agent" for the treatment of narcolepsy; it has been occasionally used for the management of inattention in adults. Its mechanism is not well known, but may have nondopaminergic-activating action on the frontal cortex. A recent meta-analysis on five RCT's showed an effect size of 0.7 on ADHD symptoms and a significantly higher incidence of decreased appetite and insomnia, but nonsignificant cardiovascular events.[6]

Nutraceutics

There is a growing interest in the roles of the n-3 polyunsaturated fatty acids (PUFAs), docosahexaenoic acid (DHA) and the precursor eicosapentaenoic acid as potential treatment for ADHD. The longest-chain n-3 PUFA DHA is the most abundant PUFA in the brain membrane phospholipids, it has important role in membrane fluidity and associated metabolic and neural activities. DHA appears to more concentrated at synapses, influencing dopaminergic, serotonergic, noradrenergic and GABAnergic neurotransmission. Recent meta-analysis suggests that omega supplementation may improve ADHD symptoms to a modest degree. Whether subnormal blood concentration should be an indication for treatment is still not clearly established.[6]

ANTIANXIETY DRUGS

Anxiety is an unpleasant emotional state, associated with uneasiness, discomfort, and concern or fear about some defined or undefined future threat. It is characterized by both psychologic and somatic symptoms. These are the group of drugs producing restful state of mind without interfering with normal mental or physical functions. These have no effect on thought control and do not produce extrapyramidal side effects.

Classification

- *Benzodiazepines:*
  - *Short-acting:* Triazolam, oxazepam, midazolam, and remimazolam
  - *Intermediate-acting:* Alprazolam, estazolam, temazepam, lorazepam, and nitrazepam
  - *Long-acting:* Diazepam, flurazepam, clonazepam, and chlordiazepoxide
- *Azapirones:* Buspirone, gepirone, and ipsapirone
- *Others:* Beta blockers—Propranolol, Sedative hypnotics—Hydroxyzine, selective serotonin reuptake inhibitors

Benzodiazepines

Benzodiazepines are selective CNS depressants which produce sedation, relieve anxiety, facilitate sleep, suppress seizures, and reduce muscle tone. Chlordiazepoxide and diazepam, the first benzodiazepines, were introduced around 1960 as antianxiety drugs and has replaced barbiturates and other similar drugs as sedative and hypnotics as well.

Mechanism of Action

Normally, a balance between excitatory inputs (mostly glutaminergic) and the inhibitory inputs (mainly GABAnergic) determines the prevailing level of neuronal activity in limbic system and reticular-activating system of brain. If the balance swings in favor of GABA, nervousness, and anxiety are reduced while sedation, amnesia, muscle relaxation and ataxia appear. In contrast, a reduction in GABAnergic activity elicits arousal, anxiety, insomnia and restlessness. GABA acts on two distinct classes of receptors:

1. *GABA-A:* Located mainly postsynaptically, they are linked with chloride ion channels, opening of which causes hyperpolarization and reduction in membrane excitability
2. *GABA-B:* These are G-protein-coupled receptors. Their activation decreases cyclic AMP formation.

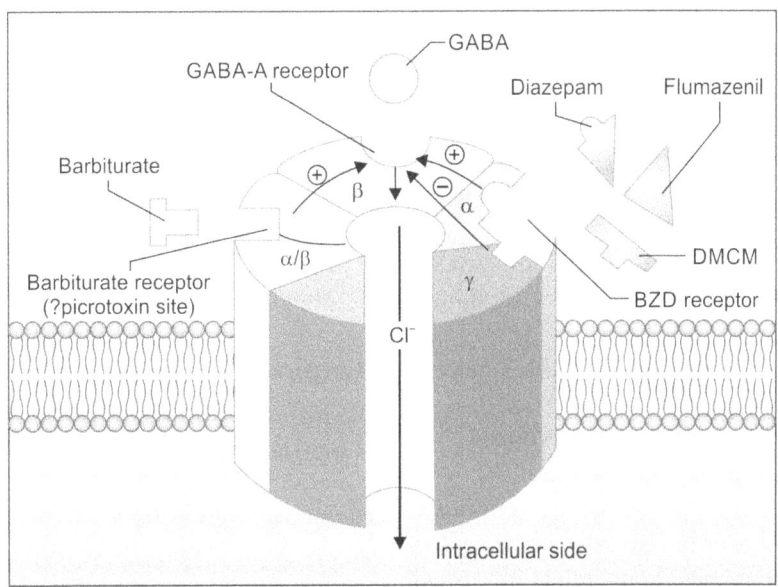

Fig. 1: Schematic depiction of GABA-A benzodiazepine chloride channel is gated by the primary ligand GABA acting on GABA-A receptor located on the beta subunit. The BZD receptor located on α and γ subunit modulates GABA-A receptor in either direction; agonists such as diazepam facilitate while inverse agonists such as DMCM hinder GABA-mediated Chloride channel opening and BZD antagonist Flumazenil blocks the action of both. The barbiturate receptor located either on α or β subunit also facilitates GABA and is capable of opening chloride channels directly as well.
Source: Tripathi KD. Antidepressants and antianxiety drugs and antipsychotic and antimanic drugs. Essentials of Medical Pharmacology, 8th edition. Jaypee Brothers Medical Publishers (P) Ltd. pp. 462-96.

They cause pre- and postsynaptic inhibition by inhibiting calcium channel opening and increasing potassium conductance.

Benzodiazepine bind to specific recognition site (Benzodiazepine binding site) on GABA-A receptor and increase the sensitivity of GABA-A receptors to GABA and thus increases the frequency of opening of opening of chloride channels, leading to hyperpolarization **(Fig. 1)**.[7]

Pharmacokinetics

There are marked pharmacokinetic variations among benzodiazepines. All the drugs can be given orally except midazolam. Some benzodiazepines are >90% protein bound (diazepam, oxazepam, and chlordiazepoxide), but no significant drug displacement reaction occurs because of their marked volume of distribution. They can cross placental barrier. Most benzodiazepines are metabolized in liver, and some of the metabolites are pharmacologically active which extend the half-life and hence duration of action, e.g., midazolam (acts through its active metabolite, hydroxymethyl midazolam); diazepam (active metabolite oxazepam); alprazolam (active metabolite, alpha-hydroxyalprazolam).

Accumulation with multiple dosing, is not clinically significant with short acting drugs but is significant with intermediate and long acting drugs. Because of longer $t_{1/2}$, withdrawal effects are milder with long-acting benzodiazepines.[7]

Doses

- *To treat anxiety:*
  - Alprazolam has anxiolytic–antidepressant effect and, therefore, is useful in anxiety associated with depression (dose: 0.25–0.5 mg, BD or TDS) or in panic disorders associated with anxiety (dose maximum up to 6 mg/day in divided doses). It is claimed to produce less drowsiness. Safety and efficacy below 18 years of age have not been established.
  - Lorazepam has been preferred for short-lived anxiety states, compulsive-obsessive neurosis and tension induced psychosomatic symptoms (dose 1-6 mg/day). It is most suitable for parenteral use also.
  - Oxazepam is used for short-lived anxiety states, preferably in those with liver dysfunction because

its hepatic metabolism is less and duration of action is short (dose 30–60 mg in three divided doses).
- Diazepam is preferred in acute panic–anxiety states associated with organic disease where sedation is also desired (dose 2–10 mg BD or TDS). Safety and efficacy in children <6 months of age is not established.
- Chlordiazepoxide is preferred in chronic anxiety states. Its active metabolite prolongs its duration of action.
  Dose: Safety and efficacy not established in children <6 years of age.
  - *>6 years:* 0.5 mg/kg/day divided 6–8 hourly.
  - *>12 years:* 25–50 mg every 6–8 hours.
- *To treat insomnia:* Benzodiazepines are hypnotics of choice, and preferred over barbiturates because they have low-abuse liability, they do not effect REM sleep and cause lesser distortion of normal hypnogram, they can be used as anxiolytic-sedative in subhypnotic dose and specific antagonist for benzodiazepines (e.g., flumazenil) can be used in case of poisoning.
  - *Transient insomnia:* Rapidly acting and rapidly eliminated drug benzodiazepine such as triazolam (0.125–0.25 mg) or temazepam (15–30 mg) at bedtime is used.
  - *Short-term insomnia:* Temazepam (15–30 mg) or flurazepam (15–30 mg) or estazolam (1–2 mg) at bedtime.
  - *Long-term chronic insomnia:* Intermittent use (with a break after every third day) of longer-acting benzodiazepines such as flurazepam (15–30 mg) or nitrazepam (5–10 mg) at bedtime is preferred because rebound insomnia and withdrawal effects are less marked with these drugs.[8]

Adverse effects
- Dose-dependent drowsiness, fatigue, disorientation, lethargy and impairment of psychomotor skills, yet, with them suicidal risk is minimal.
- Fast intravenous injection can precipitate cardiac arrest.
- Tolerance and dependence may develop after prolonged use, although mild.
- Paradoxical stimulation may occur, in rare cases, especially with flurazepam.
- Flunitrazepam, one of the tasteless benzodiazepines, misused in sexual assault or so called "date rapes", because of its sedative–amnestic properties.

Drug interactions
- Benzodiazepines potentiate the effect of other CNS depressants, such as alcohol, hypnotics, and neuroleptics.
- Smoking decreases the activity of benzodiazepines.
- Aminophylline antagonizes sedative effects of benzodiazepines.
- Enzyme inhibitors such as cimetidine and ketoconazole enhance benzodiazepine actions.

Azapirones

Buspirone is the first azapirone, a class of selective antianxiety drug.

Mechanism of Action

They act through non-GABAnergic systems. They exert their anxiolytic effects by acting as a partial agonist primarily at brain 5HT1A receptors (serotonin receptors). 5HT1A are presynaptic autoreceptors, their stimulation decreases the activity of dorsal raphe serotonergic neurons, and thus reduces anxiety.

Pharmacokinetics

It is rapidly absorbed orally, undergoes extensive first-pass metabolism (bioavailability <5%), one of its metabolite is active and is excreted both in urine and feces. $t_{1/2}$ is 2–3.5 hours.[7]

Dose and Therapeutic Effect

It is not FDA approved for use in pediatric age group.
- Buspirone (5–15 mg OD-TDS) is used in anxiety states, it is effective in mild-to-moderate anxiety, but ineffective in severe cases and those showing panic reaction.
- Buspirone in relatively higher doses is used to augment therapeutic effect of SSRI in obsessive-compulsive disorder (OCD).
- The beneficial effect in anxiety develops slowly; maximum effect may be delayed up to 2–3 weeks.

Adverse Effects

- Minor side effects: dizziness, nausea, abdominal discomfort, headache, lightheadedness, rarely excitement
- It may cause rise in blood pressure in patients on MAO inhibitors.

Drug Interaction: May potentiate the effect of other CNS depressants.

Other Anxiolytics

Propranolol

It is a nonselective beta blocker.

Mechanism of action: Many somatic symptoms of anxiety (palpitation, rise in blood pressure, shaking, tremors, gastrointestinal hurrying, etc.) are due to sympathetic overactivity, and these symptoms reinforce anxiety. Propranolol helps anxious patients troubled by these symptoms, by cutting vicious cycle and providing symptomatic relief. They do not affect the psychological symptoms such as worry, tension, and fear.

Therapeutic role in anxiety: The role of beta blockers in anxiety disorders is limited but may be used for performance or situational anxiety or as adjuvant to benzodiazepines. 20 mg of propranolol, an hour before the performance reduces the anxiety in special situations. It is not FDA approved for treatment for treatment of anxiety in pediatric age group.

Hydroxyzine

An H1 antihistaminic has sedative, antiemetic, antimuscarinic, and spasmolytic properties. It is claimed to have selective anxiolytic action but sedation is quite marked. It may be used in reactive anxiety or that associated with marked autonomic symptoms. It is not approved for treatment of anxiety in children.[7,8]

ANTIDEPRESSANTS

Major depression is an affective disorder which refers to pathological change in mood state. It is characterized by symptoms such as sad mood, loss of interest and pleasure, low energy, worthlessness, guilt, psychomotor retardation or agitation, change in appetite or sleep and suicidal thoughts.

Various hypotheses proposed for pathogenesis of depression:
1. Decrease in level or function of monoamines [serotonin (5HT), nor adrenaline (NA), dopamine (DA)]
2. Decrease in brain-derived neurotrophic factors (BDNF)
3. Abnormalities in hypothalamopituitary axis, thyroid function and sex steroid levels.[8]

Classification

- *Reversible inhibitors of MAO-A:* Moclobemide and Clorgyline
- *Tricyclic antidepressants:*
  - Noradrenaline and serotonin reuptake inhibitors: Imipramine, amitriptyline, trimipramine, doxepin, clomipramine
  - Predominantly noradrenaline reuptake inhibitors: Desipramine, nortriptyline, and reboxetine
- *Selective serotonin reuptake inhibitors (SSRIs):* Fluoxetine, fluvoxamine, paroxetine, sertraline, citalopram, escitalopram, and dapoxetine
- *Serotonin and noradrenaline reuptake inhibitors (SNRIs):* Venlafaxine, desvenlafaxine, and duloxetine.
- *Atypical antidepressants:* Trazodone, mianserin, mirtazapine, bupropion, and amoxapine.

Mechanism of Antidepressant Action (Fig. 2)

In general, all antidepressants affect monoaminergic transmission in the brain in one way or other with some other associated properties.

Tricyclic Antidepressants

For example, imipramine, desipramine, trimipramine, and nortriptyline.

Mechanism

Tricyclic antidepressants (TCAs) inhibit reuptake of noradrenaline and serotonin into their respective neurons and thus, increase their concentration in synaptic cleft. They also block muscarinic receptors, alpha-1 receptors and histaminic (H1) receptors, thus, producing side effects.

Pharmacokinetics

Tricyclic antidepressants are well absorbed orally and are highly bound to plasma proteins and are widely distributed in tissues including CNS. They are metabolized in liver. Some of them (imipramine, amitriptyline) produce active metabolites which are responsible for long duration of action. TCAs were excreted mainly in urine as active metabolites.[9]

Adverse Effects

- *Anticholinergic effects:* Dryness of mouth, blurring of vision, constipation, and urinary retention

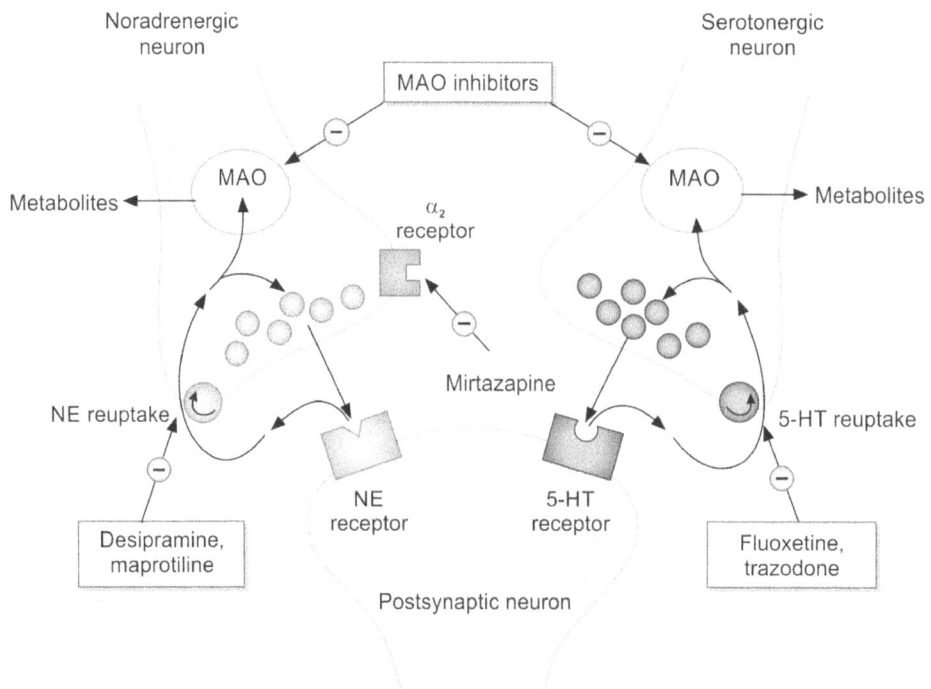

Fig. 2: Mechanism of action of various antidepressant drugs.
Source: Sedative and Hypnotic drugs. Katzung and Trevor's Basic and Clinical Pharmacology, 15th edition.

- *Adrenergic blocking effects:* Postural hypotension, tachycardia, and cardiac arrhythmia
- *H-1 blocking effects:* Sedation and confusion
- *Other effects:* Increased appetite, weight gain, rash may precipitate epilepsy.
- *Acute poisoning:* Accidental or self-attempted overdosing may endanger life. It presents as excitement, delirium, and anticholinergic features followed by muscle spasm, convulsion and coma. Respiration is depressed, hypotension, hypothermia and tachycardia. Ventricular arrhythmias are common.

Drug Interactions

- TCAs potentiate effect of sympathomimetic amines (present in cold remedies) and CNS depressants.
- Phenytoin and aspirin displace TCAs from protein-binding sites and cause transient overdose symptoms.
- SSRIs inhibit metabolism of TCA's: Dangerous toxicity may occur, if two are given simultaneously.
- MAO inhibitors: Dangerous hypertensive crisis with excitement and hallucinations, when used together.

Doses of Commonly Used TCAs

Imipramine

- *For nocturnal enuresis:*
  - *6–12 years:* Start at 10 mg and increase by 10 mg/day after 1–2 weeks, maximum dose: 50 mg/day.
  - *12–18 years:* Start 10 mg and increase by 10–25 mg/day after 1–2 weeks, maximum dose: 75 mg/day.

  Give 30 minutes before bedtime. Maximum period of treatment is 3 months. Review before giving further course.

- *Hyperactivity:*
  - *6–12 years:* 25–75 mg
  - *12–17 years:* 50–75 mg, once daily

  Start at lower doses. Doses >1.5 mg/kg given in two divided doses

- *Depression:* 1.5 mg/kg/day given orally thrice a day and increased every 3–4 days by 1 mg/kg if required, maximum dose: 5 mg/kg/day

  It is not FDA approved for pediatric age group.

Amitriptyline:
- *Depression:*
  Adolescents: 25-50 mg/day orally in divided doses initially, then gradually increases to 100 mg/day in divided doses.
  Children (off-label): 1 mg/kg/day in divided doses every 8 hourly for first 3 days, followed by 1.5 mg/kg/day oral in divided doses every 8 hours.
- *Nocturnal enuresis:* Try for 3 months
  - *6-12 years:* 10-25 mg PO
  - *12-18 years:* 25-50 mg at bedtime PO
  It is not FDA approved for pediatric age group.

Trimipramine: Depression—>12 years: 50 mg initially, maximum 100 mg/day. It is not FDA approved for use in pediatric age group.

Selective Serotonin Reuptake Inhibitors

For example, Fluoxetine, citalopram, escitalopram, and sertraline.

To overcome the drawbacks of TCAs (such as anticholinergic, cardiovascular, neurological, relatively low safety margin, and acute poisoning), newer (second generation) antidepressants have been developed since 1980's, which include both SSRIs and SNRIs.

Mechanism and advantage over TCAs: SSRIs selectively inhibit reuptake of serotonin and noradrenaline. Unlike TCAs do not block muscarinic, adrenergic and histaminic receptors, do not have cardiac side effects, do not precipitate seizures and are safer in overdose. Patient acceptability is better. Because of freedom from psychomotor and cognitive impairment, SSRIs are preferred over TCAs for prophylaxis of recurrent depression.[9]

Pharmacokinetics: They are well absorbed orally. They inhibit drug-metabolizing enzymes such as CYP2D6 and CYP3A4 and thus elevate level of TCAs, haloperidol, clozapine, warfarin, beta blockers, some benzodiazepines, and carbamazepines.

Adverse effects: Nervousness, restlessness, insomnia, anorexia, dyskinesia nausea and headache. There is increased incidence of epistaxis and ecchymosis due to impairment of platelet function.

Drug interactions:
- Elevate plasma levels of TCAs, Haloperidol, clozapine, warfarin, beta blockers and carbamazepine.
- Produces "serotonin syndrome" characterized by agitation, restlessness, rigidity, hyperthermia, delirium, sweating, twitching followed by convulsions when used along with serotonergic drugs such as MAO inhibitors, tramadol, and pethidine.

Other uses of SSRIs:
- They are now first-line drugs for trichotillomania, OCD, panic disorder, social phobia, eating disorders, premenstrual dysphoric disorder (PMDD), and post-traumatic stress disorder (PTSD).
- They are being increasingly used for anxiety disorders, body dimorphic disorders, compulsive buying and kleptomania, and premature ejaculation.

Doses of commonly used SSRIs:
- *Sertraline:* It is FDA approved for children >6 years of age.
  - *>6 years:* Initially 12.5-25 mg 24 hourly increasing slowly as required over several weeks till desired response is attained. Maximum: 200 mg/day.
- *Escitalopram:* It is FDA approved for children >12 years of age.
  - *12 to 17 years:* 10 mg orally OD. The dose may be increased to maximum of 20 mg after 3 weeks.
- *Fluoxetine:* It is FDA approved for children >8 years of age.
  - *For major depression: 8-18 years*—Initial dose 10-20 mg orally once daily. The dose should be increased to 20 mg/day after a week.
  - *Obsessive compulsive disorder: 8-18 years*—Initial dose: 10 mg orally once daily, for adolescents and higher weight children, after 2 weeks at 10 mg/day, the dose should be increased to 20 mg/day. A dose range of 20-60 mg/day is recommended.[8,9,11,12]

ANTIPSYCHOTICS

Antipsychotics also known as neuroleptic drugs are mainly used to treat all types of functional psychosis, especially schizophrenia but few of these drugs are also used in various behavioral disorders such as anxiety, aggressive behaviors, and conduct disorders. These drugs are known as neuroleptics because in normal individuals, they produce neuroleptic syndrome characterized by indifference to surroundings, psychomotor slowing, emotional quietening, and slowing of spontaneous movements. Whereas in people with psychosis, they reduce irrational behavior, agitation, aggressiveness, anxiety is relieved and hyperactivity is decreased.[10]

Classification

- *Typical antipsychotics*: Haloperidol, penfluridol, chlorpromazine, thioridazine, and pimozide
- *Atypical antipsychotics*: Clozapine, risperidone, olanzapine, quetiapine, and aripiprazole.

Mechanism of Action

Excess dopaminergic and serotonergic activity, mainly in mesolimbic pathway are thought to be responsible for psychosis; therefore, the drugs mainly target these two pathways:

1. All typical antipsychotics block dopamine receptors (D2) in mesolimbic pathway, which is considered to be overactive in psychotics, but the dopaminergic blockage does not remain restricted to mesolimbic pathway. Dopaminergic receptors in nigrostriatal and tuberoinfundibular pathway are also blocked, leading to major side effects i.e., extrapyramidal syndromes and hyperprolactinemia. They also have marked ant cholinergic and alpha-1 adrenergic-blocking effects, thus producing cardiovascular and anticholinergic side effects.
2. *Atypical antipsychotics*: They have weak D2-blocking property but potent 5HT2 (serotonergic receptors) antagonistic activity. Thus, extrapyramidal side effects are minimal.

Adverse Effects

Typical Antipsychotics

- *Extrapyramidal disturbance* is the major dose-limiting side effects, more common with high-potency drugs such as haloperidol and pimozide. Extrapyramidal effects may be categorized into:
  - *Acute muscular dystonia:* Bizarre muscle spasms, mostly involving linguofacial muscles—grimacing, tongue thrusting, torticollis, locked jaw, occur within few hours of a single dose or within few weeks. Promethazine or hydroxyzine injected IM clears the reaction within 15 minutes.
  - *Parkinsonism:* With typical manifestations, rigidity, tremors, hypokinesia, mask-like face, shuffling gait appear between 1 and 4 weeks of therapy and persist until dose is reduced. Changing the antipsychotic, especially to an atypical agent, may help.
  - *Akathisia:* Restlessness, feeling of discomfort, apparent agitation manifested as a compelling desire to move about, but without anxiety, is seen in some patients between 1 and 8 weeks of therapy. Benzodiazepines (clonazepam or diazepam) are the first choice of treatment. Propranolol may be given in nonresponsive patients.
  - *Malignant neuroleptic syndrome:* It occurs rarely, with high doses. Patient develops marked rigidity, immobility, tremor, hyperthermia, semiconsciousness, fluctuating blood pressure, and heart rate, myoglobin may be present in blood. The syndrome lasts 5–10 days after withdrawal and may be fatal. The drug must be stopped, IV dantrolene may benefit. Bromocriptine in large doses has been found useful.
  - *Tardive dyskinesia:* It occurs late in therapy, sometimes even after withdrawal of neuroleptic, manifests as purposeless involuntary facial and limb movements such as constant chewing, pouting, puffiness of cheeks and choreoathetoid movements. It is less common in children. There is no satisfactory treatment. Recently, two vesicular monoamine transporter 2 (VMAT-2) inhibitors such as dutrabenazine and valbenazine have been approved for symptomatic treatment of tardive dyskinesias.[9]
- *Other adverse effects:* Sedation, postural hypotension, palpitations, tremors, gynecomastia, galctorrhea, skin rash urticaria, teratogenicity, and cholestatic jaundice.

Atypical Antipsychotics

- *Minor side effects:* Nausea, vomiting, sedation, confusion, and delirium
- *Major side effects:* Agranulocytosis (weekly monitoring of leucocyte counts), grand mal seizures, myocarditis, extrapyramidal symptoms may develop with atypical agents, but incidence is much less.[9]

COMMONLY USED ANTIPSYCHOTICS IN BEHAVIORAL DISORDERS AND THEIR SALIENT FEATURES

Haloperidol

It most commonly used typical antipsychotic, has high potency. It used for schizophrenia, Tourette syndrome, tics, acute agitation, mood instability in autistic disorders. It is metabolized by cytochrome enzymes (CYP 3A4 and 2D6 both) and interacts with quinidine, thioridazine, and pimozide. It is extensively metabolized in liver, and therefore, it is recommended to halve the initial dose with smaller increments and at longer intervals than in patients without hepatic impairment. It is still not approved by FDA for pediatric use.

Dosing: 2-12 years—25-50 µg/day (maximum: 10 mg/day) and divided into two or three doses. *12-18 years*—0.5-2 mg/day (maximum: 60 mg/day) in two divided doses. Parenteral formulation for IM use is available.[9]

Pimozide

It is most commonly used in Tourette syndrome and tics. Because of its long half-life (48-60 hours), it is considered good for maintenance therapy in behavioral disorders, but not when psychomotor agitation is prominent. It is FDA approved for use in children >12 years of age.

Dosing: 2-12 years—Initially, 0.05 mg/kg/day orally at bedtime can be increased to 0.2 mg/kg/day orally at bedtime every 3 days; followed by 2-4 mg/day maintenance dose. *Maximum dose:* 10 mg/day. *>12 years*—Initially, 1-2 mg oral daily and increase every other day; maximum dose: 10 mg/day; followed by maintenance dose of <2 mg/kg/day or 10 mg/day; lowest dose to be chosen.[9]

Risperidone

Controlled trials suggest that risperidone is beneficial in management of disruptive behavior.[13] It is a more potent D2 blocker than clozapine, thus, extrapyramidal side effects are less only at low doses (<6 mg/day). Prolactin levels rise disproportionately during risperidone therapy. It is less epileptogenic than clozapine. It is FDA approved for treatment of schizophrenia in children >13 years of age.[14]

Dosing:
- *For aggressive behavior: 2-12 years*—0.5-2 mg/day, orally OD or BD;
  12-18 years: 1-4 mg, OD or BD.
- *Schizophrenia:* >13 years—Initially 0.5 mg/day orally in the morning/evening may be increased in increments of 0.5-1 mg/day to recommended dose of 2.5 mg/day (dose range: 0.5-6 mg/day). In case of persistent somnolence, divide daily dose 12 hourly.

Olanzapine

It is an atypical antipsychotic. It is used in children for bipolar depression, mania, schizophrenia and it is also approved for use in stuttering and eating disorders. Although it has less incidence of extrapyramidal side effects, however, it is epileptogenic, causes weight gain, glucose intolerance and elevation of serum triglycerides and agranulocytosis. It is not approved by the FDA for children <13 years of age.

Dosing:
- *Bipolar depression: 10-17 years*—2.5 mg orally in the evening and fluoxetine 20 mg orally, every evening initially, dosage adjustment if required.
- *Stuttering: <12 years*—1.25 mg orally at bedtime for 1 month, then 2.5 mg at bedtime. *>12 years*—2.5 mg orally, at bedtime for 1 month then 5 mg at bedtime.[8,9,11,12]

MISCELLANEOUS DRUGS

Desmopressin

It is used for primary nocturnal enuresis. It is a synthetic peptide analog of natural hormone arginine vasopressin, 12 times more potent antidiuretic than AVP, but has negligible vasoconstrictor activity and is also longer acting than AVP, because its enzymatic degradation is slow, $t^{1/2}$ 1-2 hours, and the duration of action is 8-12 hours. Intranasal preparations are available but bioavailability is only 10-20%. An oral formulation has been marketed with bioavailability of 1-2%, oral dose is 10-15 times higher than the intranasal dose, but systemic effects are produced and nasal side effects are avoided.

Dose for primary enuresis:
- *Intranasal:* 5-10 µg at bedtime
- *Oral:* >6 years—0.2-0.6 mg orally once daily before bedtime.[8]

Hydroxyzine

It is an H1 antihistaminic, with sedative, antiemetic, antimuscarinic and spasmolytic properties. It is researched that hydroxyzine affects the CNS by reducing production of proinflammatory cytokine, selective serotonin reuptake inhibition, and increasing GABA level. This decreases anxiety and improves behavior. Current indications include preprocedural sedation, generalized anxiety, bruxism, and sleep problems (especially in hepatic encephalopathy due to cirrhosis. Due to its immunomodulatory and anti-inflammatory actions and lack of long-term side effects, it is being researched for treatment of autism spectrum disorders. It is not approved by the FDA for these disorders.[4,9]

Dose:
- *<6 years:* 50 mg/day in four divided oral doses.
- *>6 years:* 50-100 mg in four divided oral doses. *For sedation:* 0.6 mg/kg given orally or 0.5-1.1 mg/kg IM.

N-acetyl Cysteine

It is a glutamate modulator, and is being researched for its use in trichotillomania (dose: 1,200 mg orally). Other drugs being recently tried in trichotillomania are clomipramine, fluoxetine, lamotrigine, and escitalopram. It is not approved by the FDA for this indication.[14]

GENERAL PRINCIPLES FOR PRESCRIBING PSYCHOPHARMACOLOGICAL DRUGS

- The dosing strategy of "start low and go slow, taper slowly" should be followed, particularly when using antipsychotic drugs.
- Caution and careful monitoring should be exercised while prescribing stimulants to adolescents, as there is high rate of substance misuse in this population.
- Adherence, side effects, and drug interactions should be monitored routinely and systemically. It is important to ascertain whether patient is concurrently using any psychoactive substances or complementary therapies that may interact with drugs.
- Before switching, augmenting, combining or discontinuing medications because of lack of response, it should be ensured that patient has received adequate trial (dose and duration) as well as psychosocial intervention.
- Polypharmacy should be avoided.[13]

CONCLUSION

Over the past 50 years, research in psychoactive drugs has made great strides and drugs are prescribed as part of a comprehensive treatment plan for childhood behavioral disorders but holistic management still involves combining a variety of interventions, such as cognitive behavioral therapy (CBT), behavioral modification, and social communication techniques, as well as parenting skill training, psychopharmacology, and psychosocial treatment. General prescribing principles for psychopharmacological agents should always be followed while prescribing these drugs.

REFERENCES

1. Parry TS. Assessment of developmental learning and behavioral problems in children and young people. Med J Aust. 2005;183:43-8.
2. Bagner DM, Rodríguez GM, Blake CA, Linares D, Carter AS. Assessment of behavioral and emotional problems in infancy: a systematic review. Clin Child Fam Psychol Rev. 2012;15:113-28.
3. Ogundele MO. Behavioural and emotional disorders in childhood: a brief overview for paediatricians .World J Clin Pediatr. 2018;7(1):9-26.
4. Mukherjee SB, Kaushik JS. Psychopharmacology for behaviour problems in children. Indian Pediatr. 2019;56:683-4.
5. Chan E, Fogler JM, Hammerness PG. Treatment of attention-deficit/hyperactivity disorder in adolescents: a systematic review. JAMA. 2016;315:1997-2008.
6. Judas A, Carruci S. Management and treatment of attention deficit hyperactivity disorder. Oxford Textbook of Psychiatry, 3rd edition. UK: OUP Oxford, 2020. pp. 344-54.
7. Sharma HL, Sharma KK. Anxiolytics and hypnotics. Principles of pharmacology, 3rd edition. New Delhi: Paras Medical Publisher; 2017. pp. 448-56.
8. Bertram G. Katzung, and Todd W. Vanderah. McGraw Hill, 2021, https://accessmedicine.mhmedical.com/content.aspx?bookid=2988&sectionid=250593595.
9. Tripathi KD. Antidepressants and antianxiety drugs & antipsychotic & antimanic drugs. Essentials of Medical Pharmacology, 8th edition. New Delhi: Jaypee Brothers Medical Publishers (P) Ltd; 2019. pp. 462-96.
10. Pringsheim T, Hirsch L, Gardner D, Gorman DA. The pharmacological management of oppositional behaviour, conduct problems, and aggression in children and adolescents with attention-deficit hyperactivity disorder, oppositional defiant disorder, and conduct disorder: a systematic review and meta-analysis. Part 1: psychostimulants, alpha-2 agonists, and atomoxetine. Can J Psychiatry. 2015;60:42-51.
11. Shah I. (2023). Drug index. [online] Available from: https://www.pediatriconcall.com/drugs/drugs-a-to-z. [Last accessed October, 2023].
12. David K, Maso D, Walter HJ, Urion DK. Psychopharmacology & ADHD. In: Kliegman RM, St. Geme JW III. Nelson Textbook of Pediatrics, 21st edition. Philadelphia: Elsevier. pp. 189-96, 262-6.
13. Spetie L, Rey JM. Oppositional defiant & conduct disorders, ADHD. Lewis's Child & Adolescent Psychiatry, 5th edition. Philadelphia: Wolters Kluwer; 2018. pp. 364-98.
14. Rodrigues-Barata AR, Tosti A, Rodríguez-Pichardo A. N-acetylcysteine in the treatment of trichotillomania. Int J Trichology. 2012;4(3):176-8.

Chapter 29: Genetics and Behavioral Disorders

Priyanshu Mathur, Sharanpreet Kaur

INTRODUCTION

Behavioral disorders in children refer to a group of conditions that affect a child's neurological and behavioral development. These disorders can manifest as difficulties in social interactions, communication, emotional regulation, attention, learning, and other cognitive functions. Genetics can play a significant role in the development of behavioral disorders. Many behavioral disorders have a complex and multifactorial etiology, which means they result from a combination of genetic, environmental, and social factors. However, in some cases, the genetic component can be particularly influential.

Some common neurobehavioral disorders in children include: Autism spectrum disorder (ASD), attention-deficit/hyperactivity disorder (ADHD), intellectual disability (ID), specific learning disabilities (SLD), oppositional defiant disorder (ODD), conduct disorder (CD), Tourette syndrome (TS), language disorders, developmental coordination disorder (DCD), and anxiety disorders.

EPIDEMIOLOGY

Behavior disorders are relatively common worldwide, affecting a significant portion of the population. However, the prevalence can vary depending on the specific disorder, the age group studied, and the region or country being examined.

Autism spectrum disorder is characterized by challenges in communication, social interaction, and repetitive behaviors. In United States, the prevalence of ASD is estimated to be around 1 in 54 children. Autism affects more male than female individuals, and comorbidity is common (>70% have concurrent conditions). ADHD is one of the most prevalent behavior disorders in childhood. It affects approximately 5-7% of children globally. Prevalence rates may vary across countries and regions CD and ODD often emerge during childhood and adolescence. The prevalence rates for CD and ODD can vary but are estimated to be around 2-10% and 1-11%, respectively.[1-3]

ETIOPATHOGENESIS

Genetic contributions to autism are extremely heterogeneous, with many different loci underlying the disease to a different extent in different individuals. Moreover, the phenotypic expression (i.e., "penetrance") of these genetic components is also highly variable, ranging from fully penetrant point mutations to polygenic forms with multiple gene–gene and gene–environment interactions. Furthermore, many genes involved in ASD are also involved in ID, further underscoring their lack of specificity in phenotypic expression.

Twin studies have played a crucial role in understanding the genetic and environmental factors that contribute to ASD. It is worth noting that the concordance rate (both twins having ASD) among monozygotic twins is not 100%, indicating that there are additional factors, both genetic and environmental, that contribute to the development of ASD. Genetics is not the sole determinant for autism, and other factors such as prenatal and early-life environmental influences may contribute to the development and severity of the condition.

While many genes have been implicated in the risk for autism, there is no single "autism gene". Instead, there are numerous genes and genetic variations associated with ASD.

Some of the genes that have been linked to autism are:
- *SHANK3:* The *SHANK3* gene is involved in synaptic function. Mutations in the *SHANK3* gene have been associated with Phelan-McDermid syndrome, a rare

genetic disorder that can include autism as one of its features.
- *CHD8:* *CHD8* is involved in chromatin remodeling and gene expression regulation and mutation in this gene have been found in some individuals with autism.
- *SCN2A:* Mutations in the *SCN2A* gene, which codes for sodium channel protein, have been associated with a range of neurodevelopmental disorders, including autism.
- *ADNP:* Mutations in the *ADNP* gene are linked to the ADNP syndrome, which includes autism as one of its features.
- *PTEN:* Mutations in the *PTEN* gene have been associated with PTEN hamartoma tumor syndrome (PHTS), and individuals with this syndrome may also exhibit autism spectrum features.
- *NRXN1 and NLGN3/4:* Genes such as *NRXN1* (Neurexin 1) and *NLGN3/4* (Neuroligin 3 and Neuroligin 4) code for proteins involved in synaptic function and have been implicated in the genetic risk for autism.
- *MECP2:* Mutations in the *MECP2* gene are associated with Rett syndrome, a disorder that can present with autistic behaviors.
- *CDH10* and *CDH9:* These *cadherin* genes have been implicated in the risk for autism and are involved in cell adhesion and neural connectivity.
- *FOXP1:* FOXP1 is a transcription factor important for brain development and mutations in the *FOXP1* gene have been linked to developmental disorders, including autism.

It is important to note that the genetic underpinnings of autism are highly complex, and the genes mentioned above represent just a small fraction of those associated with ASD.

GENETIC MECHANISMS SEEN IN DIFFERENT BEHAVIORAL DISORDERS

Heritability: Heritability refers to the extent to which genetic factors contribute to the variation in a particular trait or disorder within a population. For some behavioral disorders, such as ASD[4] and ADHD,[5] there is evidence to suggest a strong genetic contribution. Twin and family studies have demonstrated higher concordance rates for these disorders among relatives compared to the general population.
- *Gene–environment interplay:* While genetics can predispose individuals to certain behavioral disorders, the actual expression of these disorders often depends on interactions between genes and the environment. Environmental factors, such as early life experiences, parenting styles, and exposure to stress or trauma, can modify the expression of genetic predispositions.
- *Candidate genes:* In some cases, specific genes have been implicated in behavioral disorders. For example, certain genes have been associated with an increased risk of developing schizophrenia or bipolar disorder. However, it is essential to note that these genetic associations are often complex and involve multiple genes and their interactions.
- *Polygenic nature:* Most behavioral disorders are believed to be polygenic, meaning they result from the combined effects of multiple genes, each with a small individual impact. Identifying all the contributing genes and their interactions is a challenging task, but advances in genetic research have made it possible to identify some genetic risk factors for certain disorders.
- *Epigenetics:* Epigenetic mechanisms can also influence gene expression without changing the underlying DNA sequence. These epigenetic changes can be influenced by environmental factors and play a role in the development of behavioral disorders.
- It is crucial to recognize that genetics is just one piece of the puzzle when it comes to behavioral disorders. Environmental factors, lifestyle choices, and individual experiences also significantly impact the development and expression of these conditions. Understanding the interplay between genetics and the environment is essential for a more comprehensive view of behavioral disorders and for developing effective prevention and treatment strategies. **Table 1** describes the various causative phenomenon involved in common behavioral disorders, implying the multifactoriality of the disorders.

CLINICAL FEATURES

Clinical features of behavior disorders in children can vary depending on the specific disorder and its severity. However, disruptive behaviors (temper tantrums, aggression, defiance, non-compliance with rules, and oppositional behavior), impulsivity, inattention, hyperactivity, aggression, rule violation, emotional dysregulation, social difficulties, academic challenges, poor school performance, risky behaviors (substance abuse, self-harm, delinquent activities), and sleep problems

Behavioral disorder	Various genetic phenomenon observed[4]
Autism spectrum disorder (ASD)	Heritability,[6] genetic mutations, polygenic nature, candidate genes, copy number variants (CNVs), gene expression and regulation, X-linked genes, gene–gene and gene–environment interactions
Attention-deficit/Hyperactivity disorder (ADHD)	Heritability,[7] polygenic nature, candidate genes, neurodevelopmental genes, gene–gene and gene–environment interactions, dopamine signaling pathways, epigenetic factors
Intellectual disability (ID)	Chromosomal abnormalities (as in genetic syndromes and X-linked disorders), single-gene mutations, hereditary with autosomal recessive inheritance, de novo mutations, copy number variants (CPV), epigenetic factors[8]
Specific learning disabilities (SLD)	Familial clustering, heritability, candidate genes, polygenic nature, gene expression and regulation, gene–gene and gene–environment interactions, neurodevelopmental genes, comorbidity with other disorders[9]
Oppositional defiant disorder (ODD)	Heritability, candidate genes, neurotransmitter systems, gene–gene and gene–environment interactions, epigenetic factors, comorbidity with other disorders[10]
Conduct disorder (CD)	Heritability, candidate genes, neurotransmitter systems, epigenetic factors, comorbidity with other disorders[11]
Tourette syndrome (TS)	Heritability, complex inheritance, candidate genes, copy number variations (CNVs),[12] polygenic nature, gene–gene and gene–environment interactions, sex differences
Language disorders	Heritability, candidate genes, genetic syndromes, copy number variations (CNVs), gene expression and regulation, polygenic nature, gene–gene and gene–environment interactions
Developmental coordination disorder (DCD)	Familial clustering, candidate genes, copy number variants (CNVs), polygenic nature, gene–gene and gene–environment interactions, sex differences
Anxiety disorders	Heritability, candidate genes, gene–gene and gene–environment interactions, polygenic nature, comorbidity with other disorders, epigenetic factors

TABLE 1: Genetic mechanisms observed in common neurobehavioral disorders

(difficulty falling asleep, frequent awakenings, or nightmares) are some common clinical features that may be observed in children with behavior disorders.

It is important to note that not all children with behavior challenges have a behavior disorder. The severity and persistence of these behaviors, as well as the impact on the child's daily functioning and relationships, help distinguish typical childhood behavior from behavior disorders. Proper assessment and diagnosis by qualified healthcare professionals, such as child psychologists or psychiatrists, are essential to determine the presence of a behavior disorder and develop an appropriate intervention plan.

GENETIC SYNDROMES AND BEHAVIORAL DISORDERS

Klinefelter's Syndrome

It is a genetic syndrome characterized by inheritance of an extra X chromosome which leads to poor sexual development in boys. Patients with Klinefelter's syndrome may have intellectual disabilities ranging from learning disabilities to mild mental retardation. These children may present with speech delay or other learning disabilities such as dyslexia; scholastic performance may be poor in these kids. Behavior of these children is also affected; they may be shy and immature, or sometimes may have aggressive and antisocial behavior. In a study by Bruining et al., these children were found to have high incidence of ASDs and ADHD. Klinefelter's syndrome can be diagnosed by karyotyping revealing XXY genotype in the affected children. This disorder can be diagnosed prenatally as well by assessment of fetal cells in amniotic fluid collected by amniocentesis. These children may require special attention for speech and language development and individualized education program (IEP) for extra help in study. Antisocial and aggressive behavior requires behavioral management therapy.[13]

Down Syndrome

Children with Down syndrome may have behavioral problems such as hyperactivity, aggression, disobedience, inattention, and impulsivity in addition to intellectual and learning disability. An Indian study showed the prevalence of behavioral problems in children with Down syndrome to be 55% as compared to 12.5% in control group which comprised of unsocialized disturbances of conduct in 37.5%, sleep disturbances in 15%, ADHD in 12.5%, and enuresis in 12.5% cases from the study group. Tics, pica, and self-mutilation were other disturbances reported. Other than that, children with Down syndrome have also been reported to suffer from depressive disorders (with psychosis), anxiety, and obsessive-compulsive disorder.[14,15]

Prader–Willi Syndrome

Prader-Willi syndrome (PWS) is a rare neurodevelopmental genetic disorder which is caused by a loss of paternally expressed imprinted genes on chromosome 15q11.2-q13. Genetic subtypes of PWS include paternal deletion (del) of the 15q11.2-13 region (65%), maternal uniparental disomy (UPD) (~30%) and less commonly, an imprinting center defect (3–5%). The disorder is associated with a characteristic behavioral phenotype that includes severe hyperphagia and a variety of other behavioral challenges such as temper outbursts and anxiety. These patients also suffer from obsessive–compulsive behaviors, rigidity, and social cognition deficits. Whereas infants with PWS may have difficulty feeding; in late childhood, these patients develop a persistent and unregulated desire to eat (hyperphagia), which is a hallmark feature of this genetic disorder. Unless access to food is strictly controlled, an overwhelming drive to eat coupled with decreased energy expenditure leads to morbid obesity in these individuals. PWS-associated hyperphagia has overlap with several other conditions, including binge-eating disorder; however, it is distinguished from these conditions by its presence in early childhood as well as physiological studies have suggested that hyperphagia in PWS likely is related to a pathological defect of satiety. Intense hyperphagia can lead to undesirable behavior like food sneaking/food theft, eating food left on other people's plates, eating food that is normally considered unacceptable (e.g., food scraps, food in the trash, raw food) or non-food items (e.g., dirt, grass, soap), getting up at night to look for food, taking very large bites of food, and eating very fast. In later stages of life, these individuals may suffer from anxiety and severe depression which may or may not be related to eating disorders in these individuals. The Hyperphagia Questionnaire for Clinical

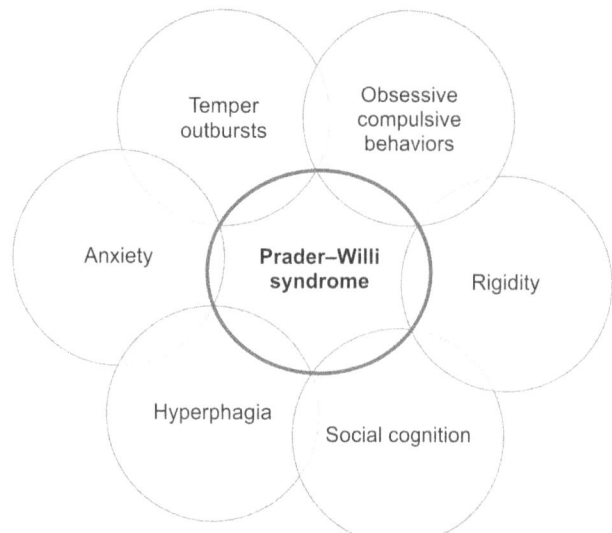

Fig. 1: Interrelated behavioral problems observed in individuals with PWS.
(PWS: Prader–Willi syndrome)
Source: Adapted From: Behavioral features in Prader–Willi syndrome (PWS): consensus paper from the International PWS Clinical Trial Consortium.[16]

Trials (HQ-CT) is a 9-item scale that helps in assessing the severity of specific hyperphagic behaviors including food seeking and food-related preoccupations by assessing distress and adaptive impairment related to hyperphagia. **Figure 1** shows multiple interrelated behavioral problems observed in individuals with PWS.[16]

Fragile X Syndrome

Fragile X syndrome (FXS) is an X-linked dominant disorder caused by expansive cytosine-guanine-guanine (CGG) trinucleotide repeats in the fragile *X mental retardation 1 gene (FMR1)* located in chromosome Xq27.3. It has been noted to be the leading cause of inherited intellectual disabilities. The children with this disorder face 3 issues, i.e., physical, behavioral/psychological and developmental. Common behavioral issues that are observed in these children are ADHD, ASD, anxiety, aggressiveness, intellectual disabilities, and developmental delay.[17]

Angelman Syndrome

Angelman syndrome is a genetic disorder caused by a deletion or mutation of the *UBE3A* gene. Individuals with Angelman syndrome often exhibit developmental delays, intellectual disabilities, and hyperactivity, which can include autistic-like behaviors.

22q11.2 Deletion Syndrome (DiGeorge Syndrome or Velocardiofacial Syndrome)

This syndrome is caused by a deletion on chromosome 22 and can result in a range of physical and developmental issues, including speech and language delays, social challenges, and an increased risk of autism spectrum disorder.

Tuberous Sclerosis Complex

Tuberous sclerosis complex (TSC) is caused by mutations in either the *TSC1* or *TSC2* genes and can lead to the formation of noncancerous tumors in various organs. Many individuals with TSC also exhibit social and communication difficulties, including features of autism.

Chromosome 16p11.2 Deletion/Duplication Syndrome

Deletions or duplications of a specific region on chromosome 16p11.2 have been associated with an increased risk of autism and developmental delays.

DIAGNOSIS

The diagnosis of behavioral disorders in children involves a comprehensive evaluation by healthcare professionals and mental health specialists. The multimodal assessment may require information from different sources, including parents, teachers, direct observations, and psychological testing, to obtain a comprehensive understanding of the child's behavior. It typically follows a structured and systematic process that includes the following steps:

- Initial assessment (child's medical history, developmental milestones, and any existing physical health conditions) by pediatrician, family physician, or primary care provider.
- Behavioral screening (standardized questionnaires) by healthcare providers.
- Parent and teacher interviews for assessment of child's behavior at home, school, and other environments.
- Behavioral observations (direct observations) by child psychologists or behavioral therapists 5. Diagnostic criteria (DSM-5).

In some cases, additional psychological testing may be conducted to assess cognitive abilities, emotional functioning, and other aspects of the child's behavior.

Types of Genetic Tests

There is no single genetic test that can detect all genetic conditions. The approach to genetic testing is individualized based on medical and family history and suspected clinical diagnosis. Genetic tests may be broadly classified in to three categories shows in **Table 2**:

1. Molecular tests (DNA sequencing to determine nucleotide order): Molecular tests include single-gene testing (only one concerned gene is tested), genetic panel testing (multiple genes related to particular condition are tested), genomic testing (all genes in the DNA are tested in whole-exome sequencing

	TABLE 2: Type of genetic tests.	
1.	Molecular tests	Employs DNA Sequencing to determine nucleotide order • *Single-gene testing:* Single gene tests look for changes in only one gene. Single gene testing is done when your doctor believes you or your child has symptoms of a specific condition or syndrome, or when there is a known genetic mutation in a family • *Panel testing:* A panel genetic test looks for changes in many genes in one test. Genetic testing panels are usually grouped in categories based on different kinds of medical concerns • *Large-scale genetic or genomic testing:* There are two different kinds of large-scale genetic tests; – *Exome sequencing* looks at all the genes in the DNA (whole exome) or just the genes that are related to medical conditions (clinical exome) – *Genome sequencing* is the largest genetic test and looks at all of a person's DNA, not just the genes Exome and genome sequencing are ordered for people with complex medical histories. Large-scale genetic tests can have findings unrelated to why the test was ordered in the first place (secondary findings)[18]
2.	Chromosomal tests	DNA is packaged into structures called chromosomes. Some tests look for changes in chromosomes rather than gene changes. Examples of these tests are *karyotype* and *chromosomal microarrays*[19,20]
3.	Gene expression	Genes are expressed, or turned on, at different levels in different types of cells. Gene expression tests compare these levels between normal cells and diseased cells because knowing about the difference can provide important information for treating the disease

and all concerned genes are tested in clinical exome sequencing).
2. Chromosomal tests (look for changes in chromosomes): Chromosomal tests include karyotyping and microarrays
3. Tests of gene expression.

TREATMENT

The treatment of behavior disorders in children often involves a multidisciplinary approach, addressing various aspects of the child's well-being, and can include the following components:
- Behavioral interventions (applied behavior analysis, cognitive behavioral therapy, and parent–child interaction therapy)
- Parent training and support
- School-based interventions
- Medications
- Social skills training
- Supportive Services (occupational therapy, speech therapy, or play therapy).

In addition, for some behavior disorders, such as anxiety and depression, cognitive interventions which aim to identify and challenge negative thought patterns and promote healthier cognitive processes may be employed.

Early identification and intervention are crucial for improving outcomes. Starting treatment as soon as possible can prevent the escalation of behavior issues and promote positive development. It's important to remember that each child is unique, and there is no one-size-fits-all approach to treating behavior disorders. Treatment plans should be tailored to the child's specific needs, strengths, and challenges. Regular monitoring and ongoing communication between all members of the treatment team are essential to assess progress and make necessary adjustments to the intervention plan. The involvement and support of parents and caregivers throughout the treatment process are crucial for successful outcomes.

Potential Therapeutic Targets for Future

Autism is a complex neurodevelopmental disorder with a multifactorial etiology, meaning it results from a combination of genetic, environmental, and possibly epigenetic factors. While there has been significant progress in understanding the genetics of autism, developing a gene therapy for ASD is a highly complex and challenging endeavor due to the heterogeneity of the condition. It is important to note that research into the genetic basis of autism is ongoing, and new insights may lead to potential therapeutic targets in the future **(Fig. 2)**.

The therapeutic interventions in ASD are aimed at rescuing haploinsufficiency of individual genes in cases of loss-of-function mutations and could be developed to target all three levels of the central dogma of molecular biology: DNA, mRNA, and protein. Examples of such interventions include genome editing with CRISPR at the genetic level, antisense oligonucleotides (ASOs) at both, the transcriptional and post-transcriptional level, and the use of small-molecule drugs to target molecular pathways at the translational, or protein level.[21]

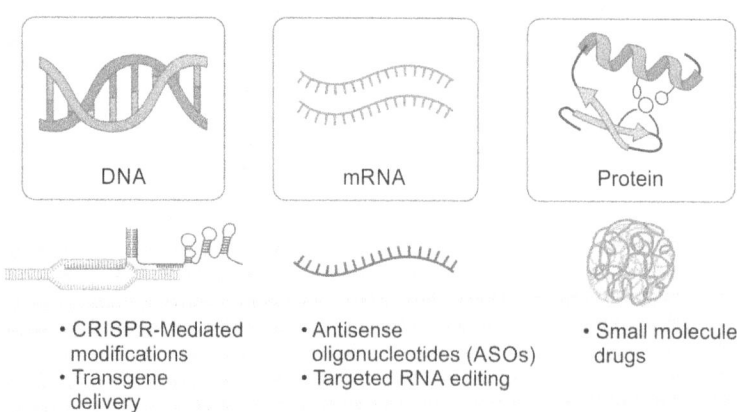

Fig. 2: Potential therapeutic targets for ASD at different levels of the Central Dogma of Molecular Biology. (ASD: autism spectrum disorder.)
Source: Adapted from: Therapeutic strategies for autism: targeting three levels of the central dogma of molecular biology. Transl Psychiatry. 2023;13:58.

Prevention: Top of Form

Preventing behavior disorders in children involves a combination of strategies that promote healthy development, early identification of risk factors, and the implementation of effective interventions. While not all behavior disorders can be completely prevented, early intervention and supportive environments can significantly reduce the risk and severity of these disorders.

Prenatal Diagnosis

Prenatal diagnosis techniques, such as prenatal genetic testing and screening, are primarily used to identify chromosomal abnormalities, genetic conditions, or certain birth defects in the developing fetus. They are not designed to predict or prevent behavioral disorders because most of the behavioral disorders do not result from a single genetic mutation or chromosomal abnormality that can be reliably detected through prenatal testing. The role of prenatal diagnosis and termination in subsequent pregnancies is limited only in those families, where previous siblings had confirmed genetic defect as an underlying cause of behavioral disorders with poor neurodevelopmental outcome and quality of life despite treatment. As behavioral disorders put a lot of toll on the family and in various societies around the world, these disorders are still considered a social taboo, prenatal diagnosis of these disorders may help such families. Yet, we have a long way to go in developing valid and clinically useful prenatal genetic diagnostic tests to help these families.

Multiple researches are going on to identify proposed biomarkers for ASD risk which include genetic and biochemical findings in blood or urine, placental pathology and maternal autoantibody profiles, although none has yet shown definitive predictability to identify these disorders. However, there is ongoing accelerated research into the neurobiology of ASD and with the increasing capabilities to screen large numbers of bioactive compounds, examine the entire genome, and simultaneously analyze large data sets; we may soon find some clinically useful and valid biomarkers. Similarly, a lot of research is going on ADHD patients regarding identifying candidate genes responsible for the disorder, as well as on pharmacogenetics to identify which drug would provide the best results in these cases. With advances in genetics, neurobehavioral imaging studies, and identification of biomarkers, soon we may have better approaches for early identification of these behavioral challenges and timely intervention. Also, with advancing pharmacogenetics, it would be easier to identify the most effective drug in an individual case and get better results.

CONCLUSION

Multiple researches are going on to identify proposed biomarkers for ASD risk, which include genetic and biochemical findings in blood or urine, placental pathology and maternal autoantibody profiles, although none has yet shown definitive predictability to identify these disorders. However, there is ongoing accelerated research into the neurobiology of ASD and with the increasing capabilities to screen large numbers of bioactive compounds, examine the entire genome, and simultaneously analyze large data sets; we may soon find some clinically useful and valid biomarkers. Similarly, a lot of research is going on ADHD patients regarding identifying candidate genes responsible for the disorder, as well as on pharmacogenetics to identify which drug would provide the best results in these cases. With advances in genetics, neurobehavioral imaging studies, and identification of biomarkers, soon we may have better approaches for early identification of these behavioral challenges and timely intervention. Also, with advancing pharmacogenetics, it would be easier to identify the most effective drug in an individual case and get better results.

REFERENCES

1. Salari N, Ghasemi H, Abdoli N, Rahmani A, Shiri MD, Hashemian AH, et al. The global prevalence of ADHD in children and adolescents: a systematic review and meta-analysis. Ital J Pediatr. 2023;49:48.
2. Mohammadi MR, Salmanian M, Keshavarzi Z. The global prevalence of conduct disorder: a systematic review and meta-analysis. Iran J Psychiatry. 2021;16(2):205-25.
3. Canino G, Polanczyk G, Bauermeister JJ, Rohde LA, Frick PJ. Does the prevalence of CD and ODD vary across cultures? Soc Psychiatry Psychiatr Epidemiol. 2010;45(7):695-704.
4. Bai D, Yip BHK, Windham GC, Windham GC, Sourander A, Francis R, et al. Association of genetic and environmental factors with autism in a 5-country cohort. JAMA Psychiatry. 2019;76(10):1035-43.
5. Freitag CM, Rohde LA, Lempp T, Romanos M. Phenotypic and measurement influences on heritability estimates in childhood ADHD. Eur Child Adolesc Psychiatry. 2010; 19:311-23.

6. Freitag CM, Staal W, Klauck SB, Duketis E, Waltes R. Genetics of autistic disorders: review and clinical implications. Eur Child Adolesc Psychiatry. 2010;19:169-78.
7. Banaschewski T, Becker K, Scherag S, Smoller JW, Goralnick JJ, Holmgren MA, et al. Molecular genetics of attention-deficit/hyperactivity disorder: an overview. Eur Child Adolesc Psychiatry. 2010;19:237-57.
8. Iwase S, Bérubé NG, Zhou Z Kasri NN, Battaglioli E, Scandaglia M, et al. Epigenetic etiology of intellectual disability. J Neurosci. 2017;37(45):10773-82.
9. Plomin R. Genetic factors contributing to learning and language delays and disabilities. Child Adolesc Psychiatr Clin N Am. 2001;10(2):259-77, viii.
10. Mikolajewski AJ, Taylor J, Iacono WG. Oppositional defiant disorder dimensions: genetic influences and risk for later psychopathology. J Child Psychol Psychiatry. 2017;58(6):702-10.
11. Salvatore JE, Dick DM. Genetic influences on conduct disorder. Neurosci Biobehav Rev. 2018;91:91-101.
12. Domènech L, Cappi C, Halvorsen M. Genetic architecture of Tourette syndrome: Our current understanding. Psychol Med. 2021;51(13):2201-9.
13. Klinefelter's Syndrome. [online] Available from: https://www.nelsonpatientinstructions.com/Forms/KlinefeltersSyndrome.pdf. [Last accessed October, 2023].
14. Fidler DJ, Most DE, Philofsky AD. The Down syndrome behavioural phenotype: Taking a developmental approach. Down Syndrome: Res Pract. 2009;12:37-44.
15. Bhatia M, Kabra M, Sapra S. Behavioral problems in children with Down syndrome. Indian Pediatr. 2005;42:675-80.
16. Schwartz L, Caixàs A, Dimitropoulos A, Dykens E, Duis J, Einfeld S, et al. Behavioral features in Prader-Willi syndrome (PWS): Consensus paper from the International PWS Clinical Trial Consortium. J Neurodevelop Disord. 2021;13:25.
17. Davidson M, Sebastian SA, Benitez Y, Desai S, Quinonez J, Ruxmohan S, et al. Behavioral problems in fragile X syndrome: a review of clinical management. Cureus. 2022;14(2): e21840.
18. Lazaridis KN, Schahl KA, Cousin MA, Babovic-Vuksanovic D, Riegert-Johnson DL, Gavrilova RH, et al; Individualized Medicine Clinic Members. Outcome of whole exome sequencing for diagnostic odyssey cases of an individualized medicine clinic: The Mayo clinic experience. Mayo Clin Proc. 2016;91(3):297-307.
19. Miller DT, Adam MP, Aradhya S, Biesecker LG, Brothman AR, Carter NP, et al. Consensus statement: chromosomal microarray is a first-tier clinical diagnostic test for individuals with developmental disabilities or congenital anomalies. Am J Hum Genet. 2010;86(5):749-64.
20. Manning M, Hudgins L; Professional Practice and Guidelines Committee. Array-based technology and recommendations for utilization in medical genetics practice for detection of chromosomal abnormalities. Genet Med. 2010;12(11):742-5. Erratum in: Genet Med. 2020;22(12):2126.
21. Hong D and Lakoucheva LM. Therapeutic strategies for autism: targeting three levels of the central dogma of molecular biology. Transl Psychiatry. 2023;13:58.

Chapter 30: Cognitive Behavior Therapy

S Sitaraman, Swati Ghate

INTRODUCTION

Research in neuroscience has established that our thoughts, emotions, and actions are intricately intertwined.[1] The effect of a change in either of the three resonates on the rest of the two.

Cognitive behavioral therapies (CBTs) are based on the premise that addressing the thoughts and changing them favorably may be put to use in shaping the desirable emotional states and behaviors and vice versa. Since behavioral and mental health issues abound in children and especially in adolescents, CBT has a unique place in pediatric and adolescent practice.

DEFINITION

Cognitive behavioral therapy is a psychotherapeutic method that aims to reduce psychological distress and dysfunction, by exploring and addressing how the integration of a client's thoughts, feelings, and behaviors are contributing to the presenting problem.[1]

Cognitive behavioral therapy helps in converting undesirable behavior or mental states of the clients to more favorable and desirable counterparts by analyzing and rectifying the underneath cognitive processes.

ORIGIN OF COGNITIVE BEHAVIORAL THERAPY

Till the middle of the twentieth century, Freud's psychoanalytical approach and Skinner's behavioral approach formed the basis of psychotherapeutic assistance provided to help people in distress.

The psychoanalytical approach is "inward looking" and heavily depends on searching the root cause of the present distress in the experiences of remote past. The behavioral approach focuses objectively on the observable behavior and works on the principle that desirable behaviors can be learned and undesirable behaviors can be unlearned by manipulating their antecedents and consequences. These therapy types have many limitations. Some of them are that they require a lot of time to show the effect, they need multiple sessions to accomplish the desired goals, and the clients are rather passive outside of the therapy sessions. The behavioral therapeutic techniques rely a lot on the external environmental factors which are rather difficult for the therapist to intervene.

In the latter half of the twentieth century, psychologists like Dollard and Miller (1950) and Homne (1965) introduced the concept that it is primarily what we think about ourselves and the world around us that brings about our behavior. Dr Albert Ellis was one of the pioneers in the field of using this "cognitive approach" who postulated that it is our core beliefs and irrational thoughts that cast their shadow on our emotions.

American psychiatrist Dr Aron T Beck and his associates studied in details the thought processes of patients suffering from depression. They found a consistent pattern of thinking in most of the patients, which could correlate and explain their low mood and typical behaviors. They addressed these thoughts and tried changing them to get the desired outcome behavior.

This was very different from the then prevalent notion that "passive hostility against self" is the root cause of depression. Dr Beck and his associates (Beck and Hollon, 1977), in a double-blind controlled trial demonstrated that depressed patients have less hostility than normal population and by addressing their thoughts, depression can be as effectively treated as antidepressants.[2]

This started a new era of applying concepts of cognitive theory of psychology to address mental health concerns. The cognitive theories use personal attributes of the patient, his own higher mental functions (such as the thoughts, beliefs, perceptions, values) to resolve his problems.

For example, if an obese person bears a thought that "I shall not be able to attain my desired weight", he will have no motivation to get up for workout. If his thought is converted to a more productive thought like "I shall try for a minimal weight reduction of 1 kg", then there are chances that he may want to give it a try.

After Ellis and Beck, many other psychologists tried different cognitive techniques as therapeutic interventions and successfully generated evidence for their application in various clinical settings.[1] These therapeutic interventions, which address higher mental processes in bringing out desired behavior, are collectively placed under the umbrella term "cognitive behavioral therapy". Important among them are rational emotive behavior therapy (REBT; Dr Albert Ellis, 1962), dialectal behavior therapy (DBT; Linehan, 1993), assistance commitment therapy (ACT; Hayes, 2004), and problem-solving therapy (D'Zurilla and Nezu, 2006).[1,3-6]

HOW IS COGNITIVE BEHAVIORAL THERAPY CONDUCTED?

Let us see Beck's CBT as a prototype and learn about its practical utility in pediatric office practice through an example of a depressed adolescent.

Shrawan is a 16-year-old boy from an educated family who was brought to a pediatrician for low mood, reluctance to attend the school, remaining aloof, not eating well since past 1 month after he failed in a class test. He showed nonsuicidal self-injurious behavior since last 1 week.

A detailed psychosocial history was taken using the HEEADSSS (home, eating, education, activities, drugs, suicidality, sexuality, safety, spirituality) to know about his strengths and weaknesses.

PRINCIPLES OF COGNITIVE BEHAVIORAL THERAPY

Upon an experience (which could be an event or a thought in itself), everyone generates automatic thoughts in response. These thoughts then decide how we feel about the experience and what actions we chose to take. When these thoughts are positive, one feels good and engages in productive, meaningful behavior whereas if the thoughts generated are negative, one goes in a negative state of mind (feels depressed, anxious, angry, etc.). Then he indulges in behaviors that are nonproductive or even harmful to self or others.

Cognitive behavioral therapy believes that the dysfunctional thoughts and beliefs are the root cause of emotional and behavioral states observed in people with mental health challenges. Such thoughts are generally irrational and could be about self, the world, or the future. They are labeled as the "negativity triad."

- *Negative view of self:* Worthlessness
- *Negative view of the world:* Helplessness
- *Negative view of the future:* Hopelessness

Cognitive behavioral therapy claims that these thoughts are amenable to changes and that results in change in the mental frame and resultant behaviors. These thoughts are supposed to arise out of the core beliefs that the individual is harboring in his mind. The core beliefs are also called "schema" and are the images about self and others that are formed over experiences since early years of life. For example, in a family of academic achievers, the child might have a schema that "success equates to exam scores," whereas a boy from a poor family might have a core belief that "one is successful if one can earn for life by hook or crook."

Shrawan's thought analysis

Let us see how we can figure out what is going on in Shrawan's mind with the CBT lens.

Event—thought—emotional consequences/behavior

The antecedent triggering event in his case is failing an exam. When he was asked to elaborate, and open his mind, in a nonjudgmental and empathetic way, he spelt out his thoughts and emotions. That gave an insight into his behavior.

- *Failure:* I am not worthy of anything —sad mood/poor self-care
  - Worthlessness—I shall not be able to accomplish anything—school refusal
  - Worthlessness—I am no good and my friends will ridicule me—remains aloof
  - Worthlessness—I am not worthy of living—I should die—suicidal behavior
- *Failure:* No one will ever understand me—sad mood, anger, irritability
  - Helplessness—teachers and friends will not help but reject me—school refusal
  - Helplessness—no one loves me—remains away from family
  - Helplessness—I cannot live alone and neglected—suicidality
- *Failure:* I shall never be able to succeed—hopelessness
  - Hopelessness—whatsoever I might try, I cannot succeed—school refusal

- Hopelessness—no one would ever appreciate me—distances self from others
- Hopelessness—the future is dark and painful—suicidal ideations

Thus, in CBT, the client and therapist together first identify these thoughts. The therapist then tries to disprove them before the client by making him verify his own thoughts. He is then taught to replace them with more realistic and less distressing thoughts through various techniques.

Eliciting the core beliefs behind the thoughts: Shrawan belonged to a family where scores in formal education were highly appreciated and expected. Everyone was a high achiever. So, he had developed some schemas since his early childhood, which were then probed.

Shrawan's core beliefs:
- Failure is not acceptable. I must pass in every examination.
- Once a failure, always a failure.
- No one bothers about a person who has failed.

COGNITIVE ERRORS

The negative thoughts are automatic, habitual, involuntary, and difficult to control.

They are at the superficial conscious level and can be elicited through systematic psychoevaluation. Underlying these faulty thoughts are "cognitive errors" or a distorted thinking pattern. Some of them are as follows:
- *Overgeneralization:* Depending on one negative event, the client concludes that everything is going wrong in whole of his life. Shrawan failed in one exam, and he thought that his entire life is a failure.
- *Maximization:* Exaggerating mistakes and shortcomings. "I am a big fool who couldn't handle a small challenge as a class test."
- *Minimization:* Belittling one's efforts and achievements. "I passed in other subjects. So what? Anyone can do that!"
- *Dichotomous thinking:* All-or-none law, thinking in extreme polarities. "If I fail in exams, I shall be good for nothing." (Another example: "If I am not tall, I cannot have a good personality.")
- *Arbitrary inference:* Jumping to negative conclusions without adequate evidence to support the belief. "Teacher failed me deliberately." (Another example: "My friend did not talk with me today. He does not like me anymore. He will break our friendship.")
- *Selective abstraction:* Focusing on negative and ignoring the positive. Shrawan ignored that he has passed all other tests except one and all the while focused on the failure. (Another example: A student might just remember his teacher's scolding while keeping aside his teaching skills. "My teacher doesn't know anything other than punishing me.")
- "Mustitis": Adding must to all desirable things: I must pass, there is no other go. (Another example: "I must have a scooter" rather than "I would like to have a scooter.")

COGNITIVE BEHAVIORAL THERAPY SESSIONS

Cognitive behavioral therapy sessions are highly structured and preplanned with specific agenda for each one. Unless there are comorbidities, generally 5–20 sessions of 45 minutes each suffice.[1] While the thoughts are being worked upon, the behavioral component is also taken care of. Activities are recorded and monitored. The aim is to reduce negative behaviors (such as crying spells, poor self-care, avoidance to take challenges) and promote positive behaviors (such as healthy lifestyle, pleasurable activities, mingling, etc.). This is done by targeting SMART (specific, measurable, attainable, rewarding, time-bound) goals which are set in collaboration with the client.

The therapy is conducted under three broad headings:
1. *Collaborative empiricism:* Establishing an agreement on therapy goals/rapport building
2. *Cognitive techniques:* Eliciting/testing automatic thoughts, identifying/testing maladaptive assumptions, reconstruction of thoughts
3. *Behavioral techniques:* Scheduling and monitoring activities, mastery and pleasure tasks, graded task assignments, role play.

PROCESS OF COGNITIVE BEHAVIORAL THERAPY

Let us now go stepwise with Shrawan in his journey of CBT.
- CBT focusses on here and now and works on the present problems rather than the past or the future. (Shrawan has low mood and suicidal thoughts. So they were focus of addressal.)
- It requires willingness and an active participation of the client. (He was willing for therapy sessions.)

- The client is given psychoeducation about his mental health problems and about the basics of CBT. (Shrawan was shared scientific information on what is depression and what is CBT.)
- The client needs to identify, vocalize, and prioritize his problems. (Shrawan shared his troubling thoughts: I am a total failure. No one loves me.)
- He is encouraged to gather information about his thought processes in different settings in an unbiased manner. The therapist acts as the facilitator. (Shrawan was asked to contemplate and enlist in what other areas of life he has succeeded till now? Making a list of loving gestures by family/friends.)
- Together, the client and the therapist identify the client's beliefs and expectations. (Shrawan had coined his success with his parents' love for him and his purpose to stay alive: "I should pass every exam so that I make everyone happy or else I should die.")
- Hypotheses to be tested are then formulated. (His hypothesis was "failing in an exam necessitates ending the life.") The client is encouraged to test the hypothesis in the real world. (He was asked to explore his roles other than a student—a son, a brother, a player, a friend, etc.)
- Structured sessions are conducted that focus on skill building of the client for initiation of activities starting with very small goals. (Activity scheduling, motivating, and rewarding for the same: Shrawan was ready to take dinner with the family and call a friend in the next 3 days. He was advised to reward himself by listening to his favorite song, after achieving each small goal.)
- *Pleasure and mastery activities:* Client is directed toward activities that he has some mastery on and the ones he enjoyed earlier. (Shrawan agreed to try his hands on his flute, which he had learned in hobby classes.)
- Home assignments are given. These involve record keeping of the automatic thoughts/emotions/behaviors/mood level (on a scale of 1-10) and other relevant details. (A weekly sheet was made for Shrawan.)
- Therapists try to bring forth the connect between all these variables to the client. (Shrawan was shown that his mood score was higher when he engaged himself in his hobby and mingled with family.)
- Identifying the cognitive errors in the automatic thoughts (Overgeneralization and catastrophizing were identified by Shrawan.)
- Identifying the distorted core belief ("It is a must to pass every exam." He came out with this as a wrong belief.)
- Restructuring of thoughts. (Shrawan was asked to reconstruct a positive and rational thought: "Exams are not a do or die situation." "One should find out difficulties in studies, get help and try his best." "There is always another chance to prove yourself.")

STRENGTHS AND AREAS OF APPLICATIONS OF COGNITIVE BEHAVIORAL THERAPY

Culture fair nature: CBT is a well-researched, evidence-based therapy that has proven effective for clients from multiple backgrounds. Hence, it is applicable to almost all culture settings.

Ease of administration: CBT can be conveniently carried out in an online digital mode. It can also be administered as a group intervention for individuals who have the same concerns, either for self-enhancement or for their mental health problems.

For healthy individuals: Through CBT, the client learns to recognize and label his own and other's emotions and thus his emotional quotient (EQ) increases, which is so very important for success. Cognitive restructuring helps in replacing irrational/negative thoughts by rational/positive thoughts making it useful as a mental well-being strategy that helps in self-enhancing and personality development, for healthy individuals as well.

For children and adolescents: It can be used as a mental health promotive and anticipatory tool kit. Various personality dimensions such as self-esteem, self-efficacy, and interpersonal relationships get better with this skill set. Life skills such as interpersonal skills, communication skills, and problem-solving skills improve, and there are less chances of engaging in high-risk behaviors.

Cognitive behavioral therapy is a statistically proven useful tool for adolescents and children over 7 years of age for various mental health concerns.[7] Before 7 years of age, children find it difficult to comprehend their emotions and seek help or participate actively in such a demanding process.

COGNITIVE BEHAVIORAL THERAPY IN PSYCHOLOGICAL ISSUES

Cognitive behavioral therapy is most widely used for treating adolescent depression and anxiety, as a monotherapy or in adjunct with pharmacological therapy.[7] CBT finds its application in depression, various forms of anxiety, including panic attacks, obsessive-compulsive disorder (OCD), and post-traumatic stress disorder (PTSD). For adolescents with suicidality and recurrent and chronic self-harm, CBT has been the psychotherapy of choice. Children and teenagers who are victims of abuse and trauma have been benefited by CBT. Children with externalizing and violent behaviors such as attention-deficit hyperactivity disorder (ADHD) and substance abuse are helped by this technique. CBT has been shown to be effective in diverse challenges such as anger management, body dysmorphic disorder, eating disorders, schizophrenia, and obesity. It has been recommended by the National Institute for Health and Clinical Excellence (NICE) guidelines, UK, for most of these mental health problems.[7] For children above 8 years of age and adolescents suffering from mild depression without comorbidities, the NICE recommends CBT as the first-line therapeutic intervention.[7]

Some classroom-based studies have demonstrated that cognitive interventions are useful in managing undesirable behavior in children as young as 5 years of age.[7]

CONCLUSION

Cognitive behavioral therapy is a structured therapy and counselors need training to carry it out successfully. It requires active participation of the client in and out of the sessions. Homework assignments are an integral part of the process. It is not appropriate for people seeking a more unstructured, insight-oriented approach that does not require their strong participation. CBT is primarily cognitive in nature and not usually the best approach for people who are intellectually limited or who are unmotivated to change. Cognitive behavioral therapy is demanding for both the client and the counselor. It takes around 6–20 sessions to be really helpful.

REFERENCES

1. Lazović N. Cognitive behavioral therapy with children. Zbornik radova Uciteljskog fakulteta Prizren-Leposavic. 2018;173-87.
2. Rush AJ, Beck AT, Kovacs M, Hollon SD. Comparative efficacy of cognitive therapy and pharmacotherapy in the treatment of depressed outpatients. Cognitive Therapy and Research. 1977;1:17-38.
3. David D. Rational emotive behavior therapy in the context of modern psychological research. Available from: https://albertellis.org/rebt-therapy-in-the-context-of-modern-psychological-research/
4. Development of DBT. Available from: https://www.dbt-training.co.uk/what-is-dbt/development-of-dbt/
5. Hayes SC. Acceptance and commitment therapy, relational frame theory, and the third wave of behavioral and cognitive therapies. Behavior Therapy. 2004;35(4):639-65. Available from: https://www.sciencedirect.com/science/article/abs/pii/S0005789404800133
6. Nezu MA, Nezu CM, D'Zurilla TJ. Problem-Solving Therapy. In: Kazantzis N, Reinecke MA, Freeman A (Eds). Cognitive and Behaviour Theories in Clinical Practice. Gullford Publications, New York ; 2010. pp. 76-113.
7. Halder S, Mahato A. Cognitive Behavior Therapy for Children and Adolescents: Challenges and Gaps in Practice. Indian J Psychol Med. 2019;41:279-83.

Index

Page numbers followed by *b* refer to box, *f* refer to figure, *fc* refer to flowchart, and *t* refer to table.

A

Abuse, victims of 243
Accidental aggression 163
    management 165
Accidents 104, 185
Acetylcholine 127
Acquired immunodeficiency syndrome 65
Addictive disorders 3
Adenosine 127
Adjustment disorder 78, 80, 94, 164
Adolescent-friendly clinics 201
Adrenergic blocking effects 226
Adrenocorticotropic hormone 128
Adventure therapy 206
Aggression 194, 195, 233
Aggressive behavior 160, 163, 194
    complications 164
    continuity of 164
    differential diagnosis 164
    drug therapy 166
    etiopathogenesis 163
    incidence 160
    prognosis 166
    types of 160, 162*t*
Agoraphobia 81
Airway 102
Akathisia 228
Alarm therapy 175
Alcohol withdrawal symptoms 100
Alcoholism, prevention of 101
Alimemazine 220
Alpha-2 agonist 219, 221
Alprazolam 100, 220, 222, 223
Alternative communication systems 214
Alternative therapy 24, 25*f*
American Academy of Sleep Medicine
    Guidelines 128*t*
Amitriptyline 118, 219
Amphetamine 103, 218
Anaphylaxis 81
Angelman syndrome 234
Angry 89
    pattern of 160
Anorectal manometry 177
Anorexia nervosa 106, 107, 109, 111
    severity of 107*t*
Anosmia 115
Antianxiety drugs 222
Antiasthmatic agents 81
Anticholinergic drugs 176

Antidepressants 225, 239
    action, mechanism of 225
    drugs 58, 59, 59*t*, 226
Antidotes 102
Antihistamines 81, 220
Antipsychotics 227, 228
    atypical 29, 219, 228
    typical 228
Antiseizure medications 30
Antisense oligonucleotides 236
Antisocial personality disorder 92, 161
Antistreptolysin O titers, significant
    elevation of 150
Anxiety 3, 27, 41*b*, 46*b*, 48*b*, 78, 80, 122, 150,
    193, 195, 203, 213, 217, 234, 242,
    243
    achievement 193
    child 44
    disorders 3, 17, 41, 43, 44*t*, 46*t*, 78, 81,
        82*fc*, 83*t*, 143, 217, 231, 233
        complications 83
        follow-up and prognosis 83
        management of 82
        prevalence 41
        primary prevention of 83
        public health burden of 50
        treatment of 48, 49*t*
        types of 83
    scale, multidimensional 44
    screening tool for 43
    specific screening tools 44
    types of 42
Anxiolytics 225
    agents 82
Appetite disturbance 55
Aripiprazole 29, 118, 181, 219, 228
Arm-drop test 117
Arrhythmia, cardiac 81
Art therapy 206
Artificial intelligence 21
Assistance commitment therapy 240
Asthma 81
Astrocytes 11
Ataxia 115, 116
Atomoxetine 38, 219, 221
Attention-deficit hyperactivity disorder 1,
    8, 18, 30, 33, 34*b*, 36*t*, 37*t*, 38*b*, 39,
    39*b*, 45, 49, 56, 73, 74, 81, 93, 94,
    143, 150, 164, 200, 213, 217, 220,
    231, 233, 243

adverse effects of medications 39
clinical features 33
comorbidities and associated
    conditions 36
diagnosis 34
drugs for 218
etiopathogenesis of 33
management of 37
medications for 38
prevalence estimates of 33
symptoms of 213
Augmentation strategies 76
Autism 13, 213, 231, 236
    diagnostic tools 17*t*
    modified for 15
    screening tools 16*t*
Autism spectrum disorder 1, 4, 8, 10, 11,
    14*b*, 15*t*, 16, 18*fc*, 21, 21*f*, 22*t*, 25,
    26, 30, 31, 73, 143, 150, 220, 231,
    233, 236*f*
    development, modern theories of 10
    diagnostic evaluation 8
    etiopathogenesis 8
    management of 21
    neurobiology of 237
    pharmacological management of 26
    risk of 235
Azapirones 222, 224

B

Back pain 122
Bacteroides 70
Barbiturates 100, 223
Bardley home for problem children 218
Basal ganglia 115
Behavior
    activation, medication-induced 58
    addiction 214
    aggressive 160, 163, 194
    argumentative 160
    defiant 160
    disorders 1, 2, 194, 200, 210, 212, 217-
        219, 231-233, 236
        classification of 3
        clinical features of 232
        diagnosis of 235
        management of 5
        mobile-related 212
        neurobiology of 2
        pharmacology of 217

prevalence of 1, 217
prevalent 231
treatment of 218, 236
gratification 179
interventions 37, 236
management therapy 233
masturbatory 179
observations 235
patterns, long-term 164
problems 4, 193, 194
prevention of 5
rating scales 36
repetitive 26
screening 235
self-injurious 55, 240
symptoms 122
techniques 241
therapy 151, 180
rational emotive 240
treatment, family based 205
typical 239
Benzodiazepines 100, 103, , 220, 222, 224, 228
use of 49
Beta-adrenergic blocking agents 82
Binge eating disorder 106, 107, 109, 111
Biopsychosocial factors 163
Bipolar disorders 3, 62, 94, 196, 203, 232
Bizarre muscle spasms 228
Blinded randomized controlled trials 31
Blindness 115
Blood
loss, excessive 2
pressure 50
Bodily distress, disorders of 3, 121
Body
dysmorphic disorder 119, 120
focused repetitive behaviors 147
mass index 107t
Bowel cleaning 177
Bradycardia, severe 110
Brain 12
damage 13
development 13, 88
function 13
lesion 13
stimulation techniques 59
tumors 81
Brainstem 127
Breastfeeding, absence of 179
Breath, shortness of 81
Breath-holding spells 167, 168t
clinical features 167
diagnosis 167
differential diagnosis 167
etiology 167
treatment 167
Breathing 102
deep 46
disorders, sleep-related 128, 129
support 102

Breathlessness 115
Broken mirror theory 11
Bruxism 156
Bulimia nervosa 106, 107, 109, 111
severity of 107t
Bumetanide 30
Bupropion 29, 49, 59, 83
Buspirone 219

C

Cadherin genes 232
Caffeinism 81
Callous 94
Candidate genes 232
Cannabidiol 30, 31
Cannabis 103
Carbamazepine 118
Cardiac monitoring 102
Cardiovascular system 102
Caretaker interview 164
Catatonia 3
Central hypersomnolence, disorders of 130, 130b
Central nervous system 11, 102, 218
disorders 81
Chemical agents 13
Chest
pain 81, 196, 122
tightness 87
Child-centered play therapy 123
Childhood behavioral problems, assessment of 4
Children's appercention test 81
Children's separation anxiety scale 45
Children's Yale-Brown obsessive-compulsive scale 74, 75
Chlordiazepoxide 100, 222, 224
Chlorpromazine 219, 228
Chocking, feeling of 81, 196
Chromosomal tests 235, 236
Chromosome 16p11.2 deletion syndrome 235
Circadian rhythm sleep-wake disorders 3, 128
Citalopram 29, 49, 50, 76, 82, 83, 124, 219
Clomipramine 29, 76, 83
Clonazepam 82, 83, 100, 118, 220, 222, 228
Clonidine 29, 49, 151, 166, 219, 221
Clozapine 67, 173, 219, 228
Cocaine 100, 103
Codeine 100
Cognitive distortion 47, 47t
Cognitive-behavior
cluster 55
models 115
therapy 24, 46b, 47t, 49, 58, 74, 82, 89, 95, 103, 111, 117, 118, 123, 124, 186, 196, 198, 202, 203, 203f, 204, 218, 239-243
applications of 242
effectiveness of 204

origin of 239
principles of 240
process of 241
types of 203
use of 144
treatment 75
Cold medicines 81
Collaborative empiricism 241
Communication 211, 231
technology-assisted 214
Communicative behavior, nonverbal 14
Community, role of 66
Comorbidities, treatment of 151
Competence enhancement skills training 101
Complementary therapy 24, 25f
Complex sleep apnea syndromes 129
Conduct disorders 56, 87, 160, 161, 200, 217, 231, 233
assessment of 94, 96fc
behavioral problems of 193
clinical presentation 93
comorbid conditions 93
diagnostic criteria 93
differential diagnosis of 94, 94t
epidemiology 92
etiopathogenesis 92
management of 95, 96fc
prevention 97
prognosis 96
Constipation 173
Contactin-associated protein 2 genes 150
Contingency management 47, 103
Control functional pathways 12
Conversion disorder 114, 115f, 116t, 119
clinical features 115
complications 117
diagnosis 116
epidemiology 114
etiopathogenesis 114
prognosis 117
symptoms of 115t
treatment of 117, 118t
Coping skills 198
Cough 122
Counselling 202
practice of 201
COVID-19 1
Culture fair nature 242
Cyanotic breath-holding spell 167t
Cyberbullying 163, 214
Cyclic adenosine monophosphate 31
Cyproheptadine 133
Cystitis 173
Cytochrome enzymes 228
Cytosine-guanine-guanine 234

D

D-cycloserine 76
De Novo copy-number variations 12
Deafness 115

Death 64
Deep brain stimulation 76
Deep learning models 21
Dehydration 110
Delinquency 195
Delirium 81
Dendritic morphogenesis 11
Deoxyribonucleic acid methylation 9, 12
Depressed mood 55
Depression 3, 27, 55, 56t, 57, 122, 139, 193, 196, 200, 203, 213, 226, 227, 239, 242
   development of 59
   disorders 3, 94, 217, 196
      etiology 56
      major 70
   episode 55b, 56
   exogenous 54
   risk of childhood 56
   severity of 56
   treatment of 57
Desipramine 219
Desmopressin 176, 229
Detoxification 103
Developmental coordination disorder 231, 233
Dexamphetamines 218
Dexmethylphenidate 30
Dextroamphetamine 30
Diabetes
   insipidus, acquired 173
   mellitus 173
Dialectical behavior therapy 103, 203
Diaphoresis 81
Diazepam 100, 118, 220, 222, 223f, 224, 228
Diffusion tensor imaging 69
DiGeorge syndrome 235
Digital
   connectivity 211
   parenting 211
   skills, development of 211
Dimensional Yale-Brown Obsessive-Compulsive Scale 75
Diphenhydramine 220
Direct current stimulation 21
Disability 102, 179
   nature of 140
Discomfort 179
Discrete trial training 22
Disfluency 143
   typical 142, 143
Disruptive behaviors 27
   problems 4
Disruptive mood dysregulation disorder 87
Dissociative disorders 3, 120
Distraction 213
Distress 79
   abdominal 196
Divalproex sodium 30
Dizziness 115, 122

DNA hydroxymethylation 12
Dopamine 127
Dorsal raphe nucleus 127
Dorsolateral hypothalamus 127
Double vision 115
Down syndrome 233
Doxepin 219
Duloxetine 59, 83
Dysarthria 115
Dysfunctional voiding 173
Dyskinesia 150
Dysphonia 115
Dystonias 115, 116

E

Eating attitudes test 106
Eating disorders 70, 106-109, 109t, 110t, 217
   epidemiology 106
   examination questionnaire 108, 109
   management principles 111
   screening tool for 108
   sleep-related 132
   type of 109
E-cigarettes 100
Electrocardiogram 50, 75
Electroconvulsive therapy, need for 76
Electroencephalogram 17, 139, 180
Electroencephalographic abnormalities 28
Electrolyte
   disturbance 110
   imbalance 110
Elimination disorders 3
Emotional disorders 3, 44, 217
   prevalence of 217
Emotional distress 164
   index of 45
Emotional dysregulation 150
Emotional neglect 179
Emotional regulation 231
Empathy, lack of 94
Encephalopathy 81
Encopresis 173, 176
   classification 176
   evaluation 177
   investigations 177
   pathophysiology 176
   risk factors 177
   treatment 177
Endocrine factors 10
Energy 87
Enuresis 173
   classification 173
   diagnosis 174
   management 175
   pathophysiology 174
   prevalence 173
   primary 173
   risk factors 174
   secondary 173
      causes of 173b
Epigenetics 232

Epilepsy 28
Epileptic seizures 150
Episode, mixed 197
Escitalopram 59, 76, 82, 83, 118, 124, 181, 219
Estazolam 222
Excellent mental health 200
Excitation 11
Excoriation disorder 70, 120
Exercise
   aerobic 91
   rehabilitation 187
Expressive aggression 163
   management 165
Extracellular signal-regulated kinase 31
Extrapyramidal disturbance 228
Eyes 122

F

Facial flushing 180
Factitious disorders 3
Fainting episodes 122
Family accommodation scale 75
Family psychoeducation 197
Family therapy 82, 123, 187, 205
   forms of 205
Fast track program 97
Fatigue 122
   syndrome, chronic 115, 120
Fear disorders 3
Feeding
   disorders 3, 106, 109t
   issues 27
Fentanyl 100
Fetal microenvironment 8
Fingertip test 116
Fluency disorders 142
   pathophysiology 143
   pharmacological management 145
   remedial measures and treatment 144
Flumazenil 224
Fluoxetine 29, 48, 49, 59, 76, 82, 83, 118, 124, 219
Flurazepam 222
Fluvoxamine 29, 48-50, 76, 124, 219
Fluvoxin 124
Focal weakness 115, 116
Food and Drug Administration 112, 124
Food scraps 234
Foreign accent syndrome 115
Foster open communication 215
Fragile X
   and tuberous sclerosis complex 28
   mental retardation
      1 gene 234
      protein 31
   syndrome 234
Freud's psychoanalytical approach 239
Freudian theory 163
Frontal brain electrical activity 92
Functional family therapy 205
Functional neurological disorder 114, 114b

G

Gabapentin 118
Gait disorder 115, 116
Galctorrhea 228
Gamma-aminobutyric acid 127
　A 30
　　benzodiazepine chloride channel 223*f*
Gasoline 100
Gastrointestinal issues 27
Gastrointestinal microbiome, etiology of 70
Gastrointestinal tract 102
Gender incongruence 120
Gene
　environment interplay 232
　expression 235
　therapy 236
Generalized anxiety disorder 3, 43, 50, 78, 80, 122
Genetic 88
　disorders 231
　models 12, 13
　modifications 13
　syndrome 233
　tests, types of 235, 235*t*
Genital irritation 179
Genomic testing 235
Gepirone 219
Global developmental delay 137
Glue 100
Glutamate decarboxylase 1 12
Glutamatergic and gamma-aminobutyric acidergic receptor 11
Glutamine inhibitor, use of 82
Good behavior game 101
Gratification disorder 179, 180, 180*t*
　clinical features 179
　diagnosis 180
　epidemiology 179
　etiology 179
　management 180
　predisposing factors 179
Guanfacine 29, 151, 166, 219, 221
Guru Shishya Parampara 201
Gynecomastia 228

H

H-1 blocking effects 226
Habit disorders 4, 147
　classification 147
Hair
　plucking 120
　pulling disorder 70, 120
Hallucinations 78, 84, 85
Hallucinogens 100
Haloperidol 83, 118, 219, 228
Hamartoma tumor syndrome 232
Hashish 100
Headache 122
Health education 202, 202*t*

Hearing
　disturbances 116
　loss 121
Heart
　block 173
　pounding 196
　rate 109
　　accelerated 196
Hemifacial spasm 150
Heritability 232
Higher mental processes 240
Hirschsprung disease 177
Histamine 127
Histidine decarboxylase gene 150
Histone
　deacetylase inhibition 13
　modification 12
Home, education, activity, drugs/diet, sexuality, suicidality/depression assessment 109
Hookahs 100
Hoover's test 117
Hormonal theory 163
Hostile aggression 163
　management 165
Household aerosols 100
Humanistic theory 163
Hydrocodone 100
Hydroxymethylcytosine 12
Hydroxytryptamine 56
Hydroxyzine 82, 83, 220, 222, 225, 228, 229
Hyperactivity 226, 233
Hyperkinetic movement disorders chorea 150
Hyperphagia 55, 234
Hypersomnia 55
　idiopathic 130, 131
Hypersomnolence disorders 3, 128
Hypertension 50
Hyperthermia 102
Hyperthyroidism 81, 173
Hypnotherapy 118
Hypnotics 100
Hypochondriacal disorder 119
Hypochondriasis 119, 120, 122
Hypocretin 127
Hypoglycemia 81
Hypokalemia 110
Hyponatremia 110
Hypophosphatemia 110
Hypotension 110
Hypothalamic-pituitary-adrenal axis 200
Hypothalamus 127
Hypothermia 110
Hypoxemia disorders, sleep-related 129
Hypoxic damage 10
Hysterical conversion disorder 114

I

Idiopathic infantile dyskinesia, benign 179
Imipramine 83, 176, 219

Immune system components 149
Immunity, impaired 11
Impulse control disorders 3, 70, 150
Inappropriate compensatory behaviors, frequency of 107*t*
Incontinence, subtypes of 174*fc*
Infectious disease 104
Inhalants 100
Inhibitors 219
Injury, increased risk of 164
Insomnia 128
　classification of 128*b*
　disorder 3
　　chronic 128, 129, 224
　　short-term 128, 224
　　transient 224
Instrumental aggression management 163, 165
Insufficient sleep syndrome 130
Intellectual development, disorders of 3
Intellectual disability 17, 88, 137, 143, 217, 231, 233, 234
Intelligence, Binet Kamat test of 138
Interleukin 6 13
Intermittent explosive disorder 94, 160
International Children's Continence Society 174*t*
International Classification of Sleep Disorder 128*b*
Internet 65
　addiction 214
　gaming 186
　　disorder 183
　use disorder, prevalence of 183
Intoxication 102
Ipsapirone 219
Irritability 55, 80, 87
　behaviors 27
Irritable mood 89, 160
Isolated epileptiform discharges 28

J

Joint attention 23

K

Kleine–Levin syndrome 130, 131
Kleptomania 166
Klinefelter's syndrome 233

L

Lamotrigine 30
Language
　barrier 201
　delays 217
　disorders 231, 233
　paradigms 23
Lead
　neurotoxicity 163
　poisoning 81
Learning disability 17, 137, 139, 143

Learning disorders 137, 138t, 139t
  clinical features 138
  diagnosis 138
  etiopathogenesis 138
  evaluation 138
  prevention 140
Legal issues 104, 164
Legal system 100
Levetiracetam 30
Limbs 122
Lin Zexu's efforts 98
Lisdexamfetamine 30, 219
Lithium 118
  prophylaxis 67
Liver function tests 110
Lorazepam 82, 83, 100, 220, 222, 223
Love affairs 64
Lumbosacral area 177
Lysergic acid diethylamide 100

M

Macrophages, perivascular 11
Magnetic resonance imaging, functional 69
Malnutrition, acute medical complications of 110
Manic episode 197
Marijuana 100
  nonpsychotropic component of 30
Mass media 65
Mastery activities 242
Masturbatory activity 179
Maternal alcoholism 163
Maternal uniparental disomy 234
MECP2 gene 232
Medication-assisted therapies 103
Medications, adverse effects of 39
Medicine, alternative 21
Memory
  deficits 115
  function, impaired 100
Menace reflex 116
Menstrual pain 122
Mental disorders 194
  diagnostic and statistical manual of 3b, 14, 18, 57, 114
Mental functions 239
Mental health 242
  disorders 164
  necessitates 207
  resources 66
  services, school-based 198
Mental illnesses 194
Mental practices 72
Metabolism, inborn errors of 138
Metformin 31
Methadone 100
Methamphetamines 100
Methylphenidate 30, 219, 218, 221
  short-acting 38
Microbiota-gut-brain axis 12
Microglia 11

Midazolam 222
Migraine 81
Mind, theory of 1
Mindfulness 46, 186
Mineral supplements 111
Mirror test 116
Mirtazapine 59
Mitochondrial dysfunction 13
Mitogen-activated protein kinase 31
Mobile addiction
  risk factors for 184t
  treatment of 215
Mobile disorder 210, 212
Mobile phone
  advantages of 211
  excessive 210
  problem 185
  use 210, 213
    scale, problematic 185
Mobile phone addiction 183
  diagnosis 184
  epidemiology 183
  etiopathogenesis 183
  prevention 187
  treatment 186
Modafinil 222
Modus operandi 62
Molecular biology, central dogma of 236f
Molecular tests 235
Monitor and track usage 215
Monoamine oxidase 152
Monosymptomatic nocturnal enuresis 173
Monotony 179
Mood
  behavior, low 239
  disorders 3, 164, 196
  stabilizers 118
Morphine 100
Motivation 166
Motor tic 148
  disorder, chronic 148
Mouth-dissolving tablet 176
Movement disorder
  sleep-related 128
  stereotypic 70
Multisystemic therapy 206
Muscle tension 80
Muscular dystonia, acute 228
Mutism 115
Myalgic encephalomyelitis 120
Myoclonus 115, 116

N

N acetyl cysteine 76, 230
Narcolepsy 130
Narcotic drugs 100
National Institute for Health and Clinical Excellence 243
National Institute of Open Schooling 140
Nausea 81
Neonatal intensive care unit 2

Neural migration, impaired 11
Neurobehavioral disorders 233t
Neurobiological models 13, 115
Neurobiology studies 200
Neurochemicals 127
Neurocognitive disorders 3
Neurodevelopmental disorders 1, 3, 8, 33, 111
Neurogenic bladder, acquired 173
Neuroleptic syndrome, malignant 228
Neurological dysfunction, frontal-striatal-thalamic model of 69
Neuropeptide hypocretin 127
Neuropsychiatric disorders 163
Neuropsychiatric syndrome, pediatric acute-onset 70
Neurotransmitter 56
  theory 163
Neurovegetative cluster 55
Nightmare 133
  wetting, classification of 174t
Nitrazepam 222
Nocturnal enuresis 226, 227
Nocturnal seizures, suspicion of 132
Nomophobia 214
  questionnaire 185, 191
Noncoding ribonucleic acid 12
Nondopaminergic medications 221
Nonepileptic seizures 115
Nongovernmental organizations 201
Nonmonosymptomatic enuresis 173
Nonpharmacological therapy, goals of 21f
Nonrapid eye movement 131
  parasomnia, treatment of 132
Nonstimulants 219
Nonsuicidal self-injury 61, 62, 62t, 63
  causes 61
  disorder, diagnostic criteria for 62
  management of 63
  prevalence 61
  risk factors 61
Norepinephrine 124, 127
  reuptake inhibitor 50, 124
Nortriptyline 83, 118
Nucleotide order 235
Numbness sensation 196
Nutraceutics 222

O

Obsessive-compulsive disorder 3, 17, 27, 30, 50, 69, 73-76, 76b, 78, 80, 152, 200, 217, 220, 227, 243
  assessment 72
  clinical features 71
  differential diagnosis 74
  epidemiology 69
  etiology 69
  management 74
  pharmacotherapy of 74
Obstructive sleep apnea 129, 173
Occupational therapy 23

Odoribacter 70
Olanzapine 219, 228, 229
Omega-3 fatty acids 10
Opioids 103
    painkillers 100
Oppositional defiant disorder 56, 87, 88, 94, 160, 194, 231, 233
    classification of 89
    complications 89
    management of 89
    managing symptoms 91
    prevention 90
Optokinetic test 116
Oral alpha-adrenergic agonist drugs 151
Orthostatic hypotension 109
Oscillospira 70
Osmotic-release oral system 38
Oxazepam 220, 222, 223
Oxidative stress 10, 13
Oxybutynin 176
Oxycodone 100
Oxygen, supplemental 102
Oxytocin 30, 31

P

Pain 122
    disorder 119
Paint thinners 100
Pallid breath-holding spell 167*t*
Palpitations 81, 87, 196, 228
Pamoate 220
Panic attacks 243
Panic disorder 3, 42, 81, 122, 196
Paralysis 116
Paraphilic disorders 3
Parasomnia 128, 131, 133
    classification of 131*b*
Parent training 165
Parental control apps, use 215
Parental influence 211
Parental psychiatric illness 163
Parent-focused therapy 111
Paresthesia 116, 121
Parkinsonism 228
Paroxetine 49, 50, 76
Pediatric autoimmune neuropsychiatric disorders 70, 81
Peer
    influence 211
    interview 164
    rejection 164
    support 186
Penetrance 231
Penetration disorder 120
Penfluridol 228
Persistent somatoform pain disorder 119
Personality disorders 3
Pervasive disorders 217
Pharmacotherapeutic agents 76*t*
Pharmacotherapy
    principles of 26
    role of 218

Phelan-McDermid syndrome 231
Phencyclidine 100
Phenotypic expression 231
Pheochromocytoma 81
Phobia 3, 42, 78, 83*t*
    clinical features 78
    epidemiology 78
    etiopathogenesis 78
    specific 78, 79, 196
Phosphodiesterase-4D inhibitors 31*t*
Physical abuse 94
Physical fights 87
Physical injury 194
Physical therapy 23
Pimozide 83, 219, 228, 229
Pivotal response training 22
Poisoning, acute 226
Policymakers, role of 66
Polygenic nature 232
Poor socioeconomic status 177
Porphyria 81
Positive Parenting Program 95
Posterior thalamus 127
Post-traumatic stress disorder, diagnosis of 93
Postural hypotension 228
Postviral fatigue syndrome 120
Poverty 64
Practice digital detox 215
Prader-Willi syndrome 234
Prazosin 133
Prebiotics 31
Probiotics 31
Problem-solving therapy 240
Productivity apps, use 215
Progressive muscle relaxation 46
Promethazine 228
Propranolol 82, 222, 225
Psychiatric disorders 62, 121, 194
Psychodynamic approach 123
Psychodynamic models 115
Psychodynamic psychotherapy 82, 118
Psychoeducation 47, 59
Psychogenic nonepileptic seizures 116
Psychological management 45, 74
Psychological stress 173
Psychological testing 163
Psychological treatment 123
Psychomotor skills 8
Psychopharmacological drugs 230
Psychopharmacological treatment 187
Psychopharmacology 217, 218
Psychostimulants 220
    medications 30
Psychotherapeutic method 239
Psychotherapy 58, 82, 89, 153, 177
Psychotic disorders 3
Psychotropic substances 100
PTEN gene 232
Puberty 54

Q

Quetiapine 219, 228

R

Rapamycin, mammalian target of 11
Rapid eye movement 131, 133
Rashtriya Kishor Swasthya Karyakram 101
Recognize problem 215
Reelin gene mutation 11
Relaxation techniques 90
Relaxation training 47
Religious scrupulosity 69
Remimazolam 222
Resilience 198
Respiratory factors 157
Respiratory system 102
Restless leg syndrome 134, 150
Restlessness 80
Rett syndrome 30
Reward therapy 175
Riluzole 76
Risperidone 29, 118, 181, 219, 228, 229
Rumination disorder 106, 108, 111, 170
    causes 170
    clinical features 170
    complications 171
    differential diagnosis 171
    epidemiology 170
    laboratory examination 171
    pathophysiology 170
    prognosis 172
    treatment 171
Rutter's child behavior questionnaire 138

S

Schizophrenia 67, 95, 232
    spectrum 3
School policy 187
School-based Prevention Programs 101
SCN2A gene 232
Sedation 228
Sedative hypnotics 222
Seizure 28, 168*t*, 180, 180*t*
    disorder 173
Selective abstraction 241
Selective mutism 41, 43, 78, 79, 196
Selective reuptake inhibitor
    nonadrenaline 221
    norepinephrine 48
    serotonin 9, 30, 48, 50, 58, 74, 75, 82, 124, 151, 166, 173, 222, 227
Self-efficacy 198
Self-esteem, low 164
Self-soothing 179
Sensation smothering 81
Sensory
    integration therapy 23
    loss 116
    sensitivities 213
Separation anxiety disorder 42, 78, 79, 196

Index

Serotonergic medications 29
Serotonin 56, 127
    syndrome 227
Sertraline 49, 50, 59, 76, 82, 83, 219
Serum
    electrolytes 110
    estradiol levels 110
Sex addiction 186
Sexual abuse 93, 179
Sexual dysfunctions 3, 120
Sexual obsessions 71
Sexual pain 120
Shaking 196
SHANK3 gene 231
Shopping addiction 186
Shortness of breath, sensations of 196
Shrawan's core beliefs 241
Shrawan's thought analysis 240
Signature test 116
Single-gene
    disorders 12
    testing 235
Skills, practicing new 203
Skin picking disorder 70
Skinner's behavioral approach 239
Sleep
    behavior disorder 133
    disorder 17, 27, 127
        classification of 128
    disruptions 212
    disturbance 80, 184, 213
    functions of 128
    mechanism of 127
    paralysis, recurrent isolated 134
    problems 232
    terror 132
Sleep-wake disorders 3
Sleepwalking 132
Small-molecule drugs 236
Smartphone addiction 183, 185*t*
    scale-short
        form 185
        version 192
    symptomatology of 186*t*
Smartphone penetration 210
Smartphone use
    excessive 184
    problematic 183
Social ability 207
Social anxiety
    disorder 42, 78, 79, 195
    scale 44
Social behavior, disorders of 150
Social communication 15, 214
Social interaction 15, 214, 231
Social learning theory 163
Social media, rise of 211
Social phobia 3. 78, 79
Social resistance skills training 101
Social skills
    groups 24
    impaired 212

Social smile, lack of 14
Social worries anxiety index 45
Somatic pain 124*t*
Somatic symptom 3, 119
Somatoform autonomous dysfunction 119
Somatoform disorder 119
    classes of 119
    clinical presentation 121
    diagnosis of 121, 122
    differential diagnosis 122
    epidemiology of 120
    etiology of 120
    treatment 122
Specific learning
    disabilities 137, 231, 233
    disorder 74
Speech 217
    and language
        pathologist 144
        therapy 23
    behavior 145
    characteristics 142, 143
    development, disorders of 4
    loss of 121
    symptoms 116
Spence children's anxiety scale 45, 72
Sphincters loose tone 177
Stigma barriers 201
Stimulants 103, 166, 218, 219
Stomach pain 122
Stranger anxiety, absence of 14
Streptococcal infections 70
Streptococcal throat 73
Streptococcus pyogenes 78, 81
Stress 3
    disorder
        acute 78, 79
        post-traumatic 3, 78, 79, 121, 214, 217, 220, 243
    family related 179
    level of 106
    reduction interventions, mindfulness-based 46
Stressor-related disorders 3
Sublingual tablets 176
Substance abuse 98, 164, 232
    disorder 56, 101*t*, 103
    management of 102
    prevalence 98
    prevention of 101
    risk factors 99
    screening of 101
    signs of 99
    symptoms of 99
    types of 99
Suicidal deaths 64
Suicidal ideation 62
Suicidal intent nonsuicidal self-injury 61
Suicidality, increased risk for 55
Suicide 61, 62, 62*t*, 63, 64, 65, 104, 165
    adolescence 64
    causes of 64
    old age 64

Sulforaphane 31
Swallowing disturbances 115
Swallowing symptoms 116
Sweating 180, 196
Synaptogenesis, impaired 11
Systemic desensitization 82
Systemic lupus erythematosus 81

T

Tachycardia 81, 109
Tardive dyskinesia 228
Tearing reflex 116
Temazepam 222, 224
Temper tantrums 87, 160
    clinical features 168
    management 168
Temperament 88
Textaphrenia 214
Textiety 214
TGuard 155
    appliance 155*f*
Thalamocortical circuits 115
Thematic apperception test 81
Therapeutic communities 103
Therapy sessions 241
Thioridazine 228
Thumb-sucking 154
Tic
    classification of 148*t*
    disorder 120, 147, 150, 150*t*, 152*t*
        primary 149*t*
        transient 148
    treatment of 151*fc*
    types of 148
Time management and productivity 213
Tingling 87
    sensation 196
Tobacco 100
Toilet training 177
Tourette syndrome 120, 147, 148, 150, 231, 233
    clinical course 148
    epidemiology 148
    etiology 149
Tourette-tic disorder 81
Toxic exposures 9
Toxicity 100
Trained professionals, shortage of 201
Transcranial magnetic stimulation 21, 76
Trauma 3, 93
    victims of 243
Traumatic events, reminders of 196
Trazodone 220
Trembling 196
Tremors 87, 115, 116
Triazolam 222
Trichotillomania 70, 152
Tricyclic antidepressants 49, 219, 225
Trifluoperazine 219
TSC1 gene 235
TSC2 gene 235

Tuberomammillary nucleus 127
Tuberous sclerosis complex 235
Tumor necrosis factor alpha 13
Tunnel vision 115

U

UBE3A gene 234
Urethral obstruction, acquired 173
Urge syndrome 173
Urotherapy 175

V

Valproic acid 9, 173
Vanderbilt assessment scales 44
Velocardiofacial syndrome 235
Venlafaxine 59, 83

Verbal behavior intervention 23
Vesicular monoamine transporter 2
    inhibitors 228
Vigorous exercise 91
Violence 194
    prevention 198
Violent images 198
Vision, poor 122
Visual disturbances 116
Vitamins 111
Vocal tic disorder, chronic 148
Vocal tics 148

W

Weapon, use of 94
Whole-brain voxel-based morphometry 69

X

XXY genotype 233

Y

Yale global tic severity scale 75

Z

Zaleplon 100, 220
Ziprasidone 219
Zolpidem 100, 220

EU GSPR Authorised Reprsentative
Logos Europe, 9 rue Nicolas Poussin
1700, La Rochelle, France
Phone: +33 (0) 6 67 93 73 78
E-mail: contact@logoseurope.eu

www.ingramcontent.com/pod-product-compliance
Ingram Content Group UK Ltd.
Pitfield, Milton Keynes, MK11 3LW, UK
UKHW051823100825
461745UK00019B/388